Progress in Anatomy 3

THE ANATOMICAL SOCIETY OF GREAT BRITAIN AND
IRELAND

Progress in Anatomy

Volume 3

Editors: V. Navaratnam & R. J. Harrison
Assisted by F. Beck, J. A. Gosling, R. L. Holmes & B. A. Wood

CAMBRIDGE UNIVERSITY PRESS
CAMBRIDGE
LONDON   NEW YORK   NEW ROCHELLE
MELBOURNE   SYDNEY

Published by the Press Syndicate of the University of Cambridge
The Pitt Building, Trumpington Street, Cambridge CB2 1RP
32 East 57th Street, New York, NY 10022, USA
296 Beaconsfield Parade, Middle Park, Melbourne 3206, Australia

First published 1983

Printed in Great Britain at the Pitman Press, Bath

Library of Congress catalogue card number: 81-643926

British Library Cataloguing in Publication Data

Progress in anatomy.
Vol. 3

1. Mammals – Physiology
I. Navaratnam, V.   II. Harrison, R. J.
III. Anatomical Society of Great Britain
and Ireland
599.01   QL739.2

ISBN 0 521 24953 8
PP

Contents

Preface

This is the third volume in the series of research reviews by leading anatomists and it emphasises that in a variety of biological problems, ranging from sub-cellular mechanisms to recognition of species, the interpretation of structure is a central and essential component. Several chapters in this volume are devoted to neuronal organisation and these exemplify how a variety of anatomical approaches are helping to unravel the intricacies of a particularly complex system. The Anatomical Society of Great Britain and Ireland has been much encouraged by the contributions to this series and looks forward to further impetus during the run up to the XIIth International Anatomical Congress to be held at the Barbican, London, in August 1985. It is hoped that further volumes will ensue from the proceedings of the Congress. Once again, we are much indebted to Mr D. A. McBrearty for his skilled editorial assistance.

Department of Anatomy
University of Cambridge

V. Navaratnam
R. J. Harrison

1 The pars intermedia of the pituitary gland

BRIAN WEATHERHEAD

Department of Anatomy, School of Medicine, University of Leeds, Leeds LS2 9JT, UK

INTRODUCTION

This review of the pars intermedia of the pituitary gland is not intended to be either historical or exhaustive. It is largely restricted to a consideration of the literature of the last decade and is an attempt to describe some of the more significant advances made in our understanding of this lobe of the pituitary, especially where they can be related to its morphology.

The earlier literature has been well surveyed in various chapters of the three volume series entitled *The Pituitary Gland* (Donovan & Harris, 1966), and more recently the monograph of the same name by Holmes & Ball (1974) provides an excellent comparative account of the vertebrate pituitary gland in general. Howe (1973) has compiled a review of both the structure and function of the mammalian pars intermedia. The proceedings of a Ciba Foundation Symposium (No. 81) devoted to 'Peptides of the Pars Intermedia' (Evered & Lawrenson, 1981) communicate the views of a number of authors on the origin, processing and function of the secretory products of the pars intermedia. All these texts will repay consultation.

PEPTIDES OF THE PARS INTERMEDIA: NOMENCLATURE

It is impossible to deal with almost any aspect of the most recent data concerning the pars intermedia without an appreciation of our burgeoning knowledge of its peptide secretory products. It has long been established that a number of these peptides share, with small interspecific variations, a common amino acid sequence in parts of the molecule. The sequence Tyr-X-Met-X-His-Phe-Arg-Trp-X is found for example in adrenocorticotrophic hormone (ACTH), melanocyte-stimulating hormone (MSH) and β-lipotrophic hormone (βLPH) (Eberle, 1981). More recently it has been revealed that these and related peptides are derived from a single protein precursor molecule commonly referred to as pro-opiomelanocortin, a name which indicates that the precursor gives rise to peptides with opioid, melanotrophic and adrenocorticotrophic activity. Nakanishi *et al.* (1979), employing DNA cloning and nucleotide sequence analysis techniques, have described the complete nucleotide sequence of a 1091 base pair cloned cDNA which encodes the bovine mRNA for pro-opiomelanocortin. From this sequence they have been able to derive the amino acid sequence of pro-opiomelanocortin and define the precise locations of its component peptides (Fig. 1.1).

These component peptides have, in general, been named according to the first biological activity associated with the peptide even though the biological significance

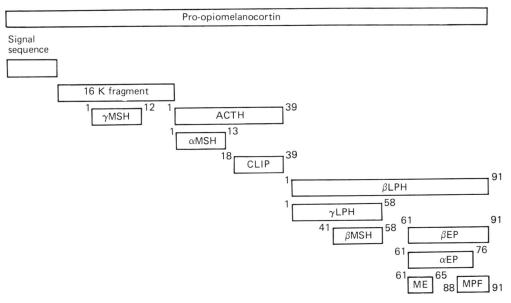

Fig. 1.1. Diagram to show the relationships of some of the more important peptide sequences derived from pro-opiomelanocortin (the lengths of the peptide fragments are not drawn strictly to scale). Abbreviations: MSH, melanocyte-stimulating hormone (melanotrophin); ACTH, adreno-corticotrophic hormone; CLIP, corticotrophin-like intermediate lobe peptide; LPH, lipotrophic hormone; EP, endorphin; MPF, melanotrophin-potentiating factor; ME, methionine-enkephalin (sequence present in pro-opiomelanocortin but normally derived from other precursors: see text).

of such activity may be seriously doubted in some species. The first peptide with a particular biological activity to be isolated is designated the α form; if related molecules with similar activity are subsequently isolated from the same species they are named β, γ, etc. Where the amino acid sequence of the peptide is known precisely, this nomenclature can be supplemented by adding as subscripts the numbers of the amino acid residues that they contain according to a convention whereby the N-terminal amino acids of ACTH and βLPH are identified as number 1. Thus ACTH is ACTH$_{1-39}$, the synthetic ACTH employed therapeutically (Synacthen, Ciba) is ACTH$_{1-24}$ and the first MSH isolated and sequenced is αMSH$_{1-13}$ (Fig. 1.1). If necessary further subscripts can be added to indicate the species from which the peptide derives, thus taking account of interspecific variations in amino acid sequence: e.g. human β-lipotrophin would be β_{human}LPH$_{1-91}$. Whilst on occasion cumbersome, this convention is at least unambiguous.

MORPHOLOGY OF THE PARS INTERMEDIA

The pars intermedia shows a surprising variety of form and size. Amongst rodents, for example, it occupies less than 1% of the total pituitary volume of the garden dormouse (*Eliomys quercinus*) but more than 25% of that of the jird (*Meriones crassus*). In some vertebrates it is entirely absent as, for example, in the cetaceans, the armadillo and certain fossorial reptiles. When present it may vary in appearance from that of an epithelial lining to the hypophysial cleft only a few cells thick, to more massive, lobulated structures where the hypophysial cleft has disappeared. In man it is found in the foetus but in the adult it regresses to a series of follicles and cysts. It is generally described as avascular especially in its simplest epithelial form where it is associated with capillaries lying between it and the subjacent pars nervosa, the plexus intermedius of Benda. Where the pars intermedia is well developed it may be penetrated by capillary loops arising from this plexus intermedius or by vessels that drain through the pars intermedia to adjacent venous sinuses.

The reader interested in the comparative anatomy of the pars intermedia is referred to the accounts by Hanstrom (1966), Wingstrand (1966a, b) and Holmes & Ball (1974). It should be said as a preface to further consideration of this tissue that, given the welter of morphological form, our understanding of the physiology of the pars intermedia and its secretions is based upon a pitifully small selection of vertebrates and that the extrapolation of findings and conclusions concerning the more common laboratory animals to exotic species should be made with extra care.

CELL TYPES OF THE PARS INTERMEDIA

The pars intermedia contains both granular secretory cells and a number of agranular cell types. In the past the secretory cells were usually classified on the basis of their morphology and tinctorial affinities but more recently light and electron microscopic immunocytochemical identification of their contents, together with biochemical studies of the peptides that they release, has permitted their description in functional terms.

Granular cells

Melanotrophs

Melanotrophs are basophil or zeta cells that comprise the bulk of the pars intermedia and display varying degrees of PAS-positivity which probably reflects the glycosylation of pro-opiomelanocortin and some of its fragments. Ultrastructurally they appear as large polygonal cells possessing the normal complement of organelles to be found in cells engaged in the elaboration, storage and release of peptide and protein hormones. Their rough endoplasmic reticulum is usually well developed forming short, parallel arrays or whorl-like formations with expanded cisternae and is associated with a prominent Golgi apparatus. The granules found in the Golgi fields are small, 150–250 nm, and electron dense with a distinct limiting membrane. Secretory granules are found throughout the cytoplasm; those lying progressively further from the Golgi fields seem to undergo a maturation which involves an increase in granule size, to as much as 450 nm in diameter, and a loss of electron density which often reveals a fibrillar substructure to the granule. The membrane of these larger secretory granules is commonly incomplete and fragmented.

Granule release is presumed to occur by exocytosis. This is rarely observed in transmission electron micrographs of tissue section but has been illustrated in the sheep (Perry, Robinson & Ryan, 1981) and also observed in freeze–fracture studies of melanotrophs of the rat (Saland, 1978) and frog (Semoff & Hadley, 1978a). In some species the largest of the secretory granules lying at the periphery of the cells or close to their secretory pole seem to be associated with pale-staining vacuoles which have been interpreted as intracellular invaginations of the extracellular space. Thus, secretory granules may discharge their contents into these spaces, implicating the extracellular compartment of the gland as an important route for the egress of secretions from the melanotrophs, an attractive suggestion in view of the relative avascularity of the pars intermedia and a matter considered in a later section (see Larsson, Rodriguez & Meurling, 1979).

Cilia are occasionally described associated with these secretory cells. Hopkins (1970) has shown that lysosomes are a prominent component of melanotrophs and that they appear to increase with changes in the overall activity of the pars intermedia.

Most studies of the pars intermedia make reference to the occurrence of light and dark cells. The light cells conform to the typical description of melanotrophs given above but, in circumstances which increase the secretory activity of the gland, they are accompanied by the appearance of dark cells which possess a more electron-dense cytoplasm and may also show hypertrophied Golgi fields and numerous free ribosomes. The explanation usually offered for this phenomenon is that the two cell types represent different secretory phases of the melanotroph, but its further functional significance remains obscure. In addition to dark cells there is invariably a small proportion of cells which show signs of degeneration, appearing contracted with deeply indented nuclei and closely packed, enlarged, irregularly shaped secretory granules as well as disrupted mitochondria and dilated rough endoplasmic reticulum. Mitotic activity seems to be generally low in normal animals but can be increased in pregnancy, by gonadectomy or during osmotic stress.

The complement of organelles found in melanotrophs is not constant. Physiological or pharmacological treatments which alter the overall activity of the gland are also reflected in the ultrastructural composition of these cells. Stimulation of the pars intermedia invariably increases the fractional volume of rough endoplasmic reticulum and Golgi apparatus, coupled with a decline in the population of secretory granules. Some of these changes, particularly in the Amphibia, may be of considerable magnitude and may be detectable within a few hours of the onset of a suitable stimulus. For example, in *Xenopus laevis*, when the pars intermedia is activated by transfer of animals to an environment with a black background the fractional volume of the rough endoplasmic reticulum increases from about 4% to more than 30% over a period of 3 days. During the same period the fractional volume of the secretory granules shrinks from nearly 40% to about 10%. These changes are detectable within 8 hours of the transfer (de Volcanes & Weatherhead, 1976*a*).

Immunocytochemical studies of melanotrophs reveal that they contain antigenic determinants to most of the potential fragments of the pro-opiomelanocortin molecule with the exception of methionine-enkephalin. As an example of such studies, that conducted by Martin, Weber & Voigt (1979) on the pars intermedia of the rat is particularly instructive. These authors employed four antisera with the following properties:

1. an antiserum raised against β-endorphin$_{1-9}$ which also recognised α-endorphin, β-endorphin, βLPH and pro-opiomelanocortin but not the enkephalins;
2. an antiserum raised against ACTH which recognised ACTH$_{1-39}$ and ACTH$_{1-24}$ but not αMSH$_{1-13}$, nor ACTH$_{25-39}$ nor any other pituitary hormone;
3. an antiserum to synthetic αMSH$_{1-13}$ which did not react with ACTH$_{1-24}$ nor porcine ACTH$_{1-39}$;
4. an antiserum to methionine-enkephalin which showed minimal cross reactivity with leucine-enkephalin, βLPH$_{1-91}$ and β-endorphin (βEP).

Study of resin-embedded sections with the light microscope showed that all the secretory cells of the pars intermedia stained positively with the first three antisera but not with the fourth. Furthermore, immunostaining of consecutive ultrathin sections with either anti-ACTH (antiserum no. 2) and anti-αMSH (3) or with anti-ACTH and anti-βEP (1) antisera revealed that individual mature secretory granules reacted to both antisera. The Golgi apparatus and some of the associated small, electron-dense granules showed no such immunoreactivity. It may be concluded from this study that melanotrophs and all their mature secretory granules probably contain all three of these peptides. The absence of immunoreactivity associated with the Golgi apparatus should be interpreted with caution since the antigenic determinants of pro-opiomelanocortin recognised by different antisera may be masked in some way or in the Golgi region they may be particularly vulnerable to alteration during fixation.

Whether all these peptides are *released* from the cells of the pars intermedia during the normal secretory process is a separate problem that requires a biochemical rather than a cytological approach. This is considered in a later section, together with a discussion of the likely time course of the appearance and processing of pro-opiomelanocortin and its fragments. The final conclusion to be drawn from this study is that although melanotrophs contain the amino acid sequence of one of the enkephalins (methionine-enkephalin) they are not a significant source of these opioid peptides and, indeed, these enkephalins are probably derived from protein precursors that are quite distinct from pro-opiomelanocortin (see Brownstein, 1980).

Pro-opiomelanocortin is probably not the only peptide produced by the melanotrophs of the pars intermedia. There seems to be at least one other group of lipolytically active peptides in the pars intermedia in addition to βLPH, an admittedly poor lipotrophin, that appear to be chemically related to the neurophysins. Loren *et al.* (1980) have shown that one of these lipolytic peptides (porcine lipolytic peptide B) can be demonstrated immunocytochemically in the melanotrophs of rats, cats, sheep and pigs. The antiserum used in this study showed no cross reactivity with other peptide hormones although it did cross react with neurophysin I. Antisera raised against neurophysin I did not stain melanotrophs although they did reveal the nerve fibres in the adjacent pars nervosa. There is also evidence that the lower molecular weight forms of gastrin (gastrin 34 and gastrin 17) occur in the melanotrophs of cats and pigs although the amounts detected are small (Rehfeld & Larsson, 1981).

The physiological significance of these peptides in this location is obscure but does show that the advent of immunocytochemistry, based on the remarkable specificity of antisera that can now be prepared, may in the future tell us much more about the peptides present in melanotrophs.

Various enzyme activities can be located in the pars intermedia. Whittaker & Labella (1973) have described the occurrence of acetyl- and butyryl- (pseudo-) cholinesterases in the melanotrophs of a number of species. In the cat, rat and rabbit the melanotrophs are acetylcholinesterase-positive, strongly so in the rabbit; only in the cow are they butyrylcholinesterase-positive. Bäck, Rechardt & Partanen (1976) report that in the melanotrophs of the rat acetyl- and butyrylcholinesterase have a similar distribution. These authors have also demonstrated non-specific esterase activity which is more pronounced at the periphery of lobules. It should be noted that the distribution of acetylcholinesterase activity revealed by these histochemical studies is not suggestive of a role in neurotransmitter function. Cholinesterase and non-specific esterase with the distribution described probably represents the esterolytic properties of intracellular proteases (see Bäck *et al.*, 1976).

Neuron-specific enolase (NSE: the most acidic isoenzyme of 2-phospho-D-glycerate hydrolase) is found throughout the pituitary, particularly in the glandular cells of the pars intermedia (Schmechel, Marangos & Brightman, 1978). This enzyme has been thought by some to be a marker for cells originating in the neural crest and neuroectoderm. There is no evidence for the derivation of the pars intermedia from

these sources, apart from the rather radical and unexpected claim that in the chick the
adenohypophysis develops from the neuroectoderm of the 'ventral neural ridge'
(Takor Takor & Pearse, 1975). A more likely explanation of the presence of this
enzyme in melanotrophs is that it is a functional adaptation to the presence of the high
chloride ion concentrations, which fail to inactivate it, found in cells such as neurons
and melanotrophs, with electrically excitable membranes.

Corticotrophs

In addition to the predominant granular cell type of the pars intermedia, characterised
as melanotrophs, many mammalian species also possess scattered cells with ultrastructural features similar to those cells of the pars distalis which have been identified
as corticotrophs. The corticotrophs of the pars intermedia are smaller than the
melanotrophs, have irregular outlines and are characterised by the accumulation of
smaller electron-dense secretory granules at the cell margin. Typically these cells are
concentrated in those parts of the pars intermedia which are contiguous with the pars
distalis. In the mouse they are concentrated in the rostral part of the pars intermedia,
adjacent to the stalk of the neurohypophysis, and have granules of 200 nm diameter
(Stoeckel, Schmitt & Porte, 1981). In other species they may be found in the most
lateral parts of the pars intermedia, which show an organisation transitional between
that of the pars intermedia and pars distalis, or they may be encountered under the
marginal lining of the hypophysial cleft as in the sheep where they are 250–300 nm in
diameter (Perry *et al.*, 1981). These cells have sometimes been referred to as 'stellate
cells' thus causing unfortunate confusion with the agranular, non-secretory cells of the
same name described below.

   Immunocytochemical studies of these cells are consistent with their identification as
corticotrophs. In the mouse Stoeckel *et al.* (1981) describe these cells as reacting
strongly with an antiserum raised against $ACTH_{1-24}$ whereas the melanotrophs stain
only faintly, thus emphasising the importance of conditions of fixation and reaction for
the demonstration of different immunoreactivities. Corticotrophs show the strongest
immunoreactivity at the periphery of the cells where the secretory granules are
concentrated under the cell membrane. In the rat these cells are less numerous and
less regularly distributed than in the mouse but, nevertheless, under appropriate
conditions they can be distinguished from the melanotrophs. In the dog there are
reported to be large numbers of corticotrophs, reflecting the high ACTH content of
the dog neurointermediate lobe. This can be demonstrated by the use of antisera
directed towards the mid-portion of the ACTH molecule which do not cross react with
αMSH, βMSH, $ACTH_{1-10}$ or corticotrophin-like intermediate lobe peptide (CLIP)
(Halmi *et al.*, 1981).

PAS-positive cells

   In mammals the melanotrophs are commonly reported to be PAS-positive but in
certain teleosts they can be distinguished from a second cell type that is present in the
pars intermedia which stains even more intensely with PAS. These PAS-positive cells
do not seem to contain either ACTH or αMSH as judged by immunocytochemical
studies. They do, however, seem to share some similarities with mammalian prolactin
cells since they stain positively with antisera to human, ovine or bovine prolactin even
when the antiserum has been absorbed with teleost prolactin (see Baker, 1981). In
some teleosts these PAS-positive cells respond to changes in the environmental
background colour of the animal; in other species their activity seems to be related to

changes in ambient salinity and calcium ion concentration (see van Eys, 1980). The significance of these varied responses is considered in the last section of this review.

Agranular cells

Cleft cells

Cleft cells form a lining to the posterior margin of the hypophysial cleft, when it is present. Some authors have referred to them as 'marginal' cells, a term which is also sometimes applied to those cells associated with the margins of the lobules of the pars intermedia of some species (see below); whilst others choose to call them 'ependymal' or 'ependymal-like' cells, likening their form to the ventricular lining of the brain and perhaps implying a similarity of function with ependymal cells which has yet to be demonstrated. The cleft cells are usually restricted to a single layer, many of the cells appearing squamous in form although it is not uncommon to find interspersed amongst them round or roughly triangular cell profiles bearing microvilli and/or cilia. Scanning electron microscopical studies of the rat hypophysial cleft surface reveals four types of cell (Ciocca, 1980): some have a smooth surface, some have microvilli restricted to the margins of the cell apex, some have cilia arranged in tufts and some have microvilli distributed evenly over the surface of the cell apex. The cells with microvilli restricted to the periphery seem to be the commonest type. Cells with cilia are infrequent but in the sheep are gathered into groups (Perry *et al.*, 1981). Many of these different types of cell contain a large population of mitochondria. All these types of cell show extensive interdigitation of their lateral cell surfaces whilst their apical connections are sealed by junctional complexes, effectively preventing any of the other cell types present in the pars intermedia from making direct contact with the lumen of the hypophysial cleft.

This layer of cleft cells is sometimes described as standing on a basement membrane. Closer examination reveals that the connective tissue usually extends from the pericapillary space; it forms a more or less extensive network through the pars intermedia and comprises two distinct basal laminae, enclosing a space in which fibroblasts and occasionally capillaries can be seen. The cleft cells show no particular morphological signs of secretory activity and granules are found in them only rarely. Some of the cleft cells possess basal processes which may penetrate between the granular cells. In species in which the pars intermedia is no more than a few cells thick, these processes stretch across to end in association with the plexus intermedius. Where the pars intermedia is better developed the termination of such processes has not been described, perhaps because there is no easy way to distinguish their processes from those of other agranular cell types (e.g. stellate and follicle cells) which may be present. Some authors describe cleft cells as possessing bulbous cytoplasmic processes which extend into the hypophysial cleft and which may become particularly marked following gonadectomy, adrenalectomy or the administration of cyproterone acetate (Perry *et al.*, 1981). In this respect the cleft cells may be reflecting the overall activity of the pars intermedia rather than betraying a specific response to the experimental conditions.

It has been reported that, in the rat, these cells display cross reactivity with antisera to the protein S100 (Cocchia & Miani, 1980). This protein was thought originally to be a specific marker for neural tissues, being associated with both glial and neuronal components. Its validity as a marker of neuroectodermal derivatives may be doubted, however, in view of its reported occurrence in human skin not only in melanocytes, which are, of course, derived from the neural crest, but also in Langerhans cells which are now known to be mesodermal products of the bone marrow (Cocchia, Michetti & Donato, 1981). S100 seems to be one of a family of acidic calcium-binding proteins with an amino acid sequence and distribution similar to that of calmodulin in the rat (Bock, 1978). This might be cited as evidence for the role of agranular cells in the regulation of the ionic milieu of the pars intermedia; indeed these cells have been shown to accumulate calcium in cytoplasmic vacuoles (Stoeckel et al., 1981).

Cleft cells show strong non-specific esterase activity in the rat (Bäck et al., 1976) but do not possess neuron-specific enolase (Schmechel et al., 1978). In immunocyto-chemical studies of the pars intermedia, the cleft cells have never been described as displaying immunoreactivity to known pituitary hormones.

Folliculo-stellate cells

Some authors have described the major agranular cell population as constituting a folliculo-stellate system. Stellate cells are characterised by their numerous radiating processes which insinuate between the cells comprising the glandular parenchyma; their elongate nuclei may be found at any level through the pars intermedia. The presence of stellate cells seems to be occasioned by the degree of development of the pars intermedia since in reptiles, for example, they are only encountered where the lobe is more than a few cells thick (Weatherhead, 1978). Their processes may terminate at the plexus intermedius where it is not uncommon to find an accumulation of pinocytotic vesicles along the free margin of the cell. The cells are agranular, containing elements of agranular reticulum but little rough endoplasmic reticulum. They possess a rich population of microtubules and microfilaments. In the sheep, extensive junctional complexes have been described between adjacent stellate cells, although they are uncommon between stellate cells and glandular cells (Perry et al., 1981). Of the species investigated by Whittaker & Labella (1973) only the stellate cells of the rat show positive butyrylcholinesterase activity. These cells have no neuron-specific enolase (Schmechel et al., 1978).

The general similarity in shape between stellate cells and astrocytes has led some authors to describe them as 'glial' or 'glial-like' cells. There is a little evidence to support this notion since Stoeckel et al. (1981) have reported that in the rat they show cross reactivity with antisera to glial fibrillary acid protein (GFA). GFA is in fact a heterogenous mixture of polypeptide chains which are associated with the 8–10 nm glial filaments that are similar to intermediate filaments. GFA has been considered to be a marker for astrocytes and supposed to reflect the supportive function of these cells (Bock, 1978); its presence in stellate cells may thus reflect their similar function in the pars intermedia. Further evidence for physiological similarities between stellate cells and glial cells comes from the work of Semoff & Hadley (1978b) who have shown that in the pars intermedia of the frog there is a histochemically demonstrable adenosine triphosphatase, perhaps a Na^+,K^+ phosphatase, at the stellate cell membrane but only where such stellate cells abut other stellate cells or granular cells. Such activity could not be found at adjacent granular cell membranes. This also underlines the role that the stellate cell may play in ionic regulation. S100 protein has been reported to occur in the follicular and stellate cells of the pars distalis and pars tuberalis of the rat but not, curiously, in the pars intermedia (Cocchia & Miani, 1980).

An overall assessment of this scanty evidence suggests that it seems wiser to avoid the description of stellate cells as glial-like since it implies a similarity of function that remains to be unequivocally demonstrated.

Perryman, de Vellis & Bagnara (1980) have drawn attention to another property of the stellate cell. When the amphibian neurointermediate lobe is transplanted ectopically to the anterior chamber of the eye or maintained *in vitro*, the stellate cells become actively phagocytic and engulf surrounding cell debris. Hopkins (1971) has also described how in *Xenopus* treated with the neurotoxic sympathetomimetic analogue of dopamine, 6-hydroxydopamine, the stellate cells show (within a few days) evidence of an increase in the size and development of the Golgi as well as an increase in the presence of lysosome-like organelles. This may reflect the activity of these cells in removing dead and dying neuronal debris from the gland. Evidence of phagocytic activity in stellate cells in normal animals is uncommon but this may merely reflect the fact that the pars intermedia may not have been examined at times when its secretory activity was undergoing great changes. Certainly the stellate cells of the pars distalis show phagocytic activity in some circumstances (see Perryman *et al.*, 1980).

These morphological observations lead to the conclusion that the stellate cells may provide not merely a structural component of the pars intermedia; they may also be involved in the movement of material into and out of the pars intermedia, the regulation of the ionic milieu of the pars intermedia and at times be able to act as phagocytes.

Follicle cells surround spaces of varying size in the pituitary. These spaces may be only a few micrometres across or may be much larger spaces visible to the naked eye, especially when they are seen in the pars distalis. Benjamin (1981) has arbitrarily classified spaces in the pituitary which are larger than 50 μm in diameter as 'cysts' and has provided us with a useful survey of what is known of their occurrence, structure and function. In the pars intermedia the follicle cells that line these spaces are sealed with apical junctional complexes and it is rare to find granular cells in contact with the follicular lumen. The free surface of the follicle cell apex may be smooth or it may bear microvilli and/or cilia. Like the cleft cells, the follicle cells sometimes possess processes but it is rare to be able to trace these through the glandular parenchyma and their sites of termination remain to be described. Small vesicles may be found under the apical plasma membrane. The smaller follicles usually appear empty but larger ones may contain more or less electron-dense, colloid-like material with varying degrees of PAS-positivity: sometimes the follicular lumen is seen to contain crystalline inclusions. Generally the follicles of the pars intermedia are smaller than those of the pars distalis although the human pars intermedia is an exception in this respect. Follicles may be found throughout the pars intermedia although in some species there seems to be a predisposition for them to occur close to the border with the pars nervosa.

The embryonic origin of these follicles and cysts is undetermined. They could represent remnants of Rathke's pouch, they could arise by the accumulation and subsequent investment of extracellular fluid or they may even be due to the degeneration of groups of secretory cells when the associated agranular cells arrange themselves to form the wall of the follicle. Benjamin (1981) has surveyed the evidence for these various possibilities.

Bordering or marginal cells

In the rat there seems to be a population of cells associated with the interlobar margins of the pars intermedia. They stain strongly for non-specific esterase and Bäck *et al.* (1976) consider them to be Schwann cells associated with the interlobar connective tissue.

Miscellaneous cell types

In those parts of the pars intermedia which abut the pars nervosa but where there are no intervening capillaries of the plexus intermedius, the so-called contact zones of Eurenius and Jarskär (1975), it is possible to find pituicytes lying close to granular secretory cells but they do not, however, seem to send penetrating processes into the pars intermedia for any distance. The pericapillary space of the plexus intermedius often contains fibroblasts accompanied by fine collagen fibrils and, where these pericapillary spaces ramify the pars intermedia, fibroblasts (or fine processes presumed to belong to fibroblasts) may be seen in them.

Amongst the mobile cells which might be expected to invade the pars intermedia, eosinophil leucocytes are sometimes seen, characterised in rodent species by their unmistakable banded granules. There have also been reports of the occurrence of mast cells in the pars intermedia of the rat pituitary (Baumgarten *et al.*, 1972).

THE HUMAN PARS INTERMEDIA

In young foetuses, even at about 15 weeks of age, there is a typical pars intermedia forming a normal epithelial lining to the posterior margin of the hypophysial cleft. At this stage most of the cells present seem to be melanotrophs. Visser & Swaab (1979) describe the gradual appearance from birth to about 19 years of age of more and more typical corticotrophs as the intermediate lobe becomes less distinct. In the adult the pars intermedia is reduced to a series of follicles and cysts, accompanied by cells which invade the pars nervosa. Very few, if any, of these cells can be identified immunocytochemically as melanotrophs. Some authors, therefore, refrain from using the term pars intermedia, which they believe should only be applied to pituitaries which show evidence of secretion of MSH, preferring the less committed term 'intermediate zone'. A recent description of the immunocytochemical affinities of this area (Osamura & Watanabe, 1978) shows that most of the cells comprising follicles are arranged as a single layer of granular, cuboidal epithelial cells without a basement membrane. They stain positively with antisera to both the N-terminal ($ACTH_{1-18}$) and C-terminal ($ACTH_{17-39}$) sequence of ACTH. Interspersed amongst them, however, are cells which contain other pituitary hormones, e.g. prolactin, follicle stimulating hormone (FSH) and luteinising hormone (LH). Thyrotrophs do not seem to contribute to the follicular epithelium. The basophilic cells which invade the pars nervosa are again mainly ACTH-positive although scattered cells which react to antisera against growth hormone, prolactin, FSH, LH and even thyrotrophin are occasionally seen. In addition to these endocrine cells there are sometimes well established acini resembling salivary glands, but the cells have no secretory granules and fail to stain with antisera to pituitary hormones.

It is quite clear from biochemical studies that the human pituitary produces extremely small amounts of αMSH_{1-13}, if any at all. All of the MSH bioactivity found in human pituitary extracts can be accounted for by the melanophore-stimulating capacity of ACTH, γMSH, βLPH and γLPH. It also seems to be well established that, even though it is possible to detect βMSH sequences in the cells of the human pars intermedia, the βMSH that is found in plasma is probably not released in that form and is a degradation artefact of βLPH (Lerner, 1981 and subsequent discussion).

In anencephalics, the pars intermedia contains the same type of cells as in normal foetuses although they tend to be smaller, less numerous and not grouped together.

This suggests that the initial differentiation of the pars intermedia can occur independently of hypothalamic influences although, in the pars distalis at least, some factors of hypothalamic origin are necessary for its full development in later foetal stages (Bégeot, Dubois & Dubois, 1978).

In addition to the sellar hypophysis, the persistence of a pharyngeal hypophysis in man is not uncommon (McGrath, 1978). It represents the extracranial remnants of the stomodaeal contribution to Rathke's pouch embedded in the mucoperiosteum of the nasopharynx. In an 8 week foetus it has been shown to contain βLPH, $ACTH_{17-39}$, β-endorphin and α-endorphin immunoreactivity (Bégeot *et al.*, 1978).

PITUITARY COLLOID

Pituitary colloid, so-called because of its histological resemblance to the colloid of the thyroid gland, may be found in three distinct situations: the evidence that it has the same origin or composition in each site is not strong. Benjamin (1981) has discussed the phenomenon of pituitary colloid in general.

Cleft colloid

There is great interspecific variation in the occurrence of colloid in the hypophysial cleft. It is found for example in cows and sheep but not in pigs and horses. There may even be intraspecific variation: of two highly selected strains of rat (the Dahl strains) one shows great accumulations of colloid which enlarge the cleft, the other does not (Rapp & Bergon, 1977). Opinions regarding the origin of cleft colloid are many and not all of course implicate the pars intermedia, since the pars distalis also contributes to the margin of the cleft. Some authors declare that the breakdown products of degenerating cells in the pars distalis secondarily accumulate as colloid, others maintain that colloid is an apocrine secretory product of the cleft cells of the posterior wall of the cleft (see Benjamin, 1981, for the variety of such views). Certainly the cleft is in physiological continuity with the extracellular space of the pars intermedia since the electron-dense marker horseradish peroxidase (HRP), when injected intravenously, rapidly penetrates the pars intermedia and appears in the cleft (Stoeckel *et al.*, 1981). Since the HRP does not penetrate the apical junctional complexes of the cleft cells, they themselves must presumably be involved in the transport of HRP, which might explain the light uptake of HRP that they show and would also be consistent with histochemical findings suggesting that the cleft cells are more likely to be involved in transport rather than secretion (Vanha-Perttula & Arstila, 1970).

The staining affinities of the colloid seem to vary greatly even within the same animal. Of the contents of the colloid little is known. It has been described as having a high melanotrophic bioactivity (Andersson & Jewell, 1958) but immunocytochemical studies fail to report on the presence of peptide fragments derived from pro-opiomelanocortin. This negative evidence should probably be treated with caution since the problems of immobilising peptides and preserving immunoreactivity in non-granular form may be considerable (see discussion following Stoeckel *et al.*, 1981).

A series of studies has revealed the identity of at least one component of the colloid. Individuals of the R strain of Dahl rats, selected for its resistance to the hypertensive effects of a high salt diet, contain vast amounts of colloid compared with rats of the sister strain (S strain) which are susceptible to such diets. Polyacrylamide gel electrophoresis of colloid from the R strain reveals at least four proteins which are probably absent in the S strain, or at least present only in small amounts (Rapp & Bergon, 1977). One of these proteins, R1, seems to be related to albumen and the other three may be polymeric forms. Whatever their exact identity there is a strong inverse relationship between the amounts of R1 protein present and blood pressure. One may conclude that the R strain rat has some altered, but as yet unidentified, pituitary function related to salt metabolism. This is interesting in view of the common observation that in some species changes in salt or water metabolism or adrenal-ectomy may alter the amount of colloid in the cleft. Curiously, R strain rats fed on a high salt diet from weaning for a period of 6 weeks apparently show no increase in the amount of cleft colloid. Perhaps the changes are more transient. The presence of albumen-like factors in the cleft colloid also underlines its functional continuity with the vascular system, but whether that of the pars intermedia, pars distalis or both is unknown. Certainly colloid may, in part, originate by a process of transudation.

Follicular (and cyst) colloid

Some of the larger follicles of the pars intermedia may contain PAS-positive and electron-dense colloid. It is presumed either to originate from the follicle cells themselves, although they possess no granules, or to represent the breakdown of groups of secretory cells that become encapsulated by agranular cells. This latter possibility is raised by Horvath et al. (1974) who consider them to be transient structures in the human pars intermedia. The constitution of this colloid is largely unknown although Andersson & Jewell (1958) reported that, where such cysts invaded the pars nervosa of the goat, the colloid possessed both antidiuretic and melanotrophic bioactivity. These authors also present evidence that with the extreme development of multilobular cysts in the goat they may become continuous with the hypophysial cleft. This does not seem to be a common observation in other species.

Intracellular colloid

Material described as 'colloid-like' also occurs within the secretory cells of the pars intermedia but the literature on the subject is confusing, largely due to the differences in descriptive terminology; as usual, interspecific variation complicates the matter further. In the bullfrog (*Rana catesbiana*) accumulation of material is found within the cisternae of the rough endoplasmic reticulum. It is fairly electron dense and may reach 1–2 μm in diameter, especially in animals in which the secretion of pars intermedia peptides has been stimulated by placing animals on a black background (Saland, 1968). Such material, however, is not usually seen in the closely related *Rana pipiens*. It has been assumed to represent a direct condensation of hormonal secretory products in the rough endoplasmic reticulum, perhaps because the synthetic capacity of the rough endoplasmic reticulum in hyperactive glands exceeds the packaging capacity of the Golgi apparatus. Iturriza & Koch (1964) described material such as this as containing a carbohydrate other than glycogen, amino acids and as being weakly sudanophilic.

Cytoplasmic colloid, i.e. extracisternal colloid, seems to be generally more electron dense than that associated with the rough endoplasmic reticulum and appears as discrete, more or less globular accumulations of material. It does seem to be distinguishable from the lipid-like bodies described in *R. pipiens* by Semoff, Fuller & Hadley (1978) which are large globular structures reaching a diameter of several micrometres. These lipid-like bodies are surrounded by a halo of secretory granules, although there is no evidence of the release of secretory products from them at this site. Lipid-like bodies have also been described in *Xenopus laevis* by Hopkins (1970) but in this species the material is irregular in outline. To what extent the varied appearance of these intracellular inclusions reflects differences in the economy of the secretory cells in different species or whether they are an artefact of different experimental manipulations seems to be a matter for conjecture. There is no modern evidence that any sort of colloid contains immunoreactive peptide hormones.

INNERVATION OF THE PARS INTERMEDIA

Amongst the various classes of vertebrate the degree to which the nerve fibres penetrate the pars intermedia varies greatly. In some, e.g. lampreys (*Lampetra*), the sturgeon (*Acipenser*) and lacertilian reptiles, there seem to be no nerve fibres in the pars intermedia at all (Weatherhead, 1978). In others, various types of nerve fibre provide a supply which varies from 'scanty' to 'rich'. The usual classification of fibres is based on their staining affinities and ultrastructural appearance, the commonest terminology recognising type A, B and C fibres.

Type A fibres

Type A fibres are still referred to by some authors as neurosecretory fibres since their contents stain with the classical neurosecretory stains, i.e. Chrome Alum Haematoxylin, Aldehyde Fuchsin and Alcian Blue. Ultrastructurally the fibres are usually of large diameter and are characterised by electron-dense granules, with a closely investing membrane giving an overall diameter of 150–200 nm, and also by electron-lucent vesicles approximately 50 nm in diameter. Most authors accept that these fibres are peptidergic and recognise subtypes, A1, A2 etc., in which the size and degree of electron density of the granules seem to correspond to similar fibres containing the different nonapeptide hormones of the pars nervosa (Rodriguez, 1971). The only direct immunocytochemical confirmation of their peptidergic nature appears to be that made by van Vossel *et al.* (1977) who showed that in *Rana temporaria* there were distinct mesotocin-containing and arginine-vasotocin-containing fibres, the former being some 5–10 times more numerous than the latter. Mesotocin and arginine-vasotocin are of course the principal neurohypophysial peptide hormones of the Amphibia.

Type A fibres seem to be common in the pars intermedia of lower vertebrates, e.g. cartilaginous and bony fishes; in the Amphibia they seem to be restricted to that part of the pars intermedia which lies close to the pars nervosa. Type A fibres certainly occur in the pars intermedia of mammals: they seem to be uncommon in the monkey, sheep, mouse, cat and rat (Anand Kumar & Vincent, 1974; Perry *et al.*, 1981; Stoeckel *et al.*, 1981) but occur more frequently in the rabbit (Cameron & Foster, 1971). These fibres are apparently common in the ferret (Vincent & Anand Kumar, 1969) but scarce in the closely related mink (Weman & Nobin, 1973). In the rabbit and the mouse the fibres seem to be largely restricted to the juxta-neural margin of the pars intermedia (Jarskär, 1977) along the plexus intermedius. Only in the ferret do they seem to penetrate throughout the pars intermedia.

In lower vertebrates the type A fibres make synaptic contacts with the melano-trophs of the pars intermedia. At such sites there are accumulations of the small electron-lucent vesicles in association with thickenings of the pre-synaptic membrane: there are also electron-dense thickenings of the adjacent post-synaptic membrane of the melanotroph. In mammals, such synaptic contacts seem to occur with any significant frequency only in the rabbit and ferret. Synaptic contacts between peptidergic fibres and corticotrophs also seem to be rare in the two species in which they have been most studied, i.e. the rat and mouse (Stoeckel *et al.*, 1973), probably reflecting the generally sparse occurrence of type A fibres in these species. Peptidergic fibres are assumed to originate from the magnocellular nuclei of the hypothalamus. In amphibians, ablation of the preoptic nucleus results in the disappearance of the peptidergic terminals from the pars intermedia. In mammals, the precise origin of peptidergic fibres remains to be established. Brooks & Vincent (1977) showed that, in the ferret, lesions of the median eminence caused the degeneration of all nerve terminals in the pars intermedia. Bilateral lesions of the paraventricular nuclei failed to affect the peptidergic fibres as did lesions of the anterior hypothalamus designed to interrupt the efferent fibres of the supraoptic nucleus. Not all peptidergic neurons in the pars intermedia may contain neurohypophysial hormones since Follenius & Dubois (1979) have demonstrated methionine-enkephalin-containing axons penetrating the proximal pars distalis and pars intermedia of the carp. They seem to correspond to neurosecretory axons of the preoptico-hypophysial tract.

Type B fibres

Type B fibres are fibres which fail to stain with the classical neurosecretory stains and which ultrastructurally contain both electron-lucent vesicles about 50 nm in diameter and larger dense-cored vesicles with an overall diameter of 75–125 nm in which there is a clear halo between the granule and its investing membrane. Various lines of evidence leave no doubt that some, at least, of these fibres are aminergic. With the Falck–Hillarp technique the varicosities seen along the course of the fibres emit a yellow-green fluorescence which is characteristic of catecholamines. Baumgarten *et al.* (1972) have shown that in the pig, rat and cat the emission spectra of most of these varicosities reveal them as containing dopamine whilst a few terminals associated with the plexus intermedius contain noradrenaline and may thus be autonomic vasomotor fibres. Type B fibres also take up the electron-opaque false transmitter 5-hydroxydopamine, a property displayed by aminergic fibres in other situations.

6-Hydroxydopamine (6-OHDA), another dopamine analogue, is a known neurotoxic agent taken up by aminergic fibres and it has been shown that after its administration to *Xenopus*, the profiles of all fibres except those of type A disappear from the pars intermedia (Hopkins, 1971). In mammals, however, 6-OHDA does not remove all type B terminals (Baumgarten *et al.*, 1972), which is interesting in view of the recent report that in the pars intermedia of the rat there is a rich network of γ-aminobutyric acid (GABA) containing fibres (Vincent, Hokfelt & Wu, 1982). Perhaps some type B fibres are GABAergic. It is type B fibres which predominate in the vertebrate, especially the mammalian, pars intermedia, forming a network amongst the secretory cells and making synaptic contacts with the melanotrophs and with the corticotrophs when they are present. Many of these contacts display the full range of synaptic structure with accumulations of small electron-lucent vesicles in association with electron-dense thickenings of the pre- and post-synaptic membranes.

Terlou & Ploemacher (1973) have shown that in *Xenopus* these dopaminergic fibres originate in the paraventricular organ and also possibly in the nucleus infundibularis dorsalis. In the rat, dopaminergic fibres originate in the rostral arcuate nucleus (Björklund & Nobin, 1972).

Type C fibres

The third type of fibre to be found in the pars intermedia, type C fibres, contain only electron-lucent vesicles of 50 nm diameter. The nature of these fibres has exercised the imagination of many authors on numerous occasions. The simplest explanation is that they represent profiles of axons in which the granules typical of either type A or type B fibres happen to be absent. Indeed, Jarskär's (1977) report on the mouse pars intermedia showed that type B and type C fibres were present in approximately equal numbers but that study of serial sections revealed that some fibres originally classified as type C did in fact contain type B granules in adjacent sections. The other explanation for the existence of type C fibres is that they are cholinergic. However, in those mammals in which acetylcholinesterase has been demonstrated it does not have the distribution which would be expected if it were concerned with synaptic function, being largely confined to the nucleus and rough endoplasmic reticulum of the secretory cells in species such as the cat and rabbit (Whittaker & Labella, 1973). Choline acetylase, the enzyme concerned with the synthesis of acetylcholine, has been localised in the junctional zone between the pars intermedia and pars nervosa of the rat, where its concentration is higher than in the adjacent parts of the pituitary (Gallardo, Cannata & Tramezzani, 1980). The origin of type C fibres may be neither the magnocellular nuclei nor the arcuate nuclei of the hypothalamus, since HRP applied iontophoretically to the neural lobe of *Bufo* reveals cell bodies in the ventromedial thalamic area and in the bed nucleus of the hippocampal commissure (Pasquier, Cannata & Tramezzani, 1980).

VASCULARITY OF THE PARS INTERMEDIA

The early studies of the vascular system of the pars intermedia employed perfusions with Indian ink, or similar media, followed either by direct examination of whole mounts or by microscopical observations of relatively thick sections ($> 10~\mu$m). More recently there have been reports based on scanning electron microscopical observations of resin casts of the vascular system from which the surrounding tissues have been eroded. Another important approach has been to employ extracellular space markers such as Ruthenium Red, Lanthanum and HRP.

The extent of the vascularisation of the pars intermedia which such techniques reveal is a matter of contention. Whilst there is no doubt that it has a very much less extensive vascular bed than either the neurohypophysis or the other parts of the adenohypophysis it would be improper to call it avascular as some authors are tempted to do. In those species in which the pars intermedia consists of only one or two cell layers it is functionally no more avascular than epithelia of comparable thickness; wherever it is more extensive than this, it is always possible to find some blood vessels. The vessels which comprise the plexus intermedius may include a very few small muscular arterioles, with a tunica media made up of a single layer of visceral muscle cells, but most are fenestrated capillaries. They are invested by a pericapillary space which contains fine collagen fibrils and fibroblasts. Some, but not all, of the granular and folliculo-stellate cells of the pars intermedia abut this space. The plexus intermedius may not form a complete barrier between the pars intermedia and pars nervosa, so that nerve fibres and pituicytes may lie adjacent to granular and folliculo-stellate cells at the contact zones described by Jarskär (1977), although there seems to be little intermingling of these elements.

Where the pars intermedia is not covered by other neurohypophysial or adeno-hypophysial tissue it may bear a superficial plexus of capillaries. This is most obvious on the dorsal aspect of the lateral transitional zones between the pars intermedia and pars distalis in some species, where one may find both melanotrophs and corticotrophs lying close to penetrating vessels. In some species, where the pars intermedia is clearly lobulated, the interlobular connective tissue septa contain capillaries which are similar in structure to those of the plexus intermedius from which they must originate. Adjacent granular cells may show polarisation of their secretory poles towards these capillaries. Bergland & Page (1979) conclude, on the basis of their studies of resin casts, that there is a paucity of direct venous connections between the adenohypo-physis and the adjacent cavernous sinuses so that there must be an alternative route for the egress of venous blood, perhaps involving retrograde (i.e. hypothalamo-petal) flow of blood in the portal vessels. They allow, however, that portal vessels are not closely related to the pars intermedia, although there is no doubt that almost every conceivable vascular anastomosis in the pituitary can be demonstrated (Holmes, 1964). Thus, while there may be an important connection between the plexus intermedius and the systemic circulation via the cavernous sinuses, it should be borne in mind that blood obtained from the portal vessels of the rat actually contains higher concentrations of immunoreactive αMSH than systemic blood. Oliver, Mical & Porter (1977) showed that these high levels of portal plasma $αMSH_{1-13}$ could be partially reduced by removal of the pars distalis and almost totally abolished by either removal of the neurointermediate lobe or total hypophysectomy. They concluded that this portal αMSH must originate from the pars intermedia and pass through both the pars distalis and pars nervosa before entering retrograde channels in the pituitary stalk.

Bergland & Page (1979) have discussed in some detail the possible dynamics of the pituitary vascular bed but it is fair to point out that most of their conclusions are really applicable only to mammals. In lower vertebrates there seem to be straightforward connections between the pars intermedia and the venous drainage of the brain (see Meurling & Willstedt, 1970). Whatever the route of egress of the secretory products from the pars intermedia, there can be no doubt that the pars intermedia is freely permeable to many blood borne substances, even those of relatively high molecular weight. The pars intermedia lies outside the blood brain barrier of course and is rapidly penetrated by markers such as Ruthenium Red and HRP (MW = 40 000) introduced into the peripheral vascular system or directly into the cardiac ventricle. Perryman was the first to employ HRP in this way (see Perryman & Bagnara, 1978) and reported that within 2 minutes of injection of HRP into the cardiac ventricle of *Rana* it was distributed throughout the extracellular space of the pars intermedia. Similar speed of penetration of this extracellular compartment is seen in the lizard, *Anolis* (Larsson, 1981), in the rat (de Bold, de Bold & Kraicer, 1980) and mouse (Holmes, 1981). Following this initial dispersal, HRP then appears in coated micropinocytotic and endocytotic vesicles in both granular and stellate cells. It does not appear to be taken up by nerve terminals nor has it been traced to follicular lumina but it does enter the hypophysial cleft, probably via the cleft cells. Although HRP appears rapidly in the pars intermedia it seems to be cleared much more slowly than in either the pars nervosa or the pars distalis, in which its appearance is transient (Stoeckel *et al.*, 1981).

In the rat, extracellular space markers have revealed a system of intercellular channels. de Bold *et al.* (1980) recognise two types. Type I channels are formed where more than two granular cells join, the potential space being filled with one or more axons, or stellate cell processes or a cilium arising from one of the granular cells. Type II spaces occur only between two adjacent granular cells and rarely include any of the above elements. A system of such well defined intercellular channels as this does not seem to be of common occurrence.

A further component of the extracellular compartment of the pars intermedia revealed by HRP and electron microscopy is extensions of the perivascular space which are too small to contain capillaries, but which are recognised by their collagen content and basement membrane and which in fortunate sections can be seen to be continuous with the pericapillary space of the plexus intermedius. These spaces do not, however, seem to be extensive enough to be regarded as a functional replacement for a rich capillary network. In some cases these spaces push up under the cleft cells and may run for some considerable distance, appearing to the casual observer as a basement membrane.

One must conclude that despite the paucity of capillaries in this endocrine organ the extracellular space compartment provides an efficient route for the ingress and egress of material to and from the pars intermedia. It may be, of course, that not all the granular cells react equally promptly to calls upon the secretory reserves of the gland, those closest to capillaries providing the first secretory supplies, a suggestion supported by the electron microscopical observations of the pars intermedia of *Anolis* (Larsson *et al.*, 1979). There is no doubt that MSH can reach the systemic circulation very rapidly as evidenced by the rapid chromatic responses seen in some lizards.

CONTROL OF SECRETORY ACTIVITY IN THE PARS INTERMEDIA

The earliest studies of the functions of the pars intermedia were undertaken in Amphibia, in which it was demonstrated that ablation of the pars intermedia resulted in failure of chromatophore control, i.e. the animals were unable to show the normal skin darkening in response to transfer to a black background. The assessment of colour in lower vertebrates, often on the basis of melanophore index (Bagnara & Hadley, 1973), still provides a convenient measure of the secretory activity of the pars intermedia. In time, these indirect estimates of circulating hormone concentrations were supplemented by direct bioassay of the hormone content of the pituitary. This was usually based upon the ability of the secretions of the pars intermedia to disperse melanosomes in the melanophores of fish, amphibian or reptilian skin *in vitro*. More recently still, the specificity and sensitivity of assays have been further improved by the production of highly specific hormone antisera and the radiolabelling at high specific activity of synthetic peptide hormone standards. Thus, radioimmunoassays permit not only the precise description of the peptide fragments being measured, but also have detection levels which allow the measurement of these peptides in peripheral plasma, a feature notably absent from most bioassays.

True morphological assessments of the secretory responses of the pars intermedia range from simple measurements of changes in overall size of the gland to full stereological analyses of the fractional volumes of the various organelles of the secretory cells. Finally, it has been shown that the cells of the pars intermedia possess resting membrane potentials and that the various regulators of pars intermedia function may act by controlling the spontaneous electrical depolarisations which accompany hormone release from these cells.

Neural versus neurohumoral control

Whilst the pars intermedia of most vertebrates receives a more or less profuse innervation of various types, the exceptions to this condition in which no nerve fibres can be identified in the pars intermedia point to the possibility of neurohumoral regulation from other parts of the pituitary or the hypothalamus. The close anatomical associations between the pars nervosa and the pars intermedia and the intervening plexus intermedius provide a ready route by which neurohypophysial peptides or biogenic amines might reach the pars intermedia, the permeability of which has already been established by HRP penetration studies. Furthermore, there is evidence of connections between the plexus intermedius and the primary plexus of the median eminence (Holmes, 1964), so that hypothalamic factors probably have access to the pars intermedia too. In any consideration of the regulation of the activity of the pars intermedia it is essential not to restrict the discussion solely to the nerve fibres which directly innervate the secretory cells since other, humoral, routes may be equally important.

The hypothalamic connection

Various lines of evidence suggest that the predominant control of the pars intermedia by the hypothalamus is inhibitory. Thus, surgical transection of the pituitary stalk in amphibians results in an uncontrolled release of melanotrophins, as evidenced by the permanent darkening of the skin due to chronic melanosome dispersion within the dermal melanophores. Transplantation of the neurointermediate lobe to sites distant from the sella turcica, the capsule of the kidney and the anterior chamber of the eye being favoured sites, also results in physiological and morphological evidence of increased MSH release. These grafts may remain viable for many months, as long as 22 months according to one report (Santolaya & Rodriguez, 1977). In most cases the transplants do not become invaded by nerve fibres and the melanotrophs contain few vesicles and many rough-surfaced vesicular elements. In some cases the pars intermedia does become re-innervated, especially in chronically grafted glands, in which case the melanotrophs appear to resemble those of the pars intermedia *in situ*, suggesting that some form of inhibitory control can become re-established. Transfer of the pars intermedia to culture *in vitro* results in the development of whorl-like formations of the rough endoplasmic reticulum and evidence of continued secretion which may persist for weeks on end (Semoff *et al.*, 1978). Set against these findings, however, are pharmacological studies which suggest that there may also be mechanisms which mediate the stimulation of MSH release.

Catecholaminergic influences

It has been repeatedly demonstrated that such non-specific depleters of catecholamines as reserpine produce prolonged increases in melanophore index, corresponding to an increase in the rate of MSH release. Saland (1978) has also shown that in the rat, reserpine administration produces in the melanotrophs of the pars intermedia all the expected signs of increased secretion, with expanded areas and whorls of the rough endoplasmic reticulum as well as extensive Golgi fields. *In vitro* studies show that adrenaline, noradrenaline and dopamine all inhibit MSH release from amphibian and mammalian glands as detected by bioassays (Bower, Hadley & Hruby, 1974). Furthermore, dopamine inhibits the release of all the fragments of pro-opiomelanocortin which can be detected in the perfusate of isolated cell preparations *in vitro* (Jackson *et al.*, 1981).

The evidence for the presence of α- and β-adrenoreceptors in the pars intermedia has been summarised by Bower *et al.* (1974). Phenylephrine, an α-adrenoreceptor agonist, inhibits MSH release *in vitro* whilst dibenamine, an α-adrenoreceptor antagonist, blocks the adrenaline-induced release of MSH. Isoprenaline (isoproterenol), a β-adrenoreceptor agonist, stimulates MSH release and also abolishes the inhibitory effects of the catecholamines on MSH release. It also stimulates MSH release when infused *in vivo*. The β-adrenoreceptor antagonist propranolol, blocks the stimulation of MSH release induced by isoprenaline. It seems, therefore, that whilst α-adrenoreceptors mediate the inhibition of MSH release, β-adrenoreceptors are responsible for the stimulation of its release. Whilst most authors agree that melanotrophs possess β-adrenoreceptors, it is possible that the apparent presence of α-adrenoreceptors may in fact be due to dopamine receptors, which some believe to be related to the α-adrenoreceptor (see Bower *et al.*, 1974). Munemura *et al.* (1980) discount the presence of an α-adrenoreceptor on the grounds that the α-adrenergic antagonists, phentolamine and yohimbine, were unable to reverse the effects of dopaminergic antagonists and that while fluphenazine and phentolamine are approximately equipotent antagonists of the α-adrenoreceptor, fluphenazine is more potent than phentolamine in reversing the inhibitory effects of dopamine upon the pars intermedia.

The evidence for the presence of dopamine receptors can be summarised as follows. Dopamine itself inhibits MSH release both *in vivo* and *in vitro* (Jackson *et al.*, 1981) and furthermore it inhibits the spontaneous electrical activity which can be recorded from the pars intermedia *in vitro* (Davis & Hadley, 1978). It can also overcome the 5-hydroxytryptamine- and isoprenaline-induced release of MSH *in vitro*. Dopamine agonists such as bromocriptine reduce the proportion of rough endoplasmic reticulum and newly formed Golgi granules in melanotrophs (Stoeckel *et al.*, 1981). By contrast a dopamine antagonist, pimozide, induces skin darkening in *Anolis* (Levitin, 1980*a*) and increases the proportion of newly forming secretory granules, Golgi apparatus and rough endoplasmic reticulum in melanotrophs whilst simultaneously depleting them of mature secretory granules. It seems to produce no observable effects upon the corticotrophs of the pars intermedia of the rat (Santolaya & Ciocca, 1981). Fluphenazine reverses the inhibitory effects of dopamine (Munemura *et al.*, 1980). Reference has already been made to the neurotoxic effects of the dopamine analogue, 6-hydroxydopamine, on the aminergic terminals of the pars intermedia. The disappearance of these terminals is accompanied by ultrastructural changes consistent with enhanced hormone release, i.e. the depletion of secretory granules and an increase in the fractional volume of the rough endoplasmic reticulum and Golgi apparatus (de Volcanes & Weatherhead, 1976*b*).

It has recently been realised that dopamine receptors can be classified into two general categories D1 and D2. D1 receptors in various tissues regulate a specific dopamine-sensitive adenylate cyclase which is responsible for the production of the intracellular second messenger cyclic AMP. Stimulation of D2 receptors on the other hand does not result in enhanced adenyl cyclase activity nor in the accumulation of cyclic AMP (see Munemura *et al.*, 1980). The dopamine receptor of the pars intermedia, at least in the rat, is of the D2 type as the following observations show. Dopaminergic stimulation of the pars intermedia fails to stimulate the measured levels of adenyl cyclase or cyclic AMP; dopaminergic ergots (e.g. lergotrile) and apomorphine mimic the inhibitory effects of dopamine on both cyclic AMP formation and MSH release; specific D2 antagonists (e.g. sulpiride and metaclopramide) block the inhibitory effects of dopamine (Munemura *et al.*, 1980). The D2 receptor may well be functionally linked with the β-adrenoreceptor sharing control of common adenyl cyclase moieties. Thus, the β-adrenoreceptor is linked to adenyl cyclase through a stimulatory component, a guanyl nucleotide: the dopamine receptor may be similarly linked, but through a hypothetical inhibitory guanyl nucleotide component, so that dopaminergic agents inhibit rather than stimulate adenyl cyclase thus reducing the effective responsiveness of the β-adrenoreceptor (Cote, Grewe & Kebabian, 1981) and providing the basis for a co-ordinated control mechanism for catecholamine regulation of secretory activity in the melanotroph.

In a recent paper, evidence has been presented for an effect of dopamine on the synthetic activity of melanotrophs (Höllt et al., 1982). Chronic administration of haloperidol, a dopamine receptor blocker, to rats results in increased tissue levels of βEP and its increased release from neurointermediate lobes in vitro. This effect is accompanied by an increased synthesis of both pro-opiomelanocortin and the mRNA which codes for it.

Serotoninergic influences

Serotonin (5-hydroxytryptamine) has been shown to release MSH in some species, notably a teleost, Anguilla (Olivereau, 1978) and the lizard Anolis (Thornton & Geschwind, 1975). The evidence for the presence of serotoninergic receptors is based upon the ability of serotonin to induce darkening in animals kept in environmental conditions that would normally produce skin pallor, i.e. white backgrounds, as well as to increase the release of MSH from neurointermediate lobes incubated in vitro. Serotonin is also able to increase the normally low rate of spontaneous action potentials in the isolated pars intermedia of Anolis although it has little effect on the higher basal electrical activity of the rat (Taraskevich & Douglas, 1979). para-Chlorophenylalanine (pCPA) is an inhibitor of tryptophan hydroxylase and thus blocks the synthesis of serotonin. When administered to lizards which are subsequently transferred to a black background the normal darkening response, which is due to increased MSH release, is abolished. Similarly, serotonin antagonists, e.g. cyproheptadine or methysergide, prevent the darkening response either to serotonin itself or to transfer to a black background (Levitin, 1980b).

It seems, therefore, that in some species serotoninergic fibres, which have yet to be identified, may provide an alternative stimulatory regulation of the pars intermedia. This could be particularly important in those animals such as the lizard where a direct innervation of the pars intermedia is lacking, and where a stimulatory mechanism may have assumed a greater importance in maintaining the tonic activity of the gland. The origin of the serotonin is presumed to be from nerve terminals in the pars nervosa which abut the plexus intermedius.

GABAergic influences

The recent immunohistochemical demonstration of a rich network of γ-aminobutyric acid (GABA) containing fibres in the pars intermedia of the rat (Vincent et al., 1982), provides the anatomical basis for the observation that GABA reversibly inhibits MSH release from the pars intermedia of the frog and rat (Hadley, Davis & Morgan, 1977). Further investigation of the importance of this neurotransmitter in relation to other neural influences is clearly warranted.

Cholinergic influences

Acetylcholine stimulates MSH release from neurointermediate lobes of the frog and mouse but not from the rat (Hadley *et al.*, 1977). Since this is an effect that can be demonstrated *in vitro* it is unlikely to represent a cholinergic vasomotor influence, as some authors have suggested. However, it is not possible at present to proffer an alternative explanation.

Peptidergic influences

Encouraged no doubt by the demonstration of hypothalamic peptide-releasing factors that regulate the secretion of some of the trophic hormones of the pars distalis, many workers have sought similar peptides which regulate MSH secretion. The only group of peptides for which there is any evidence of such involvement, are claimed to be derived from the neurohypophysial peptides (see Taleisnik, 1978). The terminal tripeptide side chains of oxytocin and vasopressin, Pro-Leu-Gly—NH_2 and Pro-Arg-Gly—NH_2 respectively, have both been considered to be MSH release-inhibiting factors (MSH-IF or MIF). They can be liberated from their parent molecules upon incubation with hypothalamic microsomal preparations. The tocin ring of oxytocin (Cys-Tyr-Ileu-Gln-Asn-Cys—OH) is also thought to be further degraded to form a pentapeptide fragment (H—Cys-Tyr-Ileu-Gln-Asn—OH) which has MSH-releasing activity, i.e., it is a MSH-RF or MRF. An admirable critical review of the evidence for and against these claims has been provided by Hadley & Hruby (1977); there is little later data to substantially invalidate their conclusion that 'it is premature to suggest a role for neurohypophysial peptides in the control of MSH secretion'. In fact the literature is repeatedly punctuated by reports which fail to substantiate the status of Pro-Leu-Gly—NH_2 as an MIF. Only two groups of workers, including the original protagonists, have promoted the cause of a peptide MIF; most other authorities now seem content to identify the hypothalamic MIF with dopamine. Little is now heard of a peptide MRF.

It has been shown that thyrotrophin-releasing hormone (TRH) promotes MSH release from the amphibian neurointermediate lobe *in vitro* (Tonon *et al.*, 1980). However, it has not proved possible to demonstrate such an effect in acutely dispersed melanotrophs of the rat (Kraicer, 1977).

Miscellaneous influences

There is a circadian rhythm of immunoreactive αMSH in the plasma of the rat (Wilson & Morgan, 1979). Males maintained in 12 h light : 12 h dark photoperiods had raised levels of plasma αMSH during the scotophase, a peak occurring about 2 hours before dawn. These findings correlate well with those of Tilders & Smelik (1975) who showed earlier that the pituitary content of bioassayable MSH was low during the scotophase and peaked during mid-photophase. This rhythm was unaffected by pinealectomy, superior cervical ganglionectomy or the intravenous injection of melatonin. In contrast, Piezzi & Benelbaz (1974) showed that daily injections of large doses (1 mg/kg) of melatonin to albino rats daily for 5 days had marked effects upon the ultrastructure of the pars intermedia. In *Anolis*, melatonin had no effect on the basal rate of release of MSH from neurointermediate lobes *in vitro* but it did reduce the stimulatory effects of serotonin (Thornton & Geschwind, 1975).

In female rats there is also a diurnal rhythm in plasma MSH concentrations but only during the 2 days of pro-oestrus. The raised levels of MSH during the scotophase were absent on the nights of dioestrus and oestrus (Wilson & Morgan, 1979). Plasma MSH levels are also raised in ovariectomised rats and the administration of oestrogen to such animals is known to restore more normal levels (see Taleisnik, 1978). Several studies have shown that the long-term administration of stilboestrol to golden hamsters produces pronounced hyperplastic changes in the pars intermedia, often with the formation of cysts. Increases in plasma αMSH levels correlate with an increase in the size of the rough endoplasmic reticulum, hypertrophy of the Golgi apparatus and increased numbers of electron-dense secretory granules. In such situations neoplasia often supervenes with invasion of the pars distalis and pars nervosa (Saluja et al., 1979).

Both salt loading and sodium deprivation stimulate the mammalian pars intermedia. Schmitt et al. (1982) have shown that in mice given 2% sodium chloride in lieu of drinking water there was, within 1 day, an increase in the fractional volume of the rough endoplasmic reticulum and Golgi apparatus of the melanotrophs. These effects did not persist, however, although there was a prolonged increase in the fractional volume of the secretory granules. Interestingly, these changes could not be lessened by the dopamine agonist bromocriptine. In mice maintained on a low sodium diet a more intense, prolonged stimulation of melanotrophs was seen than was the case in salt-loaded animals. However, the effects of salt deprivation could be completely abolished by simultaneous treatment with bromocriptine. Schmitt et al. (1982) conclude that different mechanisms may be involved in the different responses to various types of osmotic stress and discuss the possibility that the pars intermedia is peculiarly well adapted, in view of its relatively poor vascularity, to monitoring changes in the ionic composition of the extracellular space.

It has been proposed that one of the means by which MSH secretion is regulated is through 'autoinhibition' or 'mass action direct feedback inhibition' whereby MSH regulates its own release. Bioassayable pituitary MSH was found to increase after a single injection of MSH, and blockade of MSH release was also seen in rat and amphibian pituitaries in vitro as the medium MSH concentration increased (see Taleisnik, 1978; Mains & Eipper, 1981); since other authors fail to find such inhibition (Hadley et al., 1977), the importance of this phenomenon is difficult to assess.

Ionic and energetic requirements for MSH secretion

Hadley & Bower (1976) have reviewed the metabolic requirements for MSH release from the pars intermedia of the frog and rat in vitro. They find that glucose in the incubation medium reversibly enhances the release of bioassayable MSH. Agents which interfere with glycolysis and the citric acid cycle all inhibit MSH release, as does cytochalasin B (an inhibitor of microfilament function).

Potassium ions have been shown to play a role in the regulation of MSH release, the precise effects depending upon the experimental preparation. Thus, in isolated cell preparations or in whole but denervated neurointermediate lobes, high potassium concentrations (45 mM) cause the simultaneous release of immunoreactive αMSH, CLIP, βEP and αEP. In intact neurointermediate lobes maintained in vitro, high potassium levels actually inhibit MSH release but this is ascribed to an indirect effect via the dopaminergic terminals remaining in the gland which release dopamine and thus inhibit MSH release (Jackson et al., 1981).

There is a sodium/potassium pump in the pars intermedia which in the frog and rat can be inhibited by cardiac glycosides such as ouabain and strophanthin-K, resulting in an inhibition of MSH release (Hadley et al., 1977). Calcium ions have been shown to be essential for both basal MSH release and stimulus–secretion coupling in the pars intermedia. Incubation of pituitaries in calcium-free medium abolishes MSH release whilst increases in intracellular calcium, as effected by the calcium ionophore A23187, enhance MSH release. In the pars intermedia of *Anolis*, spontaneous action potentials continue in sodium-free media and in the presence of the sodium channel blocker tetrodotoxin but are abolished by manganese, which blocks the calcium membrane channel. Thus, in this species, the action potentials have a considerable calcium component: in the rat, sodium plays a more dominant role (Taraskevich & Douglas, 1979).

The entry of calcium into the melanotroph consequent upon the action potential is therefore a trigger to MSH release, and it seems that the effects of calcium ions and the intracellular second messenger cyclic AMP are closely co-ordinated. Curiously, it has not proved possible to localise adenyl cyclase in the melanotrophs of the pars intermedia of the rat although it is associated with axons close to the border with the pars nervosa (Santolaya & Lederis, 1980). Both cyclic AMP and cholera toxin, an activator of adenyl cyclase, require calcium ions in order to stimulate MSH release. However, the β-adrenoreceptor agonist isoprenaline requires calcium to stimulate MSH release, but not to stimulate cyclic AMP accumulation. Since β-adrenoreceptor agonists do not increase the frequency of action potentials in the melanotrophs of the pars intermedia, and thus do not increase the entry of calcium ions, they must in some way potentiate the response of the melanotroph to the entry of fixed quantities of calcium ion, perhaps through a cyclic-AMP-dependent mechanism. Dopamine, of course, not only reduces the frequency of action potentials and therefore the entry of calcium but also reduces the rate of cyclic AMP formation, both actions serving to diminish MSH release. Tsuruta *et al.* (1982) discuss the consequences of these interactions at greater length than is possible here.

INTRACELLULAR PROCESSING IN THE PARS INTERMEDIA

This section cannot hope to deal comprehensively with the biochemistry of pro-opiomelanocortin in view of the extraordinarily rapid advances being made in the elucidation of its synthesis and processing. What will be attempted, however, is to set some of the more general aspects of hormone production by the pars intermedia in a cytological context. Some authors have examined the pars intermedia (or at least the neurointermediate lobe) itself: others have employed preparations of the pars distalis or a pituitary tumour AtT-20 which was derived from the pars distalis. Both of these latter systems have something to tell us about the pars intermedia since melanotrophs and corticotrophs generate their secretory peptides from a common precursor, pro-opiomelanocortin.

Pro-opiomelanocortin

Reference has already been made to the work of Nakanishi *et al.* (1979) which determined the nucleotide sequence of the mRNA coding for bovine pro-opiomelano-cortin. This molecule has a molecular weight of 29 259 and contains 265 amino acids. One of its important features is that it contains three repetitions of the sequence Tyr-X-Met-His-Phe-Arg-Trp-X found in the melanotrophins. One of these corresponds to αMSH, one to βMSH and the third is found in that part of the molecule whose existence was only suspected prior to the publication of its complete sequence, the so-called N-terminal, cryptic sequence. Nakanishi *et al.* (1979) proposed that this short peptide sequence be named γMSH. The pro-opiomelanocortin molecule is also characterised by pairs of basic amino acid residues, Lys-Arg. These are preferred sites for proteolysis, although the fragments so released may be further shortened by subsequent enzymatic degradation. There is some evidence that there may be more than one form of the precursor molecule coded by separate genes (see Kawauchi, Adachi & Tsubokawa, 1980; Martens, Jenks & van Overbeeke, 1982).

Synthesis of pro-opiomelanocortin

Pro-opiomelanocortin is synthesised on the rough endoplasmic reticulum. In common with other secretory proteins, it is thought to possess an N-terminal pre- or signal sequence of non-polar amino acids which may initiate attachment of the nascent peptide, ribosome and mRNA to the rough endoplasmic reticulum and ensure its transfer to the cisternae of the rough endoplasmic reticulum (see Warren, 1982). Certainly pro-opiomelanocortin synthesised in cell-free systems under the direction of mRNA reveals a pre-sequence of at least 25 amino acid residues that is removed in intact AtT-20 cells (Fig. 1.2). Precisely where the removal of this signal sequence occurs is yet to be demonstrated but 'signal peptidases' are clearly key components in secretory peptide production and are probably membrane-bound, possibly to the inner face of the rough endoplasmic reticulum (see Geisow, 1978).

Other evidence supporting the existence and importance of the signal sequence in pro-opiomelanocortin comes from the use of tunicamycin, a specific inhibitor of protein glycosylation. In AtT-20 cells treated with tunicamycin, an unglycosylated form of pro-opiomelanocortin, with a molecular weight of about 26000 (26 K), can be detected. Since the cell-free form of the precursor (in which glycosylation may occur but any signal sequence would not be cleaved) has a molecular weight of 28500 (28.5 K), these experiments support the view that the 26 K form arises by the cleavage of about 20–25 amino acids from the N-terminus of the 28.5 K precursor. The use of tunicamycin also points to the importance of glycosylation. The attachment of sugar side chains, through N-acetylglucosamine linked to asparagine residues, is one of the earliest modifications of the precursor molecule (Fig. 1.2). Varying estimates of the molecular weight of this precursor by authors using different experimental systems probably reflect differing degrees of glycosylation in the precursors they isolate. Furthermore, inhibition of glycosylation eventually produces abnormal profiles of precursor fragments. This suggests that both core and peripheral sugar side chains in some way protect certain peptide bonds, rendering them immune to non-specific protease actions (Loh, 1981). Thus, in both corticotrophs and melanotrophs the first precursor molecule which can be isolated is already glycosylated and lacks a signal sequence (Fig. 1.2).

Packaging of the precursor molecule

Transfer of the precursor molecule to the Golgi apparatus and its sequestration within the developing granule is associated with the commencement of the post-translational modification of the molecule. This probably involves the trimming back of those sugar side chains with a high mannose content by α-mannosidase and their rebuilding with peripheral N-acetylglucosamine, galactose, fucose and sialic acid residues by glycosyltransferases. Accompanying this is the initial proteolytic cleavage of the precursor that releases the large molecular weight fragments destined to undergo further cleavage. This implies that the proteolytic enzymes responsible for the cleavage reactions are co-packaged with the precursor (Herbert et al., 1980).

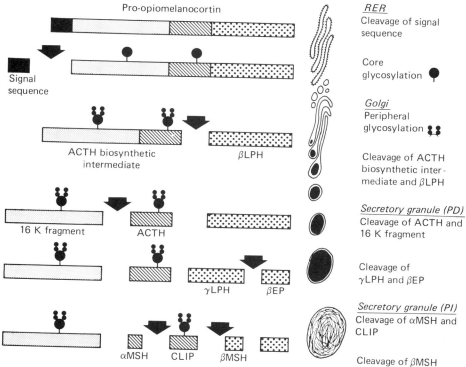

Fig. 1.2. Simplified summary schema of the post-translational processing of pro-opiomelanocortin. The arrows indicate the sequence of proteolytic cleavages which occur as the peptides pass through the cell via the rough endoplasmic reticulum (RER), Golgi apparatus and secretory granules. The processing which occurs in the secretory granules of corticotrophs in the pars distalis (PD) is continued further only in the melanotrophs of the pars intermedia (PI). For other abbreviations see legends to Fig. 1.1. Based upon information in Herbert *et al.* (1980), Mains & Eipper (1981) and Gumbiner & Kelly (1981).

The secretory granule

In secretory granules isolated from AtT-20 cells, it has been calculated that about 50% of the protein present is in the form of fragments of pro-opiomelanocortin, of which there are about 60000 copies per granule. The remainder of the protein presumably represents membrane proteins, other structural proteins and proteolytic enzymes. The granules contain almost undetectable amounts of pro-opiomelanocortin itself (Gumbiner & Kelly, 1981). Pulse–chase experiments reveal that $ACTH_{1-39}$ first appears in secretory granules 30–45 minutes after synthesis; indeed, it may be that the passage of precursor fragments from the Golgi compartment to the secretory granule compartment of the cell is the stimulus for the cleavage of ACTH from the ACTH biosynthetic intermediate. However, the time resolution of these studies is as yet inadequate to localise more precisely the process in either the Golgi or the rough endoplasmic reticulum. Further proteolysis of βLPH to βEP and γLPH almost certainly occurs in the secretory granule itself some $1\frac{1}{2}$ to 2 hours after synthesis.

Studies of rat neurointermediate lobes *in vitro* show that both ACTH and βLPH are present in very small amounts (Giannoulakis *et al.*, 1979) and thus they probably represent only obligatory transient intermediates in the production of αMSH and CLIP and of βEP, γLPH and βMSH respectively (Fig. 1.2). Presumably, therefore, these final cleavage steps are closely attendant on the preceding steps, which liberate ACTH and βLPH, in both space and time.

Further evidence from the rat pars intermedia suggests that the N-terminal cryptic sequence of pro-opiomelanocortin, which contains the γMSH heptapeptide and which is produced when ACTH is cleaved from the ACTH biosynthetic intermediate, is glycosylated but does not undergo further significant processing. This peptide seems to be released from rat melanotrophs as glycosylated variants with molecular weights of 17–19 K (Crine et al., 1980) which correspond to the partially glycosylated, so called 16 K fragment, found in AtT-20 cells (Herbert et al., 1980). There is, however, evidence that in fishes this N-terminal 16 K fragment may be further processed. In dogfish, this portion of pro-opiomelanocortin does not seem to be glycosylated in the vicinity of γMSH and a 12 amino acid form of γMSH, which may be C-terminally amidated, can be isolated (McClean & Lowry, 1981). This lack of glycosylation may be the explanation for the further processing of the N-terminal sequence, in view of the resistance to proteolysis that glycosylation confers on the molecule in the rat. It may also explain the relatively weak PAS-positivity of the melanotrophs of the pars intermedia in fish.

In summary, therefore, granules of corticotrophs contain predominantly $ACTH_{1-39}$, βLPH_{1-91}, βEP_{61-91}, γLPH_{1-58} and the 16 K fragment; by contrast, melanotrophs are able to process these peptides further and therefore contain mainly αMSH_{1-13}, $CLIP_{17-39}$, βEP_{61-91}, γLPH_{1-58}, βMSH_{41-58} and 16 K fragment.

Granule release

What little ultrastructural data there is to show that hormone release involves exocytosis, is supported by the relevant biochemical evidence. Isolated, perfused cell preparations of the rat pars intermedia release the various peptide fragments contained in secretory granules in molar proportions and the overall concentrations of these fragments in perfusates are equally affected by secretagogues such as dopamine (Jackson et al., 1981). Small but constant amounts of pro-opiomelanocortin and its higher molecular weight fragments are found in the medium bathing static i.e. non-perfused, cultures. These may simply represent an accumulation of fragments or entire precursor which have escaped intracellular processing. Their existence suggests that an alternative but minor pathway may exist for the egress of peptides from melanotrophs.

Gumbiner & Kelly (1982) have reported evidence to support such an interpretation. They have shown that AtT-20 cells produce not only ACTH and related molecules but also an endogenous leukaemia virus (MULV) which has an envelope glycoprotein that is, like ACTH, glycosylated post-translation. They find that both the virus envelope glycoprotein and small amounts of the ACTH biosynthetic intermediate reach the cell surface via a route which is distinct from that of the maturing secretory granule and which is traversed much faster. These authors conclude that some ACTH precursors escape normal proteolytic conversion and that this conversion must be specifically associated with hormone packaging into secretory granules. This interpretation would also explain why neither noradrenaline nor the cobalt ion (a calcium antagonist) significantly alters the basal release of pro-opiomelanocortin or ACTH biosynthetic intermediate from AtT-20 cells (Mains & Eipper, 1981), since both peptides would presumably have escaped being packaged into a granule and would not, therefore, be released by exocytosis, a process in which calcium ions play a key role. The stimulation of secretion by noradrenaline and its inhibition by cobalt chloride is therefore restricted to the lower molecular weight products of pro-opiomelanocortin.

Although much of the emphasis in what has gone before has been on the major proteolytic modifications of the peptides and glycopeptides derived from pro-opiomelanocortin, it should be remembered that the deletion of short sequences of amino acids at the C-terminus (or the amidation or the acetylation of the N-terminus) of peptides can lead to profound changes in their biological activity. For example, αMSH production in the pars intermedia is accompanied by inert forms of βEP which have been inactivated by proteolysis or acetylation (Smyth *et al.*, 1981). Indeed, it seems that the granular stores of αMSH are in the de-acetylated form, des-Nα-acetyl-α-MSH$_{1-13}$. Acetylation of these intragranular molecules takes place just before or during exocytosis when the fully biologically active form of αMSH (Nα-acetyl-α-MSH$_{1-13}$) is generated, perhaps under the influence of an *N*-acetyltransferase enzyme linked to either the secretory granule or the cell membrane (see Martens, Jenks & van Overbeeke, 1981).

ONTOGENETIC CHANGES IN INTRACELLULAR PROCESSING

The developmental changes in the structure of the human pars intermedia which are accompanied by the disappearance of melanotrophs have already been alluded to. In the rhesus monkey, there seems to be a dramatic switch in the synthetic repertoire of the pars intermedia at parturition. In foetal neurointermediate lobes the predominant peptides are those of low molecular weight, αMSH, βMSH, CLIP and βEP: post-partum there is a change to a peptide profile dominated by ACTH and βLPH (Silman *et al.*, 1978), suggesting that the capacity of the pars intermedia to manufacture the lower molecular weight peptides is lost. A similar situation has been described by Baker & Scott (1975) in the pars intermedia of the trout maintained *in vitro*. They have found that there is a steady decline in the capacity of the gland to synthesise and release αMSH, which is paralleled by a progressive increase in the synthesis and release of ACTH. They surmise that, in the absence of some hypothalamic influence, the proteolytic mechanisms that characterise the pars inter-media cease to function normally so that large amounts of uncleaved ACTH are available for release.

The identity of this hypothalamic influence is undetermined but it is tempting to speculate that it may be a neurotransmitter. This idea receives some support from the observations of Schmitt *et al.* (1981) who have reported that during the foetal life of the mouse the pars intermedia is not innervated and its αMSH content is almost undetectable. However, during the first post-natal week the appearance of differenti-ated, active melanotrophs coincides with an increase in the αMSH content of the gland and the establishment of its dopaminergic innervation. Perhaps the enzymes responsible for the final proteolytic cleavage steps in the pars intermedia are dopamine-dependent.

PROSPECT

It is likely that in the time that will have elapsed between the completion of this paper and its publication there will be much new information relating to pro-opiomelanocortin, especially the biochemical aspects of its synthesis and processing. It is equally likely, however, that there will be slow progress towards a full understanding of the functions of the pars intermedia. It has often been tacitly assumed that in the lower vertebrates the primary role of the pars intermedia lies in the regulation of integumentary colour change, but it probably subserves other functions too as Baker (1981) has discussed. In mammals, its function has always been enigmatic since few species show coat colour changes which might involve MSH. In fact the pars intermedia of mammals has been implicated in the regulation of lipid metabolism, in the control of sebaceous gland activity, in the regulation of both the adult and foetal adrenal gland, in aspects of intra-uterine growth, in parturition, in water and mineral metabolism and in the production of endogenous opioids. An earlier review of these possible functions by Howe (1973) has been supplemented recently by the monograph of Thody (1980).

In spite of so many accounts of the morphology, cytology and ultrastructure of the pars intermedia, the anatomist is still faced with innumerable problems. What, for example, are the cellular mechanisms involved in the co-packaging of peptides and peptidases? Could there be further processing of these small molecular weight peptide secretions by extracellular peptidases? What are the roles of the agranular cells of the pars intermedia and do they have unexpected embryological origins? Where does colloid come from, what does it contain, does it have a role to play in the normal activity of the gland? Why do follicles form and where do they come from? Why does the pars intermedia have such a sparse blood supply; is this of any special functional or developmental significance? Why are there such variations in the degree of innervation of the pars intermedia and how do the nerve terminals which contain different neurotransmitters interact? What role does the innervation of the pars intermedia play in the development of its structure and function? Mere morphological observation alone will not solve either these or other pressing questions but there is no reason why the tools and techniques at the disposal of modern anatomists should not enable them to reveal so much more of the morphological framework within which, and from which, the activity of the pars intermedia is expressed.

REFERENCES

Anand Kumar, T. C. & Vincent, D. S. (1974). Fine structure of the pars intermedia in the rhesus monkey. *Journal of Anatomy*, **118**, 155–69.

Andersson, B. & Jewell, P. A. (1958). Observations on the hypothalamo-hypophysial neurosecretory system and on variations in the structure of the pituitary of the goat. *Acta Anatomica*, **35**, 1–15.

Bäck, N., Rechardt, L. & Partanen, S. (1976). Observations on the functional cytochemistry of pars intermedia of the rat hypophysis. *Histochemistry*, **46**, 121–30.

Bagnara, J. T. & Hadley, M. E. (1973). *Chromatophores and Color Change*. New Jersey: Prentice–Hall.

Baker, B. I. (1981). Biological role of the pars intermedia in lower vertebrates. In *Peptides of the Pars Intermedia*, ed. D. Evered & G. Lawrenson, pp. 166–79. London: Pitman Medical.

Baker, B. I. & Scott, A. P. (1975). ACTH production by the pars intermedia of the rainbow trout pituitary. *General and Comparative Endocrinology*, **27**, 193–202.

Baumgarten, H. G., Björklund, A., Holstein, A. F. & Nobin, A. (1972). Organisation and ultrastructural identification of the catecholamine nerve terminals in the neural lobe and pars intermedia of the rat pituitary. *Zeitschrift für Zellforschung und mikroskopische Anatomie*, **77**, 282–98.

Bégeot, M., Dubois, M. P. & Dubois, P. M. (1978). Immunologic localisation of α- and β-endorphins and β-lipotropin in corticotropic cells of the normal and anencephalic fetal pituitaries. *Cell and Tissue Research*, **193**, 413–22.

Benjamin, M. (1981). Cysts (large follicles) and colloid in pituitary glands. *General and Comparative Endocrinology*, **45**, 425–45.

Bergland, R. M. & Page, R. B. (1979). Pituitary–brain vascular relations: a new paradigm. *Science*, **204**, 18–24.

Björklund, A. & Nobin, A. (1972). Organisation of tuberohypophysial and reticulo-infundibular catecholamine neurone systems in the rat brain. *Brain Research*, **51**, 171–91.

Bock, E. (1978). Nervous system specific proteins. *Journal of Neurochemistry*, **30**, 7–14.

Bower, A., Hadley, M. E. & Hruby, V. J. (1974). Biogenic amines and the control of melanophore stimulating hormone release. *Science*, **184**, 70–2.

Brooks, M. E. & Vincent, D. S. (1977). The effect of hypothalamic lesions on the pars intermedia of the ferret. *General and Comparative Endocrinology*, **31**, 276–86.

Brownstein, M. J. (1980). Opioid peptides: search for the precursors. *Nature (London)*, **287**, 678–9.

Cameron, E. & Foster, C. L. (1971). Some light- and electron-microscopical observations on the pars intermedia of the pituitary of the rabbit. *Journal of Endocrinology*, **49**, 479–85.

Ciocca, D. R. (1980). Scanning electron microscopy of the cleft of the rat pituitary. *Cell and Tissue Research*, **206**, 139–43.

Cocchia, D. & Miani, N. (1980). Immunocytochemical localisation of the brain-specific S100 protein in the pituitary gland of the adult rat. *Journal of Neurocytology*, **9**, 771–82.

Cocchia, D., Michetti, F. & Donato, R. (1981). Immunochemical and immunocytochemical localisation of S-100 antigen in normal human skin. *Nature (London)*, **294**, 85–7.

Cote, T. E., Grewe, C. W. & Kebabian, J. W. (1981). Stimulation of a D-2 dopamine receptor in the intermediate lobe of the rat pituitary gland decreases the responsiveness of the β-adrenoceptor: biochemical mechanism. *Endocrinology*, **108**, 420–6.

Crine, P., Seidah, N. G., Jeanotte, L. & Chrétien, M. (1980). Two large glycoprotein fragments related to the NH_2-terminal part of the adrenocorticotropin–β-lipotropin precursor are the end products of the maturation process in the rat pars intermedia. *Canadian Journal of Biochemistry*, **58**, 1318–22.

Davis, M. E. & Hadley, M. E. (1978). Hypothalamic control of pars intermedia melanophore stimulating hormone (MSH) secretion. In *Hypothalamic Hormones – Chemistry, Physiology & Clinical Applications*, ed. D. Gupta & W. Voelter, pp. 395–401. Weinheim: Verlag Chemie.

de Bold, A. J., de Bold, M. L. & Kraicer, J. (1980). Structural relationships between parenchymal and stromal elements in the pars intermedia of the rat adenohypophysis as demonstrated by extracellular space markers. *Cell and Tissue Research*, **207**, 347–59.

de Volcanes, B. & Weatherhead, B. (1976a). Early changes in the ultrastructure of the pars intermedia of the pituitary of *Xenopus laevis* after change of background color. *Neuroendocrinology*, **22**, 127–33.

de Volcanes, B. & Weatherhead, B. (1976b). Stereological analysis of the effects of 6-hydroxydopamine on the ultrastructure of the melanocyte-stimulating hormone cell of the pituitary of *Xenopus laevis*. *General and Comparative Endocrinology*, **28**, 205–12.

Donovan, B. T. & Harris, G. W. (1966). *The Pituitary Gland*. London: Butterworths.

Eberle, A. N. (1981). Structure and chemistry of the peptide hormones of the intermediate lobe. In *Peptides of the Pars Intermedia*, ed. D. Evered & G. Lawrenson, pp. 13–31. London: Pitman Medical.

Eurenius, L. & Jarskär, R. (1975). Electron microscopic studies on the neurointermediate lobe of the embryonic mouse. *Cell and Tissue Research*, **164**, 11–26.

Evered, D. & Lawrenson, G. (1981). *Peptides of the Pars Intermedia*. Ciba Foundation Symposium 81. London: Pitman Medical.

Follenius, E. & Dubois, M. P. (1979). Différenciation immunocytologique de l'innervation hypophysaire de la Carpe à l'aide de sérums anti-met-enképhaline et anti-α-endorphine. *Compte rendus hebdomadaire des séances de l'Académie des Sciences, Series D*, **288**, 639–42.

Gallardo, M. G. P., Cannata, M. A. & Tramezzani, J. H. (1980). An uneven distribution of choline acetyltransferase in the pituitary neurointermediate lobe of the rat. *Journal of Endocrinology*, **85**, 497–501.

Geisow, M. J. (1978). Snips in secreted proteins. *Nature (London)*, **272**, 308–9.

Giannoulakis, C., Seidah, N. G., Routhier, R. & Chrétien, M. (1979). Biosynthesis and characterisation of adrenocorticotropic hormone, α-melanocyte-stimulating hormone and an NH_2-terminal fragment of the adrenocorticotropic/β-lipotropin precursor from rat pars intermedia. *Journal of Biological Chemistry*, **254**, 11 903–6.

Gumbiner, B. & Kelly, R. B. (1981). Secretory granules of an anterior pituitary cell line, AtT-20, contain only mature forms of corticotropin and β-lipotropin. *Proceedings of the National Academy of Sciences of the USA*, **78**, 318–22.

Gumbiner, B. & Kelly, R. B. (1982). Two distinct intracellular pathways transport secretory and membrane glycoproteins to the surface of pituitary tumor cells. *Cells*, **28**, 51–9.

Hadley, M. E. & Bower, A. (1976). Metabolic requirements for melanophore-stimulating hormone (MSH) secretion. *General and Comparative Endocrinology*, **28**, 118–30.

Hadley, M. E., Davis, M. D. & Morgan, C. M. (1977). Cellular control of melanocyte stimulating hormone secretion. In *Frontiers of Hormone Research*, vol. 4, ed. T. van Wimersma Greidanus, pp. 94–104. Basel: Karger.

Hadley, M. E. & Hruby, V. J. (1977). Neurohypophysial peptides and the regulation of melanophore stimulating hormone (MSH) secretion. *American Zoologist*, **17**, 809–21.

Halmi, N. S., Peterson, M., Colurso, G. J., Liotta, A. S. & Krieger, D. T. (1981). Pituitary intermediate lobe in dog: two cell types and high bioactive adrenocorticotropin content. *Science*, **211**, 72–4.

Hanstrom, B. (1966). Gross anatomy of the hypophysis in mammals. In *The Pituitary Gland*, ed. B. T. Donovan & G. W. Harris, pp. 1–57. London: Butterworths.

Herbert, E., Roberts, J., Phillips, M., Allen, R., Hinman, M., Budarf, M., Policastro, P. & Rosa, P. (1980). Biosynthesis, processing and release of corticotropin, β-endorphin, and melanocyte-stimulating hormone in pituitary cell culture systems. In *Frontiers in Neuroendocrinology*, vol. 6, ed. L. Martini & W. F. Ganong, pp. 67–101. New York: Raven Press.

Höllt, V., Haarmann, I., Seizinger, B. R. & Herz, A. (1982). Chronic haloperidol treatment increases the level of *in vitro* translatable messenger ribonucleic acid coding for the β-endorphin/adrenocorticotropin precursor proopiomelanocortin in the pars intermedia of the rat pituitary. *Endocrinology*, **110**, 1885–91.

Holmes, R. L. (1964). Functional implications of the vascular pattern of the hypothalamo-hypophysial system. *Symposia of the Zoological Society of London*, **11**, 35–47.

Holmes, R. L. (1981). The pars intermedia of the mammalian pituitary gland: problems and some answers. *Symposia of the Zoological Society of London*, **46**, 223–36.

Holmes, R. L. & Ball, J. N. (1974). *The Pituitary Gland*. Cambridge University Press.

Hopkins, C. R. (1970). Studies on the secretory activity in the pars intermedia of *Xenopus laevis*. I. Fine structural changes related to the onset of secretory activity *in vivo*. *Tissue and Cell*, **2**, 59–70.

Hopkins, C. R. (1971). Localisation of adrenergic fibres in the amphibian pars intermedia by electron microscope autoradiography and their selective removal by 6-hydroxydopamine. *General and Comparative Endocrinology*, **16**, 112–20.

Horvath, E., Kovacs, K., Penz, G. & Ezrin, C. (1974). Origin, possible function and fate of 'follicular cells' in the anterior lobe of the human pituitary. *American Journal of Pathology*, **77**, 199–212.

Howe, A. (1973). The mammalian pars intermedia: a review of its structure and function. *Journal of Endocrinology*, **59**, 385–409.

Iturriza, F. C. & Koch, O. R. (1964). Effect of the administration of lysergic acid diethylamide (LSD) on the colloid vesicles of the toad pituitary. *Endocrinology*, **75**, 615–16.

Jackson, S., Hope, J., Estivariz, F. & Lowry, P. J. (1981). Nature and control of peptide release from the pars intermedia. In *Peptides of the Pars Intermedia*, ed. D. Evered & G. Lawrenson, pp. 141–62. London: Pitman Medical.

Jarskär, R. (1977). Electron microscopical study on the development of the nerve supply of the pituitary pars intermedia of the mouse. *Cell and Tissue Research*, **184**, 121–32.

Kawauchi, H., Adachi, Y. & Tsubokawa, M. (1980). Occurrence of a new melanocyte stimulating hormone in the salmon pituitary gland. *Biochemical and Biophysical Research Communications*, **96**, 1508–17.

Kraicer, J. (1977). Thyrotropin-releasing hormone does not alter the release of melanocyte-stimulating hormone or adrenocorticotropic hormone from the rat pars intermedia. *Neuroendocrinology*, **24**, 226–31.

Larsson, L. (1981). Control of the pars intermedia of the lizard, *Anolis carolinensis*. V. Extracellular transfer and cellular uptake of horseradish peroxidase in the neuro-intermediate lobe. *Cell and Tissue Research*, **214**, 1–22.

Larsson, L., Rodriguez, E. M. & Meurling, P. (1979). Control of the pars intermedia of the lizard, *Anolis carolinensis*. II. Ultrastructure of the intact intermediate lobe. *Cell and Tissue Research*, **198**, 411–26.

Lerner, A. B. (1981). The intermediate lobe of the pituitary gland: introduction and background. In *Peptides of the Pars Intermedia*, ed. D. Evered & G. Lawrenson, pp. 3–12. London: Pitman Medical.

Levitin, H. (1980a). Monoaminergic control of MSH release in the lizard, *Anolis carolinensis*. *General and Comparative Endocrinology*, **41**, 279–86.

Levitin, H. (1980b). Further evidence that serotonin may be a physiological melanocyte-stimulating hormone releasing factor in the lizard *Anolis carolinensis*. *General and Comparative Endocrinology*, **40**, 8–14.

Loh, Y. P. (1981). Processing, turnover, and release of corticotropins, endorphins and melanotropin in the toad pituitary intermediate lobe. In *Peptides of the Pars Intermedia*, ed. D. Evered & G. Lawrenson, pp. 55–78. London: Pitman Medical.

Loren, I., Schwandt, P., Alumets, J., Håkanson, R., Neureuther, G., Richter, W. & Sundler, F. (1980). Evidence that lipolytic peptide B occurs in the ACTH/MSH cells of the pituitary and in the brain. *Cell and Tissue Research*, **205**, 349–59.

McClean, C. & Lowry, P. J. (1981). Natural occurrence but lack of melanotrophic activity of γ-MSH in fish. *Nature (London)*, **290**, 341–3.

McGrath, P. (1978). Aspects of the human pharyngeal hypophysis in normal and anencephalic fetuses and neonates and their possible significance in the mechanism of its control. *Journal of Anatomy*, **127**, 65–81.

Mains, R. E. & Eipper, B. A. (1981). Co-ordinate, equimolar secretion of smaller peptide products from pro-ACTH/endorphin by mouse pituitary tumor cells. *Journal of Cell Biology*, **89**, 21–8.

Martens, G. J. M., Jenks, B. G. & van Overbeeke, A. P. (1981). Nα-acetylation is linked to α-MSH release from the pars intermedia of the amphibian pituitary gland. *Nature (London)*, **294**, 558–60.

Martens, G. J. M., Jenks, B. G. & van Overbeeke, A. P. (1982). Biosynthesis of pairs of peptides related to melanotropin, corticotropin and endorphin in the pars intermedia of the amphibian pituitary gland. *European Journal of Biochemistry*, **122**, 1–10.

Martin, R., Weber, E. & Voigt, K. H. (1979). Localisation of corticotropin- and endorphin-related peptides in the intermediate lobe of the rat pituitary. *Cell and Tissue Research*, **196**, 307–19.

Meurling, P. & Willstedt, A. (1970). Vascular connections in the pituitary of *Anolis carolinensis* with special reference to the pars intermedia. *Acta Zoologica*, **51**, 211–18.

Munemura, M., Cote, T. E., Tsuruta, K., Eskay, R. L. & Kebabian, J. W. (1980). The dopamine receptor in the intermediate lobe of the rat pituitary gland: pharmacological characterisation. *Endocrinology*, **107**, 1676–83.

Nakanishi, S., Inoue, A., Kita, T., Nakamura, M., Chang, A. C. Y., Cohen, S. & Numa, S. (1979). Nucleotide sequence of cloned cDNA for bovine corticotropin – β-lipotropin precursor. *Nature (London)*, **278**, 423–7.

Oliver, C., Mical, R. S. & Porter, J. C. (1977). Hypothalamic–pituitary vasculature: evidence for retrograde blood flow in the pituitary stalk. *Endocrinology*, **101**, 598–604.

Olivereau, M. (1978). Serotonin and MSH secretion: effect of *para*-chlorophenylalanine on the pituitary cytology of the eel. *Cell and Tissue Research*, **191**, 83–92.

Osamura, R. Y. & Watanabe, K. (1978). An immunohistochemical study of epithelial cells in the posterior lobe and pars tuberalis of the human adult pituitary gland. *Cell and Tissue Research*, **194**, 513–24.

Pasquier, D. A., Cannata, M. A. & Tramezzani, J. H. (1980). Central connections of the toad neural lobe as shown by retrograde neuronal labelling: classical and new connections. *Brain Research*, **195**, 37–45.

Perry, R. A., Robinson, P. M. & Ryan, G. B. (1981). Ultrastructure of the pars intermedia of the adult sheep hypophysis. *Cell and Tissue Research*, **217**, 211–23.

Perryman, E. K. & Bagnara, J. T. (1978). Extravascular transfer within the anuran pars intermedia. *Cell and Tissue Research*, **193**, 297–313.

Perryman, E. K., de Vellis, J. & Bagnara, J. T. (1980). Phagocytic activity of the stellate cells in the anuran pars intermedia. *Cell and Tissue Research*, **208**, 85–98.

Piezzi, R. S. & Benelbaz, G. A. (1974). Effect of melatonin on the rat pars intermedia. An electron microscopic study. *Acta Physiologica Latino Americana*, **24**, 59–62.

Rapp, J. P. & Bergon, L. (1977). Characteristics of pituitary colloid proteins and their correlation with blood pressure in the rat. *Endocrinology*, **101**, 93–103.

Rehfeld, J. F. & Larsson, L.-I. (1981). Pituitary gastrins: different processing in corticotrophs and melanotrophs. *Journal of Biological Chemistry*, **256**, 10 426–9.

Rodriguez, E. M. (1971). The comparative morphology of neural lobes of species with different neurohypophyseal hormones. *Memoirs of the Society for Endocrinology*, **19**, 263–92.

Saland, L. C. (1968). Ultrastructure of the frog pars intermedia in relation to hypothalamic control of hormone release. *Neuroendocrinology*, **3**, 72–88.

Saland, L. C. (1978). Effects of reserpine administration on the fine structure of the rat pars intermedia. *Cell and Tissue Research*, **194**, 115–23.

Saluja, P. G., Hamilton, J. M., Thody, A. J., Ismail, A. A. & Knowles, J. (1979). Ultrastructure of intermediate lobe of the pituitary and melanocyte-stimulating hormone secretion in oestrogen-induced kidney tumours in male hamsters. *Archives of Toxicology*, Suppl. 2, 41–5.

Santolaya, R. C. & Ciocca, R. (1981). Effects of pimozide on the ultrastructure of the pars intermedia in the rat. *Cell and Tissue Research*, **217**, 397–403.

Santolaya, R. C. & Lederis, K. (1980). Localisation of adenylate cyclase in the neurointermediate lobe of the rat pituitary. Ultrastructural cytochemistry. *Cell and Tissue Research*, **207**, 387–94.

Santolaya, R. C. & Rodriguez, E. M. (1977). Ultrastructure of the male rat hypophysis chronically grafted under the kidney capsule. *Cell and Tissue Research*, **179**, 271–84.

Schmechel, D., Marangos, P. J. & Brightman, M. (1978). Neurone-specific enolase is a molecular marker for peripheral and central neuroendocrine cells. *Nature (London)*, **276**, 834–7.

Schmitt, G., Stoeckel, M. E., Klein, M. J. & Porte, A. (1982). Effects of experimental hypo- or hypernatremia on the fine structure of the pars intermedia of the murine pituitary. *Cell and Tissue Research*, **223**, 641–57.

Schmitt, G., Stoeckel, M. E. & Koch, B. (1981). Evidence for a possible dopaminergic control of pituitary alpha-MSH ontogenesis in mice. *Neuroendocrinology*, **33**, 306–11.

Semoff, S., Fuller, B. B. & Hadley, M. E. (1978). Secretion of melanophore-stimulating hormone (MSH) in long term cultures of pituitary neurointermediate lobes. *Cell and Tissue Research*, **194**, 55–69.

Semoff, S. & Hadley, M. E. (1978*a*). Exocytosis in the pars intermedia as demonstrated by freeze-etching. *Journal of Cell Biology*, **79**, 374a.

Semoff, S. & Hadley, M. E. (1978*b*). Localisation of ATPase activity to the glial-like cells of the pars intermedia. *General and Comparative Endocrinology*, **35**, 329–41.

Silman, R. E., Holland, D., Chard, T., Lowry, P. J., Hope, J., Robinson, J. S. & Thorburn, G. D. (1978). The ACTH 'family tree' of the rhesus monkey changes with development. *Nature (London)*, **276**, 526–8.

Smyth, D. G., Zakarian, S., Deakin, J. F. W. & Massey, D. E. (1981). β-Endorphin-related peptides in the pituitary gland: isolation, identification and distribution. In *Peptides of the Pars Intermedia*, ed. D. Evered & G. Lawrenson, pp. 79–96. London: Pitman Medical.

Stoeckel, M. E., Dellmann, H. D., Porte, J., Klein, M. J. & Stutinsky, F. (1973). Corticotropic cells in the rostral zone of the pars intermedia and in the adjacent neurohypophysis of the rat and mouse. *Zeitschrift für Zellforschung und mikroskopische Anatomie*, **136**, 97–110.

Stoeckel, M. E., Schmitt, G. & Porte, A. (1981). Fine structure and cytochemistry of the mammalian pars intermedia. In *Peptides of the Pars Intermedia*, ed. D. Evered & G. Lawrenson, pp. 101–27. London: Pitman Medical.

Takor Takor, T. & Pearse, A. G. E. (1975). Neuroectodermal origin of avian hypothalamo-hypophyseal complex: the role of the ventral neural ridge. *Journal of Embryology and Experimental Morphology*, **34**, 311–25.

Taleisnik, S. (1978). Control of melanocyte-stimulating hormone (MSH) secretion. In *The Endocrine Hypothalamus*, ed. S. L. Jeffcoate & J. S. M. Hutchinson, pp. 421–38. London: Academic Press.

Taraskevich, P. S. & Douglas, W. W. (1979). Stimulant effect of 5-hydroxytryptamine on action potential activity in pars intermedia cells of the lizard *Anolis carolinensis*: contrasting effects in pars intermedia of rat and rostral pars distalis of fish (*Alosa pseudoharengus*). *Brain Research*, **178**, 584–8.

Terlou, M. & Ploemacher, R. E. (1973). The distribution of monoamines in the tel- , di- and mesencephalon of *Xenopus laevis* tadpoles with special reference to the hypothalamo-hypophysial system. *Zeitschrift für Zellforschung und mikroskopische Anatomie*, **137**, 521–40.

Thody, A. J. (1980). *The MSH Peptides*. London: Academic Press.

Thornton, V. F. & Geschwind, I. I. (1975). Evidence that serotonin may be a melanocyte-stimulating hormone releasing factor in the lizard *Anolis carolinensis*. *General and Comparative Endocrinology*, **26**, 346–53.

Tilders, F. J. H. & Smelik, P. G. (1975). A diurnal rhythm in melanocyte-stimulating hormone content of the rat pituitary gland and its independence from the pineal gland. *Neuroendocrinology*, **17**, 296–308.

Tonon, M.-C., Leroux, P., Leboulenger, F., Delarue, C., Jégou, S. & Vaudry, H. (1980). Thyrotropin-releasing hormone stimulates the release of melanotropin from frog neurointermediate lobes *in vitro*. *Life Sciences*, **26**, 869–75.

Tsuruta, K., Grewe, C. W., Cote T. E., Eskay, R. L. & Kebabian, J. W. (1982). Coordinated action of calcium ion and adenosine 3'5' monophosphate upon the release of α-melanocyte stimulating hormone from the intermediate lobe of the rat pituitary gland. *Endocrinology*, **110**, 1133–40.

van Eys, G. J. J. M. (1980). Structural changes in the pars intermedia of the cichlid teleost *Sarotherodon mossambicus* as a result of background adaptation and illumination. II. The PAS-positive cells. *Cell and Tissue Research*, **210**, 171–9.

Vanha-Perttula, T. & Arstila, A. (1970). On the epithelium of the rat pituitary residual lumen. *Zeitschrift für Zellforschung und mikroskopische Anatomie*, **108**, 487–500.

van Vossel, A., van Vossel-Daeninck, J., Dierickx, K. & Vandesande, F. (1977). Electron microscopic immunocytochemical demonstration of separate mesotocinergic and vasotocinergic nerve fibres in the pars intermedia of the amphibian hypophysis. *Cell and Tissue Research*, **178**, 175–81.

Vincent, D. S. & Anand Kumar, T. C. (1969). Electron microscopic studies on the pars intermedia of the ferret. *Zeitschrift für Zellforschung und mikroskopische Anatomie*, **99**, 185–97.

Vincent, S. R., Hokfelt, T. & Wu, J.-Y. (1982). GABA neuron systems in hypothalamus and pituitary gland. Immunohistochemical demonstration using antibodies against glutamate decarboxylase. *Neuroendocrinology*, **34**, 117–25.

Visser, M. & Swaab, D. F. (1979). Life span changes in the presence of α-melanocyte-stimulating hormone-containing cells in the human pituitary. *Journal of Developmental Physiology*, **1**, 161–78.

Warren, G. (1982). Stop–go proteins. *Nature (London)*, **297**, 624–5.

Weatherhead, B. (1978). Comparative cytology of the neuro-intermediate lobe of the reptilian pituitary. *Zentralblatt für Veterinärmedizin, Reihe C*, **7**, 84–119.

Weman, B. & Nobin, A. (1973). The pars intermedia of the mink, *Mustela vison*. Fluorescence, light and electron microscopical studies. *Zeitschrift für Zellforschung und mikroskopische Anatomie*, **143**, 313–27.

Whittaker, S. & Labella, F. S. (1973). Cholinesterase in the posterior and intermediate lobes of the pituitary. Species differences as determined by light and electron microscopic histochemistry. *Zeitschrift für Zellforschung und mikroskopische Anatomie*, **142**, 69–88.

Wilson, J. F. & Morgan, M. A. (1979). Cyclical changes in concentrations of α-melanotrophin in the plasma of male and female rats. *Journal of Endocrinology*, **82**, 361–6.

Wingstrand, K. G. (1966a). Comparative anatomy and evolution of the hypophysis. In *The Pituitary Gland*, vol. 1, ed. B. T. Donovan & G. W. Harris, pp. 58–126. London: Butterworths.

Wingstrand, K. G. (1966b). Microscopic anatomy, nerve supply and blood supply of the pars intermedia. In *The Pituitary Gland*, vol. 3, ed. B. T. Donovan & G. W. Harris, pp. 1–27. London: Butterworths.

2 Microscopical analysis of electrolyte secretion

J. ANTHONY FIRTH

Department of Anatomy, St George's Hospital Medical School, Cranmer Terrace, London SW17 0RE, UK

The early years of biological electron microscopy revealed an overwhelming and previously largely unsuspected world of subcellular pattern. The incorporation of this new knowledge into the main body of understanding of cell, tissue and organ function took place more quickly in some areas than in others. In protein secretion, muscle contraction and synaptic transmission the dramatic new structural findings forced radical revision of traditional concepts and suggested many new directions for integrated structural and physiological studies.

By contrast, active transport processes across epithelia proved rather resistant to any but the loosest generalisations about the relationship between structure and function. In the last ten years this picture has changed as the development and application of powerful new microscopical methods, capable of yielding direct functional information, have brought about the beginning of a coherent picture of how epithelia transport electrolytes and water. This paper examines the nature of this progress with particular reference to two leading areas of work, sodium chloride secretion and absorption and hydrochloric acid secretion; it begins with a consideration of the special structural features of salt-transporting epithelia and then describes the interplay between theoretical models and experimental studies in the attempt to reconcile the known function with observed structure.

AMPLIFICATION OF PLASMA MEMBRANE AREA AND MITOCHONDRIAL VOLUME

Ultrastructural studies on a variety of salt-absorbing epithelia, such as those of the renal convoluted tubules, and of salt-secreting epithelia, such as the salt-excreting organs of various marine and arid-environment vertebrates, show a recurrent pattern of amplification of epithelial cell plasma membrane (reviewed by Ernst, Riddle & Karnaky, 1980). The most consistent feature is amplification of the basolateral plasma membrane, abluminal to the junctional complex, although in some structures (such as the renal proximal tubules) there is also striking amplification of the luminal plasma membrane in the form of a brush border of microvilli. From the start, it seemed intuitively reasonable that cells thought to have high transcellular fluxes of ions and water should have large surface areas to accommodate sites for these fluxes. In retrospect, a particularly significant point was the realisation that the basolateral plasma membrane amplifications consisted mainly of complex pleating and interlocking of the *lateral* surfaces of the cells rather than of deep infolding of the basal surface (Thoenes & Langer, 1969). This insight opened up the possibility of a major role for the lateral intercellular spaces and their adjoining plasma membranes, a possibility which has been a recurrent theme in most subsequent models of salt and water transport.

The other obvious structural feature in actively salt-transporting epithelia is the association between the amplified and folded basolateral plasma membranes and large numbers of structurally well-developed mitochondria. The existence of a correlation between both of these structural features and the capacity for net active salt transport is demonstrable in the salt-secreting glands of marine birds. When activated by osmotic stress, the principal secretory cells of these glands show increases in both basolateral membrane complexity and mitochondrial volume in parallel with the gland's increasing capacity to secrete a hypertonic salt solution (Ernst & Ellis, 1969).

ADENOSINE TRIPHOSPHATASE ACTIVITY AND THE SODIUM PUMP

The presence of a large mitochondrial compartment in salt-transporting cells and the expansion of this compartment under conditions of increased salt transport fit well with the idea of ATP-driven active transport as the primary active process in salt transport. The role of a sodium pump identifiable with sodium–potassium-activated, magnesium-dependent adenosine triphosphatase (Na^+,K^+-ATPase) in the maintenance of the ionic differences between the intracellular and extracellular compartments is well known; the plasma membrane has a high permeability to K^+ but a low permeability to Na^+, allowing the efflux of K^+ down its concentration gradient until this is balanced by the electrical potential so created. The tendency of this membrane potential to collapse through slow leakage of Na^+ into the cell is opposed by the sodium pump which extrudes Na^+ in exchange for K^+, hydrolysing ATP in order to drive this active transport. In principle, net salt transport across an epithelium could be achieved by generating a greater active efflux of Na^+ across one cell surface than the other, resulting in passive influx of Na^+ at the other surface and accompanied by passive movement of Cl^- to maintain electroneutrality (Fig. 2.1). Net salt transport would occur provided that short-circuiting of transport through paracellular channels was prevented; the existence of tight junctions occluding the paracellular route in all salt-transporting epithelia seems to provide a structural basis for this hypothesis. A structural model of this type for salt absorption was anticipated by Koefoed-Johnsen & Ussing (1958) on the basis of short-circuit current studies on frog skin.

The evidence that a sodium pump based on Na^+,K^+-ATPase drives transepithelial salt secretion is strong, and includes the parallelism between Na^+,K^+-ATPase activity and Na^+ pumping activity in various epithelia, the capacity of similar activating ion concentrations to give half-maximal activity of both pump and enzyme, and the similar sensitivities of both enzymatic and Na^+ transport activities to specific inhibition by the cardiac glycoside ouabain. The simplest explanation of transepithelial salt transport in terms of Na^+,K^+-ATPase sites would be that the pump is orientated in the conventional way (expelling Na^+ from cells) at the surface of the cell which faces the space towards which salt is transported. Thus a salt-absorbing epithelium would have basolateral pumps (Fig. 2.1), while in a salt-secreting epithelium they would be apical (Fig. 2.2). Unfortunately this simple and elegant prediction is at variance with the morphological evidence; both salt-absorbing and salt-secreting epithelia show basolateral membrane amplification, while a most impressive example of apical plasma membrane amplification is found in a salt-absorbing epithelium, the renal proximal tubule. However, the presence of membrane amplification cannot be assumed to indicate the presence of an equal amplification

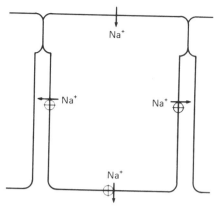

Fig. 2.1. Simple Na$^+$ extrusion model for salt reabsorption: active Na$^+$ extrusion by sodium pump at basolateral surfaces with passive Na$^+$ entry at the apical surface. Accompanying passive flux of Cl$^-$ to maintain electroneutrality is not shown. In this and all following electrolyte transport diagrams the crossed circle indicates ATPase-driven active transport, an empty circle passive coupled cotransport, and a plain arrow passive non-coupled transport.

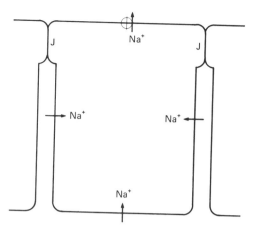

Fig. 2.2. Simple Na$^+$ extrusion model of salt secretion: active Na$^+$ extrusion by sodium pump at the apical surface with passive Na$^+$ entry at basolateral surfaces. Cl$^-$ fluxes are again not shown. Tight junctions (J) are assumed to be impermeable to electrolytes.

of pump sites. A much more important test of any model for salt transport is to determine directly in both secretory and absorptive epithelia whether the Na$^+$,K$^+$-ATPase responsible for active Na$^+$ transport is predominantly localised to the basolateral or the apical plasma membrane.

LOCALISATION OF Na$^+$, K$^+$-ATPase

The subcellular localisation of sodium pumps in salt-transporting epithelia is most directly approached by cytochemical methods, as biochemical isolation and identification of basolateral and apical plasma membrane fractions is not applicable readily to the mixed epithelial cell populations found in many salt-transporting organs. Techniques for the cytochemical localisation of Na$^+$,K$^+$-ATPase have been reviewed recently (Ernst & Hootman, 1981; Firth, 1978) and so will receive only a summary here.

Cytochemical localisation of membrane ATPases by precipitation of liberated inorganic phosphate (P$_i$) with heavy metal ions dates from the studies of Wachstein & Meisel (1957). Many of the hundreds of publications based on this technique suggest explicitly or implicitly that it localises Na$^+$,K$^+$-ATPase activity. However, a large body of evidence shows that the localisation, ion dependence, and inhibition and fixation sensitivity of reactions obtained with ATP-Pb^{2+} cytochemical methods like the Wachstein–Meisel procedure are not compatible with this idea (reviewed by Firth, 1978), although the hidden metal capture method of Chayen *et al.* (1981) may be an exception.

Specific cytochemical methods for Na$^+$,K$^+$-ATPase localisation depend on a closer examination of the characteristics of this enzyme. Na$^+$,K$^+$-ATPase has a catalytic subunit with a molecular weight of about 100 000 d, and ATP hydrolysis is carried out by a dimer of these subunits in two steps: the Na^+- and Mg^{2+}-dependent phosphorylation of a subunit, followed by K^+-dependent dephosphorylation. Various simple phosphates, such as *p*-nitrophenyl phosphate (NPP), can be hydrolysed in a K^+-dependent manner by the unphosphorylated enzyme. This principle is documented and exploited cytochemically in the elegant studies of Ernst (1972*a, b*) in which a secretory organ of high Na^+,K^+-ATPase activity, the duck salt gland, was used in the development of an ultrastructural cytochemical system specific for K^+-NPPase activity. The special features of this approach are: use of cold formaldehyde fixative with little or no glutaraldehyde to minimise inhibition of enzyme, use of NPP as substrate to avoid interference by other ATPases, and use of strontium ions (Sr^{2+}) for capture of P_i (again reducing enzyme inhibition). Use of Sr^{2+} for P_i capture necessitates incubation at high pH but, after incubation, the reaction product is stabilised and rendered electron-dense by exchange of Sr^{2+} for Pb^{2+}. This method yields a reaction located on the cytoplasmic face of the plasma membrane which is K^+-dependent and sensitive to inhibition by ouabain; these features are all appropriate for the NPPase partial reaction of Na^+,K^+-ATPase but cannot be demonstrated by Wachstein–Meisel methods.

Subsequent refinements of the NPPase approach include the use of specific inhibitors to exclude interference from alkaline phosphatases (Firth, 1974), and improvement of tissue preservation by the inclusion of very small quantities of glutaraldehyde in briefly perfused formaldehyde fixatives (Ernst, 1975). An apparent increase in sensitivity for light microscopical applications can be achieved by including 25% dimethyl sulphoxide (DMSO) in the incubation medium. DMSO acts by shifting the pH optimum of the K^+-NPPase reaction from 7.5 to 9.0, so putting it in the right range for optimal capture of P_i by metal ions not inhibitory to the enzyme. The original technique, as described by Guth & Albers (1974), appears to depend on P_i capture by Mg^{2+} and K^+ which, at high pH, can form fairly insoluble phosphates. Reaction product can be made visible by postincubation treatment with Co^{2+} or Pb^{2+}.

Our studies using the Guth & Albers' method have shown that the rather elaborate tissue preparation methods originally described are not necessary; the technique is best used on fresh, unfixed cryostat sections, and a sharp improvement in reaction product localisation can be obtained by increasing the Mg^{2+} concentration, presumably improving conditions for capture of P_i. Used in this way, the method sharply distinguishes basolateral from apical localisations and provides a reliable and simple light microscopical approach to Na^+,K^+-ATPase cytochemistry. The application of this method to kidney tissue is illustrated in Fig. 2.3. The possibilities of combining the addition of DMSO to incubation media with the advantages of direct heavy metal ion capture of P_i were not lost on Mayahara and his colleagues (1981), who used a low concentration of Pb^{2+} in an NPP–DMSO medium to give a direct ultrastructural method for localising Na^+,K^+-ATPase comparable in simplicity with the Wachstein–Meisel method; currently the Ernst and the Mayahara procedures seem to be the methods of choice for ultrastructural Na^+,K^+-ATPase localisation.

Only light microscopical methods have been used for quantitative studies at the time of writing. Both the hidden metal capture method of Chayen *et al.* (1981) and our modification of Guth & Albers' method have proved to be very suitable for quantitation using the Vickers M85a flying-spot scanning and integrative microdensitometer (Coulton & Firth, 1982). Although not easily applied to absolute quantitation of enzyme activity, this approach allows rapid, precise and easy

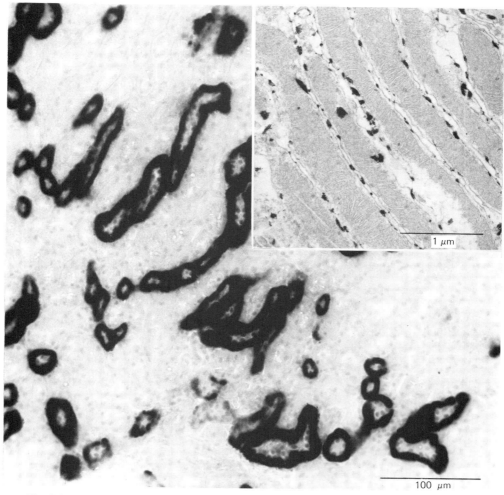

Fig. 2.3. Light micrograph of K$^+$-NPPase activity localised by a Mg^{2+} capture method to the (larger) cortical collecting tubules and (smaller) distal convoluted tubules of mouse renal cortex. Unfixed 10 μm cryostat section. Inset shows ultrastructural localisation by a Sr^{2+} capture method to the cytoplasmic surface of basolateral plasma membrane folds in a rat distal convoluted tubule.

numerical comparison between individual cells or larger structures sectioned and incubated in parallel.

A more rigorous approach to quantitative localisation of Na$^+$,K$^+$-ATPase depends on a quite different principle. In the labelled inhibitor autoradiographic method originally developed by Stirling (1972), tissue labelling with [^{3}H]ouabain is followed by washing, freeze drying, vapour fixation with osmium tetroxide and vacuum embedding in low viscosity epoxy resin. As ouabain only binds to the phosphoenzyme, it is a good marker for working enzyme; total Na$^+$-dependent binding provides a measure of the number of sodium pump sites, while the rate of binding indicates the pump turnover rate. The considerable power and flexibility of combined autoradiographic and liquid scintillation counting studies with [^{3}H]ouabain has been important to much recent progress in Na$^+$ transport studies and has been well reviewed recently (Ernst & Mills, 1980). Although the autoradiographic nature of the method effectively limits it to light microscopy, it has been shown that haempeptide-labelled ouabain has some potential as an ultrastructural label for sodium pumps; unfortunately this type of enzyme label is not suitable for quantitative studies (Mazurkiewicz, Hossler & Barrnett, 1978).

A third methodologically distinct approach to Na^+,K^+-ATPase localisation is through immunocytochemistry. This has been applied using both ferritin (Kyte, 1976) and peroxidase (Wood et al., 1977) labels. The main point about this method is its capacity to localise enzyme protein irrespective of whether catalytic or pump activity is present. In spite of its sensitivity and its value in providing independent confirmation of NPPase and [^{3}H]ouabain results, the immunocytochemical method has been little used. This is in large measure due to the technical problem of obtaining good yields of antigen from all but a few particularly favourable tissues.

Three groups of cytochemical methods are therefore available for the subcellular localisation of Na^+,K^+-ATPase in salt-transporting organs. Table 2.1 summarises the

Table 2.1. *Na^+,K^+-ATPase localisations in salt-absorbing epithelia*

Epithelium	Localisation	Original source[a]
Renal proximal and distal tubules	Basolateral	Firth, 1974; Ernst, 1975 (NPPase)
	Basolateral	Kyte, 1976 (Immunocytochemical)
	Basolateral	Shaver & Stirling, 1978 ([^{3}H]ouabain)
Eccrine sweat ducts	Basolateral	Quinton & Tormey, 1976 ([^{3}H]ouabain)
Amphibian urinary bladder	Basolateral	Mills & Ernst, 1975 ([^{3}H]ouabain)
Amphibian epidermis (stratified)	(Basolateral equivalent)	Mills & DiBona, 1977 ([^{3}H]ouabain)
Amphibian gallbladder	Basolateral	Mills & DiBona, 1978 ([^{3}H]ouabain)
Cornea	(Basolateral equivalent)	Leuenberger & Novikoff, 1974 (NPPase)
Intestinal epithelium	Basolateral	Stirling, 1972 ([^{3}H]oubain)
	Basolateral	Vengesa & Hopfer, 1979 (NPPase)
Cultured kidney cells	Basolateral	Mills et al., 1979 ([^{3}H]ouabain)

[a] Full references to these and other Na^+,K^+-ATPase localisations are found in Firth (1978) and Ernst & Hootman (1981).

localisations obtained by these means in some salt-absorbing epithelia. In all cases and with all methods, basolateral plasma membrane localisations, or equivalent inward-directed localisations in stratified epithelia, support the view that conventionally orientated sodium pumps expelling Na^+ into the lateral intercellular spaces provide the mechanism for salt uptake, assuming that passive cotransport of Cl^- and passive Na^+ entry at the apical plasma membrane can occur.

A summary of the localisations of Na^+,K^+-ATPase in some salt-secreting epithelia is provided in Table 2.2. It is striking that (with the exception of [^{3}H]ouabain localisation in choroid plexus) basolateral sodium pumps are typical of salt-secreting as well as salt-absorbing epithelia. The large numbers of systems examined, the strong biochemical validation of both NPPase and [^{3}H]ouabain methods, and the high level of agreement between results when two or more methods have been applied to the same system, make it plain that apparently identical basolateral sodium pump localisations can drive both salt absorption and salt secretion.

BASOLATERAL SODIUM PUMPS AND THE DIRECTION OF SALT TRANSPORT

This evidence on sodium pump localisation presents little difficulty with respect to salt-absorbing epithelia. Basolateral localisations are consistent with the standing

Table 2.2. *Na⁺,K⁺-ATPase localisations in salt-secreting epithelia*

Epithelium	Localisation	Original source[a]
Avian salt gland	Basolateral	Ernst, 1972 (NPPase)
	Basolateral	Ernst & Mills, 1977 ([³H]ouabain)
Turtle salt gland	Basolateral	Thompson & Cowan, 1976 (NPPase)
	Basolateral	Thompson & Cowan, 1976 ([³H]ouabain)
Iguana salt gland	Basolateral	Ellis & Goertemiller, 1976 (NPPase)
Elasmobranch rectal gland	Basolateral	Goertemiller & Ellis, 1976 (NPPase)
	Basolateral	Eveloff *et al.*, 1979. ([³H]ouabain)
Teleost gill	Basolateral	Karnaky *et al.*, 1976 ([³H]ouabain)
	Basolateral	Hootman & Philpott, 1979 (NPPase)
Teleost operculum	Basolateral	Ernst, Dodson & Karnaky, 1978 ([³H]ouabain)
Choroid plexus	Apical	Quinton, Wright & Tormey, 1973 ([³H]ouabain)
	Basolateral	Milhorat, Davis & Hammock, 1975 (NPPase)
Eccrine sweat gland	Basolateral	Quinton & Tormey, 1976 ([³H]ouabain)

[a] Full references to these and other Na⁺,K⁺-ATPase localisations are found in Firth (1978) and Ernst & Hootman (1981).

gradient osmotic flow model of Diamond & Bossert (1967) in which salt extrusion into the lateral intercellular spaces creates an osmotic flow of water which carries ions out of the basal ends of the intercellular spaces (Fig. 2.4). However, the localisation studies present a considerable problem for the interpretation of secretory epithelia. Three possible explanations of the results need to be considered:

(i) the basolateral sodium pumps in salt-secreting epithelia are concerned solely with maintenance of the intracellular ionic environment, while a different pump mechanism is responsible for transepithelial salt transport;
(ii) basolateral sodium pumps are responsible for salt secretion, but are orientated in the membrane so as to transport Na⁺ into the cell rather than out of it;
(iii) basolateral sodium pumps are responsible for salt secretion and are conventionally orientated so as to extrude Na⁺ from cytoplasm into the lateral intercellular spaces as in absorptive epithelia. Whether this results in secretion or absorption depends on aspects of cellular organisation other than the pump localisation.

The first proposal, that basolateral sodium pumps are irrelevant to salt secretion, sounds like an attempt to avoid unpalatable evidence rather than accept its implications, especially in view of the universally accepted role of the Na⁺,K⁺-ATPase sodium pump in salt absorption. The main evidence refuting such a proposal is that factors stimulating the ability to secrete salt also stimulate Na⁺,K⁺-ATPase activity to a similar extent (Fletcher, Stainer & Holmes, 1967), and salt secretion and Na⁺,K⁺-ATPase activity show parallel inhibition by ouabain (Maetz & Bornancin, 1975). The main system which might be considered as an alternative sodium pump is an ethacrynic-acid-sensitive, ouabain-insensitive and K⁺-independent electrogenic pump located at the cell apex (Proverbio, Condrescu-Guidi & Whittembury, 1975). It seems unlikely that this type of pump accounts for salt secretion, as the inhibitory effects of ethacrynic acid on salt gland secretion can be ascribed to inhibition of cellular respiration which leads to depletion of ATP (Van Rossum & Ernst, 1978).

The striking suggestion that basolateral sodium pumps in salt-secreting epithelia are reverse-polarised (so as to pump Na⁺ into the cytoplasm with passive efflux across the apical surface) forms the core of a model advanced by Diamond & Bossert (1968). However, cytochemical studies show that the catalytic site for NPP hydrolysis is at the *cytoplasmic* surface of the basolateral plasma membrane in both absorptive and secretory epithelia, while pump inhibition by ouabain in secretory epithelia leads to intracellular accumulation of Na$^+$ (evidence reviewed in Ernst *et al.*, 1980).

These considerations leave only the third possibility that salt-secreting epithelia, like absorptive systems, extrude Na$^+$ into the lateral intercellular spaces. It is now necessary to consider the mechanisms which could convert this intercellular Na$^+$ accumulation into apically directed rather than basally directed salt transport.

THE SIGNIFICANCE OF THE PARACELLULAR ROUTE

The only route to the lumen apparently available to Na$^+$ extruded into the lateral intercellular spaces of a salt-secreting epithelium is through the tight junctions near the luminal ends of the spaces. For some time it has been recognised that some tight junctions are tighter than others, and there is often a good correlation between the number of continuous junctional strands seen by thin-section and freeze–fracture techniques and the tightness of the barrier to diffusion across the junction (Claude & Goodenough, 1973). In absorptive epithelia, such as those of the renal convoluted tubules, few-stranded junctions are associated with isotonic absorption (as in proximal tubule) and many-stranded junctions with the capacity to maintain a pump-generated osmotic gradient (as in distal tubule). It is also well established that in leaky epithelia the paracellular (junctional) route is usually cation-selective because of fixed negative charges within the junction (reviewed by Diamond, 1978). It is, therefore, important to establish whether such a route may exist in salt-secreting epithelia.

The junctions of salt gland (Ellis, Goertemiller & Stetson, 1977) and elasmobranch rectal gland (Ernst *et al.*, 1981) have a simple morphology, usually consisting of a single pair of closely apposed junctional strands. The total junctional length in both organs is considerable because of extensive interlocking of the margins of the apical cell surfaces. These characteristics of junctional length and simplicity are those expected of a cation-permeable paracellular channel. Establishment of a net flux of Na$^+$ across such a junction towards the lumen requires a driving force, the nature of which is suggested by a model derived from the salt gland and rectal gland systems (Ernst & Mills, 1977; Silva *et al.*, 1977). This model is illustrated in Fig. 2.5; its essential features are as follows. Na$^+$ extrusion into the lateral intercellular spaces by basolateral sodium pumps leads to *coupled* passive entry into the cells of Na$^+$ and Cl$^-$ through a basolateral sodium chloride (NaCl) carrier. This leads to Cl$^-$ accumulation in the cells and so to Cl$^-$ efflux down its concentration gradient through apical membrane channels to the lumen. The resulting luminal accumulation of Cl$^-$ causes a lumen-negative transepithelial potential which drives Na$^+$ from the lateral intercellular spaces across the tight junction to the lumen, so completing the secretion of salt. This elegant model is supported by the experimental confirmation of various predictions it implies: frusemide, a known inhibitor of passive coupled NaCl transport, inhibits sodium pump turnover in activated salt gland cells (Hootman & Ernst, 1981), while lumen-negative potentials can be found in several salt-secreting systems and both the potential and Cl$^-$ transport under short-circuit conditions can be inhibited by ouabain or frusemide (evidence summarised by Ernst *et al.*, 1980).

UNRESOLVED ASPECTS OF SALT SECRETION

In most salt-secreting systems the application of a common set of concepts about transcellular (sodium pump and coupled passive carrier) and paracellular (lateral

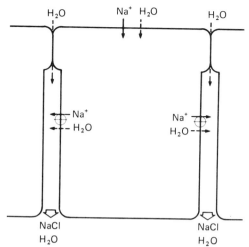

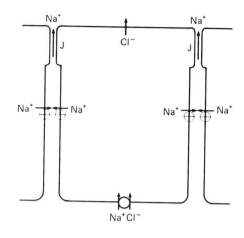

Fig. 2.4. Summary of standing gradient osmotic flow model of salt and water absorption: active Na^+ extrusion into lateral intercellular spaces accompanied by passive apical Na^+ entry leads to osmotic flow of water into lateral intercellular spaces, probably by both transcellular and para-cellular (tight junction) routes (water flows shown by broken arrows). Together with passive transcellular Cl^- movement following Na^+, this results in net salt and water flow from the lateral intercellular spaces to the subepithelial region.

Fig. 2.5. Salt secretion driven by basolateral sodium pumps. Na^+ extrusion into lateral inter-cellular spaces leads to coupled basolateral NaCl entry. Resulting intercellular Cl^- accumulation causes passive apical efflux of Cl^-, creating a lumen-negative potential which drives Na^+ flow through leaky intercellular junctions (J) to lumen.

intercellular space and tight junction) mechanisms can be used to give a reasonably adequate explanation of most experimental findings. Inevitably problems remain which defy incorporation into a simple unifying scheme. The clash between NPPase and [³H]ouabain localisations in the choroid plexus has already been mentioned. It is probably fair to point out that the NPPase localisation (Milhorat, Davis & Hammock, 1975) was on the external surface of the basolateral plasma membrane and that specific controls excluding alkaline phosphatase were not carried out. If the choroid plexus sodium pumps are apical, as is implied by [³H]ouabain autoradiography (Quinton, Wright & Tormey, 1973), this constitutes an exception to the general pattern of both isotonic and hypertonic salt-secreting epithelia. Conceivably, the early isolation of the neuroectoderm in development has allowed it to evolve its own solution to salt transport problems independently of other epithelia. The choroid plexus is something of a problem in other respects: during its embryonic development its permeability to numerous solutes declines sharply although the mean junctional strand number and the strand pattern in the tight junctions do not change significantly (Møllgård, Malinowska, & Saunders, 1976). This has been tentatively related to the presence of a system of intracellular tubules of endoplasmic-reticulum-like form (the TER); TER systems have been reported in several epithelia and have been suggested to have an important though unspecified role in salt transport in leaky isotonic salt-transporting epithelia such as renal proximal tubule, small intestinal and gallblad-der epithelia and choroid plexus (Møllgård & Rostgaard, 1978). Interesting though these morphological findings are, physiological data supporting a role for the TER in salt transport are scanty and it would be premature to make any more detailed comment. Recently a rather interesting role for at least some TER elements in water, rather than salt, transport has gained much credibility and this is discussed more extensively in the final section of this paper.

Salt-transporting epithelia are generally thought of as cuboidal, columnar or stratified and well equipped with extensive plasma membranes and complex paracellular channels. Certain atypical epithelia seem to be able to carry out polarised ion transport without the benefit of at least some of these features.

It is well known that the transfer of certain solutes between blood plasma and brain extracellular fluid is either prevented or regulated within narrow limits. One ion regulated in this way is K^+, at least part of the control of which depends on ouabain-sensitive expulsion from brain extracellular fluid to blood plasma. The well-developed multistranded tight junctions of brain capillary endothelial cells make the capillary endothelium a likely site for regulative transport, and a combined

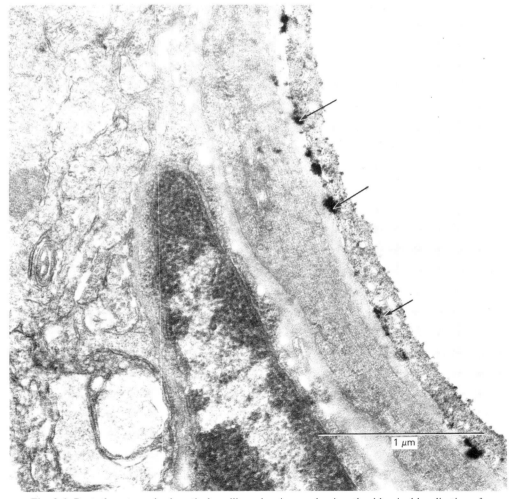

Fig. 2.6. Part of a rat cerebral cortical capillary showing predominantly abluminal localisation of K^+-NPPase activity of endothelial cell (arrows). Sr^{2+} capture method.

cytochemical and biochemical study of brain capillaries showed that the strongest K^+-NPPase and Na^+,K-ATPase activity was associated with the abluminal plasma membrane of the capillary endothelium (Betz, Firth & Goldstein, 1980; see Fig. 2.6). The probable relationship between this localisation and K^+ transport is indicated in Fig. 2.7.

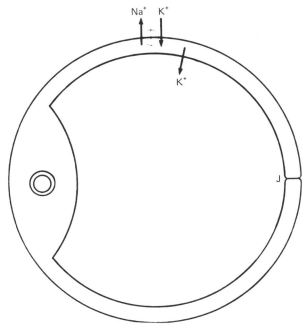

Fig. 2.7. An abluminal sodium pump in brain capillary endothelium causes a lumen-directed K^+ flux which, with a passive K^+ channel in the luminal membrane, provides a mechanism for active K^+ extrusion from brain extracellular fluid. Well-developed tight junctions (J) prevent paracellular K^+ movement.

A rather different K^+ transport problem is found in the guinea-pig placenta, in which K^+ is actively accumulated on the foetal side. Here the endothelium lining the foetal capillaries is not a major factor as it is permeable to ions and even to small proteins (Sibley, Bauman & Firth, 1982). The other continuous cellular layer, the syncytiotrophoblast, faces the maternal blood and is entirely syncytial with no lateral intercellular spaces. K^+-NPPase activity is localised to the microvillous maternal blood-facing surface of the syncytiotrophoblast (Firth, Farr & Koppel, 1979). Given a leaky endothelium and a trophoblast without lateral intercellular spaces, this is in fact the only site at which Na^+,K^+-ATPase could generate a foetus-directed K^+ transport (Fig. 2.8).

Models based on conventionally orientated Na^+,K^+-ATPase-driven sodium pumps can thus be used to explain transport of Na^+,K^+ and Cl^- across many epithelial and epithelium-like cellular layers. The realisation that basolateral extrusion of Na^+ can set up the conditions for Cl^--led salt secretion has made things simpler by eliminating the need to postulate Cl^- pumps. Unfortunately it is not possible to explain all active transport on the basis of the sodium pump, and numerous electrolyte-transporting systems still require discussion in terms of different pumps with various ionic specificities. Of these, the most thoroughly investigated is hydrochloric acid secretion

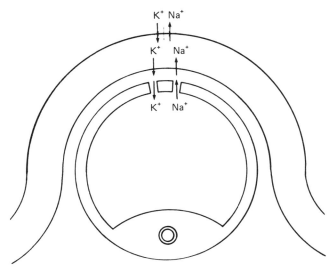

Fig. 2.8. In guinea-pig placenta a maternal-blood-facing sodium pump in the trophoblast drives foetus-directed active transport of K^+. Unlike brain, the capillaries have ion-permeable paracellular routes and so play no active role.

by the gastric mucosa. Quite apart from its practical importance, this system shows unique features which require discussion and an attempt at explanation.

THE GASTRIC PARIETAL CELL AND HYDROCHLORIC ACID SECRETION

Mammalian gastric glands provide a striking and unique example of an electrolyte-secreting gland which can create very steep ionic gradients. Hydrochloric acid (HCl) can be secreted at a concentration of 160 mM, and the transepithelial pH difference of up to 6.6 represents a huge difference in proton (H^+) concentration (Sachs & Berglindh, 1981).

This acid-secreting activity has long been ascribed to the parietal (oxyntic) cells, although conclusive evidence for this is in fact rather recent. The parietal cell shows the typical plasma membrane elaboration and large mitochondrial population of an ion-transporting cell, but these components are arranged in a unique way. The basolateral plasma membrane is rather smooth, but in the active gland the apical membrane is infolded to form microvillus-lined secretory canaliculi which extend deep into the cytoplasm (Fig. 2.9). In the inactive cell, the canalicular system is much reduced and often appears internalised in thin sections, while the cytoplasm contains an elaborate smooth membrane complex called the tubulovesicular system (Fig. 2.10).

The relationship between the tubulovesicles and the canaliculi has usually been regarded as one in which tubulovesicle membrane is incorporated into the canalicular surface by an exocytosis-like mechanism during activation and is withdrawn as secretion ends; this view is plausible in the light of morphometric studies showing that the loss of tubulovesicular membrane area during activation is matched by a corresponding increase in canalicular (apical plasma) membrane area (Helander & Hirschowicz, 1972). An alternative interpretation is that the onset of fluid secretion greatly dilates a previously collapsed canalicular–tubular system so that its continuity with the apical surface becomes obvious (Sachs & Berglindh, 1981). Preparation of

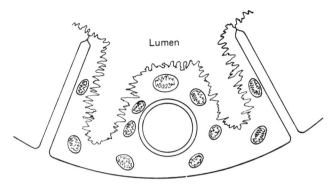

Fig. 2.9. Active parietal cell showing elaborate canaliculi continuous with lumen, and absence of tubulovesicles from cytoplasm.

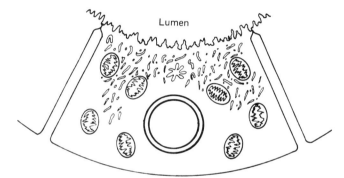

Fig. 2.10. Parietal cell in basal state, showing simple apical membrane and tubulovesicles in cytoplasm.

parietal cells by ultrafast freezing on a liquid-nitrogen-cooled copper block followed by freeze-substitution shows tubulovesicular membranes to lie very close to (but separate from) the canalicular membrane, while freeze–fracture studies show essentially similar intramembrane particle distributions in both tubulovesicular and canalicular membranes (reviewed by Ito, 1981). The issue of whether the tubulovesicles are permanently continuous with the apical plasma membrane or are intercalated into it on activation is thus unresolved, although most opinion seems to favour the latter view. Perhaps the more important point is that activation obviously involves a morphological transformation of some kind, and almost certainly involves the activity of cytoskeletal components.

GASTRIC TRANSPORT ATPases

Secretion of gastric HCl is strictly dependent on ATP, and several ion-stimulated ATPases found in gastric microsomes have been considered as possible candidates for the active transport step in acid secretion (Forte & Lee, 1977). HCO_3^--dependent ATPase was at one time looked on with interest because of the known importance of carbonic anhydrase and HCO_3^- in gastric acid secretion, but it now seems probable that this enzyme is of mitochondrial origin as it can often be eliminated by adequate purification of microsomes. Na^+,K^+-ATPase is found but at concentrations too low to

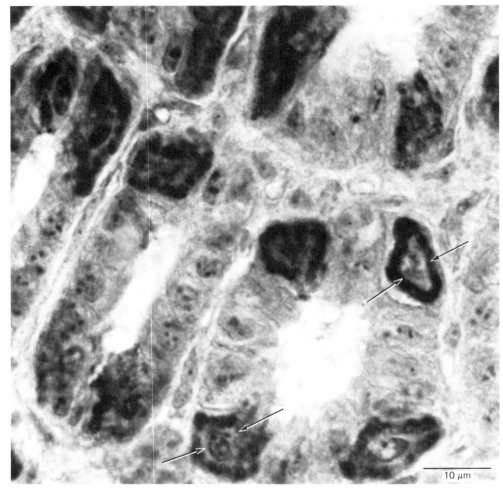

Fig. 2.11. Mouse parietal cells showing K^+-NPPase activity associated with the canaliculi (arrows). Mg^{2+} capture method on unfixed 10 μm cryostat section.

make it a credible prime mover in acid secretion although it certainly plays an important role in the overall function of parietal cells.

The most interesting and characteristic ATPase of the gastric mucosa is K^+-stimulated and Mg^{2+}-dependent but, unlike Na^+,K^+-ATPase, is independent of Na^+. This enzyme, present in very high concentrations, shows close family resemblances to Na^+,K^+-ATPase with a major protein of about 100 000 d and K^+-NPPase activity. The involvement of this K^+-dependent ATPase in acid secretion is supported by evidence showing that the membrane vesicles of enzyme-rich microsomal fractions accumulate H^+ by a K^+- and ATP-dependent mechanism (Forte, Machen & Öbrink, 1980).

These characteristics suggest that this enzyme, generally known as H^+,K^+-ATPase, is directly responsible for active secretion of H^+. However, incorporation of this enzyme into a scheme for cellular acid secretion requires information on the subcellular localisation of the enzyme, and several cytochemical studies have been directed to this end. Immunocytochemistry using peroxidase label methods with antibody raised against highly enriched microsomes, and rigorously purified, shows reaction at the microvilli of the secretory canaliculi (Sachs & Berglindh, 1981). As has already been pointed out in the context of Na$^+$,K$^+$-ATPase cytochemistry, immunocytochemical enzyme localisations can have high sensitivity and specificity but reveal little about the functional capacity of the enzyme protein. Several attempts have been made to localise gastric ATPases by virtue of their catalytic activity using metal capture methods. Koenig & Vial (1970) localised Mg^{2+}-dependent ATPase activity to the basolateral surface and HCO$_3^-$-dependent ATPase to the apical surface of toad oxynticopeptic cells using Pb^{2+}-ATP methods, but did not look for K$^+$-dependent reactions. An ultrastructural study on rat and human gastric mucosa after glutaraldehyde fixation used the Ernst method to detect NPPase activity at both the basolateral and canalicular plasma membranes of parietal cells, but did not examine K$^+$-dependence or inhibitor sensitivity of this reaction (Rubin & Aliasgharpour, 1976).

We have used a modification of the NPPase method of Guth & Albers (1974) to localise K$^+$-dependent and ouabain-resistant NPPase activity in gastric mucosa. This revealed very intense activity in parietal cells which under favourable P$_i$ capture conditions was clearly localised to the secretory canaliculi (Fig. 2.11). This activity was unaffected by ouabain and by the alkaline phosphatase inhibitor levamisole, but was sensitive to fluoride and to the sulphydryl enzyme inhibitor *p*-hydroxymercuribenzoate (Firth & Stranks, 1981). Electron microscopical localisation has so far been impeded by the enzyme's extreme sensitivity to even very brief fixation with glutaraldehyde, formaldehyde or dimethylsuberimidate.

One of the more striking features of the gastric K$^+$-NPPase reaction is that in mouse gastric glands the activity is only found in those parietal cells lying in the upper part of the gland (Fig. 2.12). Even if activity is maximised by starving the mouse for 24 h and feeding 5 minutes before killing, the parietal cells in the deeper portion of the gastric gland show no histochemical activity (Coulton & Firth, 1982). It is well established that the long-lived parietal cells originate from undifferentiated cells in the gland neck region and migrate down the gland to the base, so it was thought possible that the parietal cells of the lower segment of the gland are senescent and have lost their H$^+$,K$^+$-ATPase activity. However, succinate dehydrogenase activity is stronger in the lower segment parietal cells than in those in the upper segment, so there is no good reason for assuming that the lower segment cells are undergoing any generalised degeneration (Fig. 2.13). Enzyme protein is apparently present in all parietal cells on the basis of the immunohistochemical evidence (G. Sachs, personal communication). The basis for this difference between the immunocytochemical and catalytic cytochemical localisations of H$^+$,K$^+$-ATPase is not known, although we are currently trying to test the hypothesis that it reflects the activation state of the cell.

Whatever the basis for this finding, both immunocytochemical and NPPase cytochemical studies are in good agreement that H$^+$,K$^+$-ATPase is confined to parietal cells and is probably limited to the canalicular (apical) plasma membrane.

SECRETORY MECHANISMS IN THE PARIETAL CELL

Analysis of ion secretion by the gastric mucosa is complicated by the extreme cellular heterogeneity of this tissue. Although much has been achieved using isolated parietal cells or subcellular fractions, studies of the integrated process of acid secretion require the use of intact mucosa or, at least, of isolated gastric glands. In

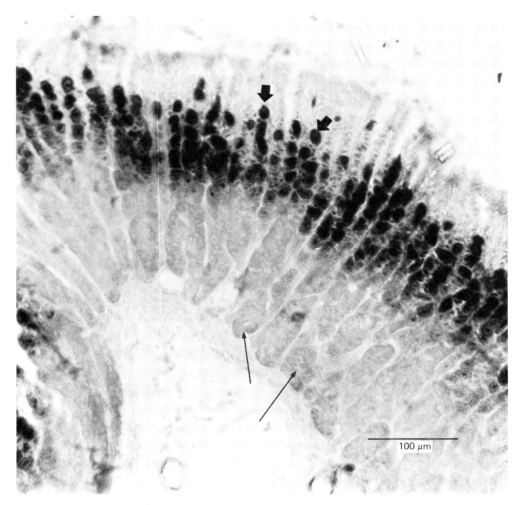

Fig. 2.12. Gradient of K^+-NPPase activity in mouse gastric glands from high activity at gland neck (short arrows) to zero activity near gland base (long arrows). Mg^{2+} capture method on unfixed 10 μm cryostat section.

these mixed epithelial cell populations it is hard to exclude the possibility that at least some of the ionic movements measured during acid secretion may derive from principal cells or mucous cells rather than the parietal cells themselves, unless decisive cytochemical evidence is available. The evidence for current ideas on ionic mechanisms in gastric hydrochloric acid secretion has received detailed discussion in two excellent recent reviews (Forte *et al.*, 1980; Sachs & Berglindh, 1981). The short summary presented here is intended only to indicate the relevance of the morphological and cytochemical features already discussed to the development of understanding of this complex epithelial system.

Cell fractionation studies on parietal cells show that H^+,K^+-ATPase and Na^+,K^+-ATPase appear in separable membrane fractions. As the cytochemical evidence supports an apical–canalicular origin for H^+,K^+-ATPase, it is probable that the main site for the relatively low total level of Na^+,K^+-ATPase is the basolateral plasma

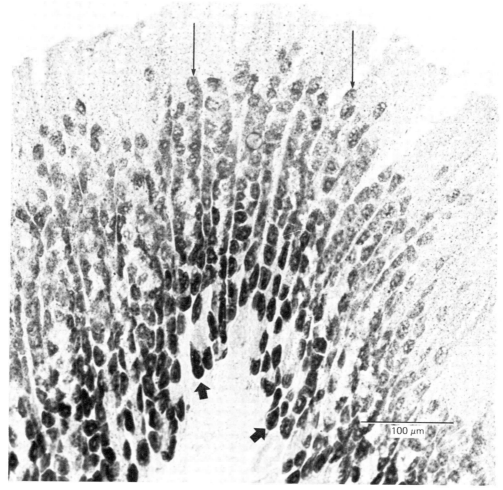

Fig. 2.13. Gradient of succinate dehydrogenase activity in mouse gastric glands from moderate activity at gland neck (long arrows) to high activity near gland base (short arrows). Nitro blue tetrazolium method on unfixed 10 μm cryostat section. (Micrograph by courtesy of Gary Coulton.)

membrane. The behaviour of the mucosa under non-acid-secreting (resting) conditions is characterised by a lumen-negative potential attributable to luminally directed Cl^- transport. This Cl^- transport in the basal state is Na^+-dependent and ouabain-sensitive, implying that it is driven by Na^+,K^+-ATPase. Probably the mechanism of this is rather similar to the Cl^--led secretion which has already been discussed at length in the context of salt-secreting glands; the main differences are the much lower level of Na^+,K^+-ATPase activity in the gastric mucosa, and the much more complex tight junctions of the gastric glandular epithelium which prevent a significant paracellular Na^+ flux (Fig. 2.14).

New mechanisms come into play during acid secretion. Active extrusion of H^+ across the apical-canalicular membrane probably involves an electroneutral exchange with K^+. The luminal K^+ needed to prime this active exchange seems to reach the lumen through passive coupled transport of K^+ and Cl^- across the canalicular membrane, the pump then acting to exchange K^+ for H^+ and so complete the HCl product. Extrusion of H$^+$ by the pump leads to an equivalent accumulation of OH$^-$ intracellularly; this is converted to HCO$_3^-$ in a reaction catalysed by carbonic anhydrase. Gastric mucosa is a rich source of carbonic anhydrase, and both immunocytochemical (Spicer, Stoward & Tashian, 1979) and catalytic cytochemical (Sugai & Ito, 1980) methods localise the bulk of this enzyme to the parietal cells. HCO$_3^-$ is secreted from the basolateral surface of the parietal cell by a passive coupled exchange for Cl$^-$, so maintaining the availability of Cl$^-$ for K$^+$-coupled extrusion at the apical-canicular membrane. These pathways of ion movement are summarised in Fig. 2.15.

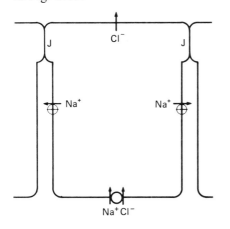

Fig. 2.14. Parietal cell in basal state: basolateral Na$^+$ extrusion by sodium pump with coupled salt (NaCl) entry maintains a high intracellular Cl$^-$ concentration favouring passive Cl$^-$ movement to the lumen. The cation-impermeability of the tight junctions (J) prevents charge neutralisation by paracellular Na$^+$ diffusion, so no net NaCl transport occurs (contrast with Fig. 2.5).

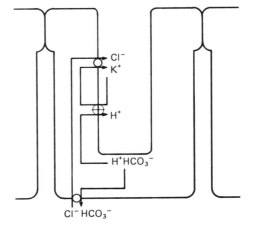

Fig. 2.15. Activated parietal cell. In addition to the basal state ion pathways (see Fig. 2.14), a coupled passive KCl carrier at the canalicular membrane provides extracellular K$^+$ to activate K$^+$/H$^+$ exchange by the canalicular membrane proton pump. Protons are derived from ionisation of water, OH$^-$ being converted to HCO$_3^-$ and eliminated by coupled exchange for Cl$^-$ at a carrier in the basolateral membrane. HCO$_3^-$ formation is catalysed by carbonic anhydrase.

COMPARISON OF BASOLATERALLY AND APICALLY DRIVEN ELECTROLYTE SECRETION

One of the most striking structural features of electrolyte-secreting epithelia, the presence of polarised plasma membrane elaboration, turns out to be a reliable guide to the location of the cation-pump ATPases which drive secretion. It is now clear that there are two main mechanisms of active cation secretion: the basolateral sodium pump associated with paracellular pathways permeable to Na$^+$ (which characterise most salt-secreting epithelia), and the more direct apical H$^+$ pump of the gastric parietal cell in which the paracellular pathway is apparently of little importance. It is interesting to speculate why two such very different systems should have evolved to achieve rather similar ends.

Basolateral localisation of gastric H$^+$,K$^+$-ATPase would not be a successful system for gastric hydrochloric acid secretion for at least two reasons. Firstly, the proton pump appears to be electroneutral. Thus the operation of the pump together with a passive K$^+$ channel and coupled HCO$_3^-$/Cl$^-$ exchange could not lead to intracellular accumulation of Cl⁻. In the absence of this, no Cl⁻ diffusion potential could develop at the cell apex and so there would be no electrical gradient to drive H⁺ movement across the tight junction to the lumen. Secondly, even if a well-developed basolateral sodium pump were also present to drive the apical extrusion of Cl⁻, the development of a Cl⁻ potential could not drive effective H⁺ secretion. The transepithelial potential required to support the observed pH gradient would be in excess of 300 mV, representing a vastly higher sodium pump turnover than that found even in extremely specialised salt secretors such as the avian salt gland. The direct apical proton pump with closed paracellular channels is really the only practicable arrangement for secretion requiring very high transepithelial ion gradients.

There does not seem to be a converse argument excluding the use of an apical sodium pump by salt-secreting epithelia, and at least in the case of the choroid plexus it is probable that an apical sodium pump is present. It is possible that the general basolateral arrangement may reflect some evolutionary economy in using the same cell polarisation for both secretion and absorption of salts; this sounds particularly plausible in relation to organs like the eccrine sweat gland and its duct (Quinton & Tormey, 1976), and the loop of Henle (Ernst & Schreiber, 1981) in which baso-laterally polarised secretory and absorptive epithelial segments probably occur in the same tubular unit.

THE CONTROL OF ELECTROLYTE SECRETION

Several of the secretory organs discussed here have well characterised and fast-acting neural or endocrine control mechanisms which can induce a change from a low basal rate of secretion to maximal activity. In the case of the avian salt gland there is a cholinergic parasympathetic innervation which intermittently stimulates secretion, not by a direct effect on the sodium pump, but indirectly by stimulation of the Cl⁻-dependent uptake of Na⁺ through the coupled carrier mechanism. This, in turn, causes a compensating increase in turnover of the sodium pump (Hootman & Ernst, 1981). This rapid intermittent activation of salt secretion should not be confused with the longer term adaptation of the gland to conditions of salt stress, which involves growth of the basolateral membrane and mitochondria and increase in number of sodium pumps. The short term neurogenic activation of the gland is not associated with increased cytochemical Na⁺,K⁺-ATPase activity as the ion gradients regulating pump turnover are destroyed by the preparative procedures for cyto-chemical incubation.

The activation of gastric acid secretion is rather more complex. The three main agonists, acetylcholine, histamine and gastrin, act through second messenger systems involving cyclic AMP or Ca^{2+}. It seems possible that histamine may act on ion transport processes through a cyclic-AMP-mediated mechanism while the other agonists both cause histamine release and also have a specific Ca^{2+}-mediated effect in bringing about the changes in parietal cell morphology associated with acid secretion. K⁺-NPPase cytochemistry shows that feeding-induced gastric acid secretion is accompanied by a very large increase in parietal cell H⁺,K⁺-ATPase activity in cryostat sections of mouse stomach (Coulton & Firth, 1982). This is rather surprising as there is no evidence that any of the agonists leading to gastric acid secretion directly stimulate the H⁺ pump. I consider that it is more likely to reflect a difference in membrane organisation between the basal and stimulated states: if the enzyme-carrying apical membrane was in the form of closed internalised tubulovesicles in the basal state, build-up of ionic gradients could soon halt coupled substrate hydrolysis, whereas gradients across canalicular membranes in the activated cell would be short-circuited as a result of freezing and sectioning during tissue preparation.

NEW MICROSCOPICAL APPROACHES TO ELECTROLYTE TRANSPORT

The main purpose of this paper has been to show how initially very separate morphological and physiological studies of electrolyte-transporting epithelia have converged to produce more powerful and satisfactory models for transport function. The forces underlying this growth have been the development of specific, biochemically validated techniques for transport enzyme localisation, new insight into the significance of the organisational features of tight junctions, and above all an increasing readiness on the part of both morphologists and physiologists to understand each other's preoccupations and to work with each other's methods. This synthesis has now reached the point where sophisticated microscopical methods are being applied to isolated cells and to intact epithelia under defined physiological conditions. Two examples should suffice to illustrate the power of these approaches.

Controversy over the behaviour of lateral intercellular spaces during salt and water absorption by leaky epithelia has never been adequately resolved by electron microscopy because changes in space width were swamped by the artefactual changes which could be generated by fixation and specimen preparation. These difficulties can be avoided by the use of high-resolution light microscopy with image intensification on living epithelial sheets mounted in miniature Ussing chambers and superfused separately on mucosal and serosal sides with solutions of defined compositions (Spring & Hope, 1979).

Dramatic optical sections of living cells at high resolution may be obtained by the now familiar technique of differential interference contrast (DIC) microscopy. A system for combined DIC and fluorescence microscopy has recently been applied to gastric acid secretion in an elegant series of studies (reviewed by DiBona et al., 1981). Examination of isolated parietal cells and isolated gastric glands under DIC microscopy shows that stimulation with histamine or dibutyryl cyclic AMP causes vacuolation or canaliculus formation in the parietal cell cytoplasm. Use of fluorescence microscopy with Acridine Orange shows that these vacuoles and canaliculi exhibit the characteristic red fluorescence of Acridine Orange under low pH conditions, while unstimulated cells and the cytoplasm of the stimulated cells show the green fluorescence typical of neutral pH. This method gives direct confirmation of the inference from morphological, cytochemical and physiological data that acid is formed at the canalicular surface of the parietal cell. The same review also demonstrates the possibility of applying these approaches to isolated, perfused segments of renal tubules. There can be little doubt that these methods are the beginning of an exciting new phase in epithelial transport studies.

A quite different but equally pleasing fusion of physiological and morphological methods has recently admitted light to the long-standing problem of the cellular basis for the vasopressin-mediated stimulation of osmotic water absorption. Freeze–fracture studies of toad urinary bladder show that vasopressin stimulation leads to the appearance of orderly clusters of intramembranous particles (IMPs) on the P face of the luminal membrane and of complementary groove patterns on the E face. The number of such clusters and the fraction of the luminal surface occupied by them both show highly significant correlation with the vasopressin-dependent increase in osmotic water flow across the bladder (Kachadorian *et al.*, 1977). Cross-fractures of bladder cells reveal tubular membrane structures which also carry the characteristic arrays of P face IMPs. After vasopressin stimulation, continuity between tubules and the luminal plasma membrane can be seen both in freeze–fracture and thin-section images, and studies of the effects of colchicine show inhibition of the fusion event and of osmotic water flow in response to vasopressin (Muller, Kachadorian & DiScala, 1980). Freeze–fracture studies of the response of the rat collecting duct to vasopressin show dose-dependent appearance of similar IMP clusters in the luminal plasma membrane of duct epithelial cells (Harmanci *et al.*, 1980). These results clearly imply that membrane channels for transcellular osmotic water flow are intercalated into the luminal plasma membrane by an exocytotic mechanism controlled by vasopressin, and that the channels may correspond to the IMPs seen in freeze–fracture images. The idea that cytoplasmic tubular elements have a role in transport, especially in isotonically transporting epithelia, recalls the morphological findings of Møllgård & Rostgaard (1978) that a well-developed cytoplasmic tubule system (the TER previously mentioned) was present in such epithelia. It seems likely that the IMP-carrying tubules of toad bladder correspond to at least a component of the TER.

This last example neatly encapsulates a recurring theme in epithelial transport studies as a whole: description of morphological entities such as folded basolateral plasma membranes or the TER in transporting epithelia can encourage speculation on possible relationships to known physiological events, but coherent models of transport processes in morphologically complex system grow from holistic experimental approaches in which morphology provides a dimensional and topological map of carefully defined biochemical and biophysical mechanisms.

I am grateful to Stephen Ernst and Colin Sibley for many helpful discussions, to Stephen Norton and Karol Bauman for artwork and photography, and to Melanie Stock for typing. Experimental work in this laboratory was supported by the Wellcome Trust and the MRC.

REFERENCES

Betz, A. L., Firth, J. A. & Goldstein, G. W. (1980). Polarity of the blood–brain barrier: distribution of enzymes between the luminal and anti-luminal membranes of brain capillary endothelial cells. *Brain Research*, **192**, 17–28.

Chayen, J., Frost, G. T. B., Dodds, R. A., Bitensky, L., Pitchfork, J., Bayliss, P. H. & Barnett, R. J. (1981). The use of a hidden metal-capture reagent for the measurement of Na^+-K^+-ATPase activity: a new concept in cytochemistry. *Histochemistry*, **71**, 533–41.

Claude, P. & Goodenough, D. A. (1973). Fracture faces of zonulae occludentes from 'tight' and 'leaky' epithelia. *Journal of Cell Biology*, **58**, 390–400.

Coulton, G. R. & Firth, J. A. (1982). Modification by feeding regime of the intensity and distribution of cytochemically localized proton transport adenosine triphosphatase activity in mouse stomach. *Journal of Physiology*, **326**, 26–7P.

Diamond, J. M. (1978). Channels in epithelial cell membranes and junctions. *Federation Proceedings*, **37**, 2639–44.

Diamond, J. M. & Bossert, W. H. (1967). Standing gradient osmotic flow: a mechanism for coupling of water and solute transport in epithelia. *Journal of General Physiology*, **50**, 2061–83.

Diamond, J. M. & Bossert, W. H. (1968). Functional consequences of ultrastructural geometry in 'backwards' fluid-transporting epithelia. *Journal of Cell Biology*, **37**, 694–702.

DiBona, D. R., Schafer, J. A., Berglindh, T. A. & Sachs, G. (1981). The use of combined difference-contrast and fluorescence optics for analysis of epithelial transport. In *Epithelial Ion and Water Transport*, ed. A. D. C. MacKnight & J. P. Leader, pp. 1–7. New York: Raven Press.

Ellis, R. A., Goertemiller, C. C. & Stetson, D. L. (1977). Significance of extensive 'leaky' cell junctions in the avian salt gland. *Nature (London)*, **268**, 555–6.

Ernst, S. A. (1972a). Transport adenosine triphosphatase cytochemistry. Biochemical characterization of a cytochemical medium for the ultrastructural localization of ouabain-sensitive, potassium-dependent phosphatase activity in the avian salt gland. *Journal of Histochemistry and Cytochemistry*, **20**, 13–22.

Ernst, S. A. (1972b). Transport adenosine triphosphatase cytochemistry. II. Cytochemical localization of ouabain-sensitive, potassium-dependent phosphatase in the secretory epithelium of the avian salt gland. *Journal of Histochemistry and Cytochemistry*, **20**, 23–38.

Ernst, S. A. (1975). Transport ATPase cytochemistry: ultrastructural localization of potassium-dependent and potassium-independent phosphatase activities in rat kidney cortex. *Journal of Cell Biology*, **66**, 586–608.

Ernst, S. A. & Ellis, R. A. (1969). The development of surface specialization in the secretory epithelium of the avian salt gland in response to osmotic stress. *Journal of Cell Biology*, **40**, 305–21.

Ernst, S. A. & Hootman, S. R. (1981). Microscopical methods for the localization of Na^+,K^+-ATPase. *Histochemical Journal*, **13**, 397–418.

Ernst, S. A., Hootman, S. R., Schreiber, J. H. & Riddle, C. V. (1981). Freeze-fracture and morphometric analysis of occluding junctions in rectal glands of elasmobranch fish. *Journal of Membrane Biology*, **58**, 101–14.

Ernst, S. A. & Mills, J. W. (1977). Basolateral plasma membrane localization of ouabain-sensitive sodium transport sites in the secretory epithelium of the avian salt gland. *Journal of Cell Biology*, **75**, 74–94.

Ernst, S. A. & Mills, J. W. (1980). Autoradiographic localization of tritiated ouabain-sensitive sodium pump sites in ion transporting epithelia. *Journal of Histochemistry and Cytochemistry*, **28**, 72–7.

Ernst, S. A., Riddle, C. V. & Karnaky, K. J. (1980). Relationship between localization of Na^+,K^+-ATPase, cellular fine structure, and reabsorptive and secretory electrolyte transport. *Current Topics in Membranes and Transport*, **13**, 355–85.

Ernst, S. A. & Schreiber, J. H. (1981). Ultrastructural localization of Na^+,K^+-ATPase in rat and rabbit kidney medulla. *Journal of Cell Biology*, **91**, 803–13.

Firth, J. A. (1974). Problems of specificity in the use of a strontium capture technique for the cytochemical localization of ouabain-sensitive, potassium-dependent phosphatase in mammalian renal tubules. *Journal of Histochemistry and Cytochemistry*, **22**, 1163–8.

Firth, J. A. (1978). Cytochemical approaches to the localization of specific adenosine triphosphatases. *Histochemical Journal*, **10**, 253–69.

Firth, J. A., Farr, A. & Koppel, H. (1979). The localization and properties of membrane adenosine triphosphatases in the guinea-pig placenta. *Histochemistry*, **61**, 157–65.

Firth, J. A. & Stranks, G. J. (1981). Gastric proton pump localization: application of triphosphatase and monophosphatase techniques. *Journal of Histochemistry and Cytochemistry*, **29**, 344–50.

Fletcher, G. L., Stainer, I. M. & Holmes, W. N. (1967). Sequential changes in the adenosinetriphosphatase activity and the electrolyte excretory capacity of the nasal glands of the duck (*Anas platyrhynchos*) during the period of adaptation to hypertonic saline. *Journal of Experimental Biology*, **47**, 375–91.

Forte, J. G. & Lee, H. C. (1977). Gastric adenosine triphosphatases: a review of their possible role in HCl secretion. *Gastroenterology*, **73**, 921–6.

Forte, J. G., Machen, T. E. & Öbrink, K. J. (1980). Mechanisms of gastric H^+ and Cl^- transport. *Annual Review of Physiology*, **42**, 111–26.

Guth, L. & Albers, R. W. (1974). Histochemical demonstration of (Na^+-K^+)-activated adenosine triphosphatase. *Journal of Histochemistry and Cytochemistry*, **22**, 320–6.

Harmanci, M. C., Stern, P., Kachadorian, W. A., Valtin, H. & DiScala, V. A. (1980). Vasopressin and collecting duct intramembranous particle clusters: a dose–response relationship. *American Journal of Physiology*, **239**, F560–4.

Helander, H. F. & Hirschowicz, B. I. (1972). Quantitative ultrastructural studies on gastric parietal cells. *Gastroenterology*, **63**, 951–61.

Hootman, S. R. & Ernst, S. A. (1981). Effect of methacholine on Na^+ pump activity and ion content of dispersed avian salt gland cells. *American Journal of Physiology*, **214**, R77–86.

Ito, S. (1981). Functional gastric morphology. In *Physiology of the Gastrointestinal Tract*, ed. L. R. Johnson, pp. 517–50. New York: Raven Press.

Kachadorian, W. A., Wade, J. B., Uiterwyk, C. C. & DiScala, V. A. (1977). Membrane structural and functional responses to vasopressin in toad bladder. *Journal of Membrane Biology*, **30**, 381–401.

Koefoed-Johnsen, U. & Ussing, H. H. (1958). The nature of the frog skin potential. *Acta Physiologica Scandinavica*, **42**, 298–308.

Koenig, C. & Vial, J. D. (1970). A histochemical study of adenosine triphosphatase in the toad (*Bufo spinuolosus*) gastric mucosa. *Journal of Histochemistry and Cytochemistry*, **18**, 340–53.

Kyte, J. (1976). Immunoferritin determination of the distribution of $(Na^+ + K^+)$ ATPase over the plasma membranes of renal convoluted tubules. *Journal of Cell Biology*, **68**, 287–318.

Maetz, J. & Bornancin, M. (1975). Biochemical and biophysical aspects of salt secretion by chloride cells in teleosts. *Fortschritte der Zoologie*, **23**, 322–62.

Mayahara, H., Fujimoto, K., Ando, T. & Ogawa, K. (1981). A new one-step method for the ultracytochemical localisation of ouabain-sensitive potassium-dependent *p*-nitrophenyl phosphatase activity in rat kidney. *Histochemistry*, **67**, 125–38.

Mazurkiewicz, J. E., Hossler, F. E. & Barrnett, R. J. (1978). Cytochemical demonstration of sodium–potassium adenosine triphosphatase by a hemepeptide derivative of ouabain. *Journal of Histochemistry and Cytochemistry*, **26**, 1042–52.

Milhorat, T. H., Davis, D. A. & Hammock, M. K. (1975). Localization of ouabain-sensitive Na-K-ATPase in frog, rabbit and rat choroid plexus. *Brain Research*, **99**, 170–4.

Møllgård, K., Malinowska, D. H. & Saunders, N. R. (1976). Lack of correlation between tight junction morphology and permeability properties of developing choroid plexus. *Nature (London)*, **264**, 293–4.

Møllgård, K. & Rostgaard, J. (1978). Morphological aspects of some sodium transporting epithelia suggesting a transcellular pathway via elements of endoplasmic reticulum. *Journal of Membrane Biology*, **40**, 71–89.

Muller, J., Kachadorian, W. A. & DiScala, V. A. (1980). Evidence that ADH-stimulated intramembrane particle aggregates are transferred from cytoplasmic to luminal membranes in toad bladder epithelial cells. *Journal of Cell Biology*, **85**, 83–95.

Proverbio, F., Condrescu-Guidi, M. & Whittembury, G. (1975). Ouabain-insensitive Na$^+$ stimulation of an Mg^{2+}-dependent ATPase in kidney tissue. *Biochimica et Biophysica Acta*, **394**, 281–92.

Quinton, P. M. & Tormey, J. M. (1976). Localisation of Na/K-ATPase sites in the secretory and reabsorptive epithelia of perfused eccrine sweat glands: a question to the role of the enzyme in secretion. *Journal of Membrane Biology*, **29**, 383–99.

Quinton, P. M., Wright, E. M. & Tormey, J. M. (1973). Localization of sodium pumps in the choroid plexus epithelium. *Journal of Cell Biology*, **58**, 724–30.

Rubin, W. & Aliasgharpour, A. A. (1976). Demonstration of a cytochemical difference between the tubulovesicles and plasmalemma of gastric parietal cells by ATPase and NPPase reactions. *Anatomical Record*, **184**, 251–64.

Sachs, G. & Berglindh, T. (1981). Physiology of the parietal cell. In *Physiology of the Gastrointestinal Tract*, ed. L. R. Johnson, pp. 567–602. New York: Raven Press.

Sibley, C. P., Bauman, K. F. & Firth, J. A. (1982). Permeability of the foetal capillary endothelium of the guinea-pig placenta to haem proteins of various molecular sizes. *Cell and Tissue Research*, **223**, 165–78.

Silva, P., Stoff, J., Field, M., Fine, L., Forrest, J. N. & Epstein, F. H. (1977). Mechanism of active chloride secretion by shark rectal gland: role of Na–K-ATPase in chloride transport. *American Journal of Physiology*, **233**, F298–306.

Spicer, S. S., Stoward, P. J. & Tashian, R. E. (1979). The immunohisto-localization of carbonic anhydrase in rodent tissues. *Journal of Histochemistry and Cytochemistry*, **27**, 820–31.

Spring, K. R. & Hope, A. (1979). Dimensions of cells and lateral intercellular spaces in living *Necturus* gallbladder. *Federation Proceedings*, **38**, 128–33.

Stirling, C. E. (1972). Radioautographic localization of sodium pump sites in rabbit intestine. *Journal of Cell Biology*, **53**, 704–14.

Sugai, N. & Ito, S. (1980). Carbonic anhydrase: ultrastructural localization in the mouse gastric mucosa and improvements in the technique. *Journal of Histochemistry and Cytochemistry*, **28**, 511–25.

Thoenes, W. & Langer, K. H. (1969). Relationship between cell structures of renal tubules and transport mechanisms. In *Renal Transport and Diuretics*, ed. K. Thurau & Jahrmarker, pp. 37–65. Berlin: Springer-Verlag.

Van Rossum, G. D. V. & Ernst, S. A. (1978). Effects of ethacrynic acid on ion transport and energy metabolism in slices of avian salt gland and of mammalian liver and kidney cortex. *Journal of Membrane Biology*, **43**, 251–75.

Wachstein, M. & Meisel, E. (1957). Histochemistry of hepatic phosphatase at a physiologic pH. With special reference to the demonstration of bile canaliculi. *American Journal of Clinical Pathology*, **27**, 13–23.

Wood, J. G., Jean, D. H., Whitaker, J. N., McLaughlin, B. J. & Albers, R. W. (1977). Immunocytochemical localization of sodium, potassium activated ATPase in knifefish brain. *Journal of Neurocytology*, **6**, 571–81.

3   The generation of cellular differences in the pre-implantation mouse embryo

W. J. D. REEVE

*Department of Anatomy, University of Cambridge, Downing Street,
Cambridge CB2 3DY, UK*

INTRODUCTION

Many scientists have attempted to categorise all embryos as being either 'mosaic' or 'regulative'. Eggs were considered to be mosaic where cell fate was specified according to the inheritance of different regions of the egg cytoplasm. Cell divisions caused a parcelling out of localised morphogenetic determinants, so that cells were destined to follow definite, inevitable lineages to particular, different prospective fates. In other types of embryo, such a rigid lineage relationship was thought to be absent, and, in these 'regulative' embryos, cellular fate was assumed to be governed by factors that operated after the cleavage of the egg. Many analyses have shown the naivety of this approach to classification. Wilson (1925) demonstrated that a regulative ability and the inheritance of morphogenetic determinants were not mutually exclusive, and it is now realised that cell lineages exist in almost all species, but that cellular interaction is also essential to subsequent development. A variable ability to regulate is superimposed upon the operation of lineage inheritance (Davidson, 1976; Graham & Wareing, 1976).

Those embryos that were considered to show mosaic development have a pattern of cytoplasmic localisations of morphogenetic determinants that is both dominant within the egg, and relatively fixed. For instance, in the extreme form of mosaic development shown by annelid and nematode embryos, the lineages operate so precisely that particular cells can be assigned to specific fates, which are often only realised several rounds of cell division later. In contrast, in regulative embryos such as those of the sea urchin and frog, the normal fate of any cell is less than its potential and is determined by the relative position of cells in the embryo. Morphogenetic determinants are present within these embryos, but their action can usually be over-ridden, enabling regulation after interference with the developing embryo.

The early pre-implantation mammalian embryo has been considered to be unique in its apparent lack of localised cytoplasmic determinants (Davidson, 1976). There are two possible reasons for the failure to detect the operation of a mosaic mechanism within the differentiating mammalian embryo: either this embryo does indeed differ from those of other multicellular organisms, or, alternatively, it shows a covert form of inheritance that is so labile as to be readily over-ridden during experimental manipulation. Thus, a lineage inheritance may exist but be dominated by a regulative ability. In this review I intend to discuss recent evidence that supports this second possibility, and therefore indicates that the differentiation of the mammalian embryo may conform to the patterns of development of other embryos.

DIFFERENTIATION IN THE PRE-IMPLANTATION MAMMALIAN EMBRYO

From the egg to the blastocyst

The development of the pre-implantation mouse embryo involves cellular proliferation, the generation of subpopulations of cells and the establishment of different lineages. After fertilisation, a series of approximately synchronous cell divisions generates an embryo of eight blastomeres. All the blastomeres have a similar spherical appearance and specialised intercellular junctions are absent. However, during the 8-cell stage, there are dramatic changes in the overall morphology of the embryo and in the structure of individual blastomeres. The 8-cell morula undergoes the process of 'compaction', in which an increase in intercellular apposition causes the intercellular spaces to become reduced and individual cells to lose their former spherical shape such that they become no longer easily identifiable (Lewis & Wright, 1935; Ducibella & Anderson, 1975). With the subsequent round of cell division, some cells become surrounded completely by their neighbours. Later those cells located in an internal position are thought to differentiate as the inner cell mass (ICM), whereas those located externally are thought to follow a different differentiative path, developing eventually into the trophectoderm of the blastocyst. At $3\frac{1}{2}$ days post-fertilisation, the 64-cell blastocyst consists of a monolayer of trophectodermal cells surrounding a fluid-filled cavity (the blastocoel) which, at one end, contains a cluster of cells, the ICM.

It is now accepted widely that cells in the expanded blastocyst are committed to either the trophectodermal or ICM lineages, and therefore have restricted developmental potentials. The results of microsurgical manipulations have demonstrated that cells in the trophectoderm develop to form the giant cells and chorionic ectoderm, whereas those in the ICM are destined to form the embryo proper and all extra-embryonic mesoderm and endoderm (Rossant & Papaioannou, 1977). Furthermore, the ICM and trophectodermal tissues show biochemical, structural, physiological and behavioural differences (Johnson, Handyside & Braude, 1977). Cells of the trophectoderm are phagocytic, secrete fluid, transport ions and macromolecules and stimulate a decidual response; cells of the ICM have more adherent surfaces and show greater sensitivity to cytotoxic drugs and high temperature. The cells of the two tissues have distinctive antigens and enzymes. In fact, differences can be detected between the supposed precursors of ICM and trophectoderm, the inside and outside cells respectively of the morula, as regards their thymidine labelling indices, sensitivities to radiation and polypeptides synthesised.

A crucial problem in mammalian development concerns the generation of different types of cells. How do differences arise between these inside and outside cells, and what causes the differentiation of the first two tissues, ICM and trophectoderm?

How do the two cell populations of the blastocyst arise?

The notion that ICM and trophectoderm may inherit different cytoplasmic determinants from the egg is old but the evidence remains poor (Dalcq, 1957). It was claimed that a cytoplasmic asymmetry could be identified in the unfertilised egg of the rat and mouse: the denser, dorsal cytoplasm was richer in ribonucleoproteins; the ventral cytoplasm appeared more vacuolated, and contained higher levels of mucopolysaccharides, acetalphosphatides and acid phosphatases. It was further suggested that this unequal distribution in the egg, followed by cleavage, could generate differences in the content of cells. Although the orientation of the first cleavage division could not be related consistently to the axis of polarity within the fertilised egg, it did relate to the cleavage planes of the second and third divisions. At the 8-cell stage, so it was claimed, four larger blastomeres contained predominantly the vacuolated cytoplasm, whereas the four smaller cells were rich in ribonucleoproteins. These larger cells spread over and enveloped the smaller cells, after which the two groups became increasingly divergent, representing presumably the ICM and trophectodermal lineages. Unfortunately, subsequent studies have failed to detect cellular differences in the 8-cell embryo, and there is no support for Dalcq's observations on cellular behaviour at this stage. Moreover, even the asymmetries described by Dalcq have not been confirmed (Solter, Damjanov & Skreb, 1973), and those asymmetries in the fertilised egg that have been identified have not been demonstrated to be critical to subsequent development (Johnson, 1979, 1981).

An alternative basis for the early differentiative events in the mammalian embryo was suggested by studies of the development of the rabbit embryo and its isolated cells. It was proposed that the egg contains an organising centre, the presence of part of which is needed for isolated cells from the 4-cell embryo to form normal blastocysts (Seidel, 1960). However, the results of similar experiments with isolated cells of the mouse embryo could not be explained on this basis. An unequal segregation of factors from the egg ought to cause a progressive segregation of the potentials for forming either ICM or trophectoderm in the isolated blastomeres of later developmental stages. However, the incidence of trophectodermal-like vesicles formed from cells isolated from 4-cell embryos was increased compared with that observed from blastomeres isolated from 2-cell embryos. This observation, together with the fact that the timing of 'cavitation' did not appear to be affected by the disaggregation of an embryo into single cells, and appeared therefore to be intrinsic to each cell, led Tarkowski & Wroblewska (1967) to propose an epigenetic, inside–outside hypothesis. It was argued that the differentiative decision depended on the response to relative position of cells in the morula. The different micro-environments were regarded as being critical in causing inside cells to form the ICM, whereas cells exposed to outside conditions formed the trophectoderm. The increased proportion of trophoblastic vesicles derived from cells isolated from later developmental stages arises from these embryos having a lower cell number, and hence no enclosed cells, at the time of commitment.

There is now much evidence to support a relationship between cellular position within the compacted mouse morula and the differentiation of the ICM and trophectodermal lineages of the blastocyst (Herbert & Graham, 1974). The evidence includes approaches in which subpopulations of cells are identified within the embryo. One approach has been to inject a marker, commonly an oil droplet, into cells of the morula and cleavage-stage embryos. The location of the oil droplet in the blastocyst that developed depended on the site of earlier intracellular injection. The central cytoplasm of 2- and 4-cell stages appeared in both the inside and the outside cells of the later blastocyst, whereas the peripheral cytoplasm was later detected only in the trophectoderm. In a second approach, chimaeras were formed from embryos that differed either in their electrophoretic variant isomers of glucose phosphate isomerase or in whether or not they had been labelled previously with radioactive thymidine (McLaren, 1976). Cleavage-stage embryos were aggregated to form chimaeras in which the cells of one type of embryo were placed primarily in an inside position, and those of another type were on the outside of the aggregate. Despite minimal mixing of blastomeres, regulation in subsequent development results in the cellular aggregate forming a single blastocyst that can be examined for the location of the marked cell(s). Embryos placed in an inside position contributed disproportionately to the ICM, whereas those positioned externally tended to develop to trophectoderm.

It has also been possible to disaggregate labelled and unlabelled embryos into single cells, and reaggregate the blastomeres so that the position of the labelled cells within the aggregate can be varied. An inside position in the aggregate favoured the formation of the ICM and its derivatives, whereas an outside position led to trophectodermal derivatives (Hillman, Sherman & Graham, 1972). The experiments in which the position of a labelled blastomere was varied within an aggregate of unlabelled cells were extended by Kelly (1975, 1977), who surrounded single blastomeres from either the 4-cell (1/4 cells) or 8-cell (1/8 cells) embryo with six or four genetically distinct 'carrier' 1/8 cells, respectively. These chimaeras were cultured *in vitro*, transferred to the uteri of pseudopregnant females, and examined later (using glucose phosphate isomerase and coat colour markers) for the contributions made by the two types of blastomeres to particular tissues in the foetus and young animal. For one particular embryo, the fate of each of the four 1/4 blastomeres – in combination with 'carrier' blastomeres – was traced, and each made a substantial contribution to embryonic tissues. Further evidence against a rigid segregation of cytoplasmic determinants during cleavage, leading to a restricted developmental potential, was provided by the octet pair experiments in which each of two sibling 1/8 cells was surrounded by four 1/8 cells. The totipotentiality of both cells of an octet pair argues against a segregation at division of the 1/4 cell to two 1/8 cells (2/8 couplet), and in favour of the generation of the ICM and trophectoderm at some time after compaction.

The differentiation of the blastocyst

The evidence presented above makes it seem likely that some feature of cellular position within the compacted mouse morula is critical for the differentiation of the ICM and trophectoderm, but the mechanism by which position is translated to fate has been unclear. It was proposed that the event of compaction may have a role in defining the conditions whereby cells detect their relative position (Ducibella & Anderson, 1975; Ducibella, 1977). At compaction, the cells of the 8-cell embryo develop gap and focal tight junctions, and in the late morula these apical tight junctions form the zonula occludens. This impermeable barrier prevents the access, for instance, of both immunoglobulin and lanthanum tracer to the inside cells, and allows the generation and maintenance of the blastocoelic cavity. Interpretations of the inside–outside hypothesis have stressed the differences between the inside and outside micro-environments, and their dependence on the existence of the zonula occludens (Graham, 1971; Ducibella & Anderson, 1975); nevertheless, the permeability seal is imperfect in the early morula since the zonula occludens is established only at the later 32-cell stage, and access by antibody is reduced only when the blastocoel has formed. Moreover, there is evidence that the inside micro-environment alone is not crucial to the generation of an ICM.

It has been possible to prevent compaction, and thereby demonstrate that a period of prolonged compaction is not essential to the morphogenesis of the blastocyst. For instance, the Fab fragment of an anti-teratocarcinoma (F9) antiserum prevented compaction in 2-cell embryos cultured for 50 hours to form grape-like structures of 30 or more cells. After washing away the antibody and reimplantation into foster mothers, these embryos produced live offspring (Kemler *et al.*, 1977). A whole anti-F9 antiserum was shown subsequently to inhibit compaction (Ducibella, 1980).

The culture of mouse embryos in a rabbit antiserum raised against the embryonal carcinoma cell line LS5770 also prevented compaction (Johnson *et al.*, 1979). If the embryos were removed from the antiserum and allowed to compact before they had passed beyond the 32-cell stage, normal blastocysts developed. With more prolonged decompaction, the embryos accumulated fluid intracellularly but did not compact when restored to control medium. The antibody therefore prevents compaction but allows cell interaction, cell division and fluid accumulation. Although compaction is a prerequisite for the formation of the zonula occludens and the blastocoelic cavity (Ducibella *et al.*, 1975), this period of increased cellular apposition can be delayed for up to 18–20 hours without preventing the morphogenesis of the overt ICM and trophectoderm of the blastocyst (Johnson *et al.*, 1979). Thus, prolonged compaction does not appear to be essential to the differentiation of these two lineages.

Perhaps the most cogent argument against the critical requirement of a specialised internal micro-environment for the differentiation of these two tissues has arisen from experiments in which a morula has been injected into the blastocoel of a giant blastocyst (Pedersen & Spindle, 1980). Several morulae were aggregated and allowed subsequently to form a large blastocyst. A zona-enclosed 8-cell embryo was then injected into the blastocoel, and itself developed to form a typical blastocyst. The totipotential cells of the 8-cell embryo were not induced to form ICM alone, as might be expected if the internal micro-environment were responsible for providing the cues for the generation of the ICM. However, the fate of the injected morula differed if its zona pellucida had been removed previously. Blastomeres of the morula could then make contact with cells lining the blastocoel and the injected morula developed to form a cluster of cells rather than a blastocyst. This result suggests that cell fate is governed critically by cellular interactions rather than by a distinct inside micro-environment.

The acceptance of an inside–outside hypothesis need not, of course, necessarily imply the existence of distinct inside and outside micro-environments. Nonetheless, variants of the hypothesis that relate position in the morula to the differentiative response, without implicating the zonula occludens, have seldom been considered seriously (Johnson, 1979). There are, however, other differences between inside and outside cells, apart from their respective micro-environments. First, the two cell types differ in the proportions of their plasma membranes that are apposed with those of other cells; the surfaces of inside cells are completely apposed with those of other cells, whereas an outside cell has a region of exposed membrane. Second, presumptive ICM and trophectodermal cells might be distinguished by inherited differences in the localisation of newly inserted membrane (Izquierdo, 1977), or by the quality and distribution of their intercellular junctions. At compaction, focal tight and gap junctions form between cells (Ducibella & Anderson, 1975; Magnuson, Demsey & Stackpole, 1977). Prior to this stage, only sister blastomeres of a mitotic cleavage show any exchange of cytoplasmic molecules, owing to the connection of a mid-body or strand of cytoplasm that is the residuum of the previous mitotic division. However, the development of gap junctions at the 8-cell stage results in all cells becoming both ionically- and dye-coupled (Lo, 1980). Later, other junctions develop and the trophectodermal cells of the blastocyst are connected by gap junctions, desmosomes and tight junctions. However, ICM cells possess only gap junctions, except at their areas of contact with trophectodermal cells where desmosomes and focal tight junctions can also be identified (Ducibella *et al.*, 1975; Magnuson *et al.*, 1977).

There is at present no clear evidence as to the way in which cells detect inside or outside position. However, in the absence of evidence for an alternative differentiative mechanism, involving presumably the unequal inheritance of morphogenetic determinants, much speculation has focussed on the nature of the different cues given to cells in different relative positions. Although the inside–outside hypothesis has usually been interpreted from a micro-environmental standpoint, the identification of the cues perceived by cells in the distinct inside and outside micro-environments is still awaited.

Meanwhile, recent observations have revealed polarised features in the individual blastomeres of the 8-cell embryo, and have defined criteria for identifying two distinct cell types in the early 16-cell embryo (Handyside, 1980, 1981). Individual 1/8 blastomeres have been shown to possess structural elements, which might be inherited at division to the 16-cell stage, and the role of which may possibly be analogous to those of the putative cytoplasmic morphogenetic determinants of other embryos. These observations have been incorporated into the polarisation hypothesis (Johnson, Pratt & Handyside, 1981; Johnson et al., 1983) which represents a significant challenge to the notions of control over differentiation in the pre-implantation mouse embryo that have prevailed for several years.

POLARISATION AT THE 8-CELL STAGE
Surface features of polarity

Prior to compaction, the individual blastomeres of 2-, 4- and 8-cell embryos bind fluorescent lectins and antibodies uniformly over their entire surface. However, during the 8-cell stage, a pole of ligand-binding sites becomes restricted to the apical, normally outward-facing surface of each blastomere (Handyside, 1980). This pattern of labelling has a different basis to that of the observed 'capping' or redistribution of membrane components induced in other cell types by the binding of multivalent ligands; it may be revealed by labelling in the presence of metabolic inhibitors, such as sodium azide, or by labelling with several different mono- and multivalent ligands, regardless of fixation of the cells with 4% paraformaldehyde either before or after labelling. These treatments inhibit the capping of receptors on other cell types, but do not prevent the increased ligand binding in the polar regions of the blastomeres. These poles of ligand binding can be explained purely in terms of an increased surface area of membrane due to microvilli in this region (Calarco & Epstein, 1973; Ducibella et al., 1977; Reeve & Ziomek, 1981). Thus, whereas the individual blastomeres of 4- and early 8-cell embryos have a uniform distribution of microvilli (Fig. 3.1), cells from decompacted 8-cell embryos reveal an outward-facing pole of ligand binding that appears to correspond with a similar pole of microvilli (Figs. 3.2 and 3.3).

The examination of blastomeres isolated from pre-, peri- and post-compact 8-cell embryos has suggested a progressive reduction during the 8-cell stage in the size of the polar area of intense fluorescent labelling on each blastomere. Cells isolated from early 8-cell embryos tend to label uniformly and have a uniformly sparse covering of microvilli (Fig. 3.4a), whereas those from compact embryos usually reveal tight poles both of fluorescent-ligand binding sites and of microvilli (Fig. 3.4b).

The induction of this polarised surface phenotype appears to be independent of the cell flattening occurring at compaction. Thus, polarisation not only precedes overt cell flattening, but also occurs under conditions in which cell flattening is prevented by agents such as low calcium, anti-embryonal carcinoma antibody, concanavalin A and cytochalasin D (Pratt et al., 1982). Mere cellular contact for more than 2 hours

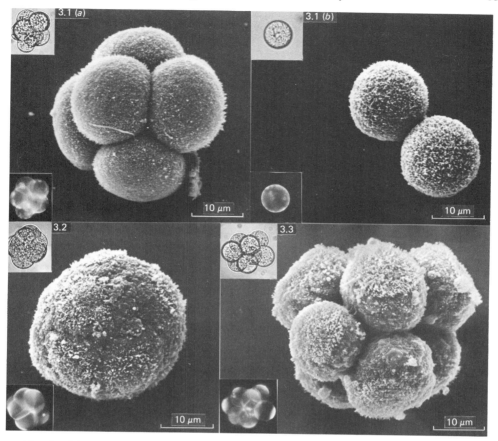

Figs. 3.1–3.3. Each figure includes a fluorescence photomicrograph with a bright-field comparison and a SEM photomicrograph.

3.1.(*a*) A newly formed 8-cell embryo and (*b*) its dissociated cells label uniformly with fluorescent ligand, and have a uniform distribution of microvilli over their entire surface.

3.2. The exposed surface of a compacted 8-cell embryo binds fluorescent ligand and appears microvillous, but with non-microvillous areas adjacent to regions of intercellular apposition.

3.3. Each blastomere of a decompacted 8-cell embryo has an area of intense fluorescent-ligand binding that coincides with a microvillous pole on the normally exposed surface of the embryo. Note that fluorescent poles on some cells are outside the focal plane.

appears sufficient to induce a blastomere from an 8-cell embryo to polarise. Moreover, it is the asymmetry of the contact that determines the axis of polarity, and causes the microvillous pole of a blastomere to develop opposite to the sites of intercellular contact.

Pairs of 8-cell blastomeres are connected generally by the mid-body that remains from the previous mitotic division. When these blastomeres are separated soon after their formation, with their relative positions altered such that the mid-bodies of both blastomeres are directed away from the site of intercellular contact, the microvillous poles are generated subsequently in the areas of the mid-bodies (Ziomek & Johnson, 1980; Fig. 3.5). Despite rotating each blastomere through 180°, the positions at which the microvillous poles developed relative to the region of intercellular contact were unchanged; the cue of intercellular contact, rather than the preformation of specific membrane components, seems to dictate the axis of polarity. Furthermore, in an

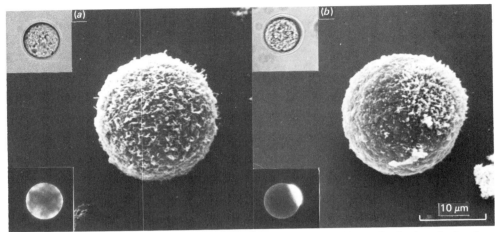

Fig. 3.4. (a) Dissociated cells of early 8-cell embryos have uniform distributions both of fluorescent-ligand binding sites and of microvilli. (b) Blastomeres isolated from late compacted 8-cell embryos have polarised patterns of labelling with fluorescent ligand and microvilli concentrated at one pole of the cell.

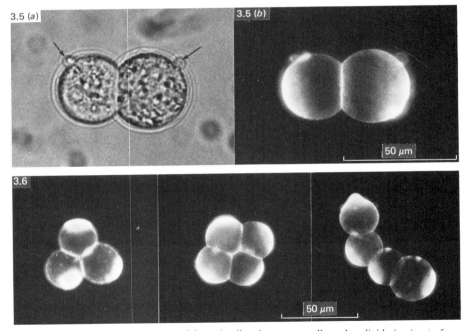

Figs. 3.5 and 3.6. Blastomeres isolated from 4-cell embryos were allowed to divide *in vitro* to form couplets of 8-cell blastomeres. After separation of the two blastomeres of each couplet, it was often possible to identify on each blastomere the remnants of the midbody.

3.5(a) When the blastomeres were rotated through 180° and reaggregated, these remnants (arrowed) faced outwards. (b) After a few hours, the pole of ligand-binding sites in each blastomere developed opposite the point of intercellular contact.

3.6. Blastomeres were isolated from early 8-cell embryos and reaggregated. The fluorescent-labelled pole of each blastomere developed in the position most distant from the overall sum of the intercellular contacts.

aggregate of blastomeres, the position of the pole in each 1/8 blastomere is governed by the combined cueing influence of the surrounding blastomeres, such that the microvillous poles that develop are directed outwards from the cluster of cells (Fig. 3.6.).

It has further been demonstrated that the induction of polarity shows specificity (Johnson & Ziomek, 1981*a*). A newly formed 1/8 cell that is aggregated with a companion blastomere from 2-, 4-, 8- or 16-cell stages develops a microvillous pole opposite to the point of intercellular contact. However, this ability to induce polarity declines with blastomeres from 4- and 2-cell embryos and is not significant with fertilised or unfertilised eggs. The capacity to induce polarity seems therefore to develop during the 2-cell stage, and may be a consequence of the first major transcription of embryonic genes. The induction of polarity appears to depend on neither cell flattening nor the presence of specialised intercellular junctions since blastomeres isolated from 2- and 4-cell embryos can induce polarity, despite the absence of communication via specialised gap and tight junctions (Goodall & Johnson, 1982).

The polarised surface phenotype is stable. Moreover, once the initial intercellular contact of at least 2 hours has established the position of subsequent pole formation, that axis of polarity cannot be altered. Two points have so far emerged concerning the response of the polarising blastomere. First, polarisation is more rapid in smaller than in larger blastomeres. Second, considerable reorganisation of the surface phenotype occurs in the presence of cytochalasin D or Colcemid, suggesting that microtubules and cytochalasin-D-sensitive microfilaments are not involved in the fundamental stages of the polarisation (Pratt *et al.*, 1982).

Cytoplasmic features of polarity

The histochemical staining of the cytoplasmic distributions of ingested horseradish peroxidase (HRP) has revealed a polarised organisation within individual blastomeres of the 8-cell embryo (Reeve, 1981*a*). HRP has proved a useful tracer in studies of endocytosis, but, in previous published data on pre-implantation embryos, HRP pulses were short and provided information mostly on uptake patterns at the cell surface.

The 4-cell and early 8-cell mouse embryos show a low level of ingestion of HRP and, even after prolonged pulses of at least 3 hours, the enzyme appears confined largely to the cytocortex (Fig. 3.7). However, endocytosis increases during development and, in each blastomere of the later compact 8-cell stage, the ingested enzyme becomes localised to a region of the cytoplasm underlying the apical pole of microvilli (Figs 3.8 and 3.9). Thus, the cytoplasmic polarity occurs on an axis identical to that of the polarised surface phenotype. Moreover, isolated cells show the same polarised cytoplasmic distribution of ingested vesicles. Cell flattening is not related causally to the distribution of HRP since similar patterns of staining were shown by blastomeres that were isolated from intact embryos before their culture in HRP and by cells derived from intact embryos that had been cultured in HRP. The restricted localisation of HRP-containing vesicles is shown by most blastomeres of compact 8-cell embryos and its occurrence in the cells of a minority of precompact 8-cell embryos is consistent with the generation of cytoplasmic polarity before overt cell flattening. There is no obvious ultrastructural basis for the restricted localisation of HRP, but in other cell types the location of the reaction product is thought to coincide with the Golgi apparatus.

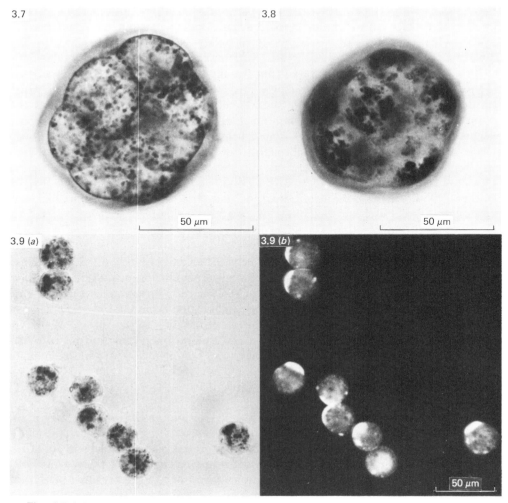

Figs. 3.7–3.9. The precompact 8-cell embryo (3.7) has a dispersed distribution of ingested HRP. The compact 8-cell embryo (3.8) shows the restricted cytoplasmic localisation of HRP peripheral to the nucleus of each cell.

Isolated blastomeres of a compact 8-cell embryo, stained (3.9*a*) for the distribution of ingested HRP and (3.9*b*) with fluorescent ligand, before embryo disaggregation. Each pole of fluorescent-ligand binding overlies a restricted cytoplasmic localisation of stain.

Nuclear features of polarity

Fluorescent labelling with 4',6-diamidino-2-phenylindole (DAPI) and Hoechst 33258 identifies the nuclei within blastomeres (Reeve & Kelly, 1983). A photographic superimposition technique enables an accurate assessment of nuclear distribution both in intact embryos and in isolated blastomeres. The fluorescence photomicrograph of the nucleus may be superimposed on a bright-field photomicrograph of exactly the same area, but of reduced density, thereby revealing both the nucleus and the outline of the cell.

During the period of compaction, the nuclei migrate towards the bases of individual cells of the 8-cell embryo. The nuclei of precompact 8-cell embryos were located in a peripheral position (Fig. 3.10*a*), whereas compact 8-cell embryos had nuclei more clustered to the centre of the embryo. This difference in nuclear clustering was independent of the cellular shape changes associated with compaction since it was also apparent after decompaction following exposure of precompact and compact embryos to calcium-depleted medium (Fig. 3.10*b*). Furthermore, the majority of blastomeres isolated from these embryos retained a basal nucleus located away from the apical pole of microvilli (Fig. 3.11). The migration of the nuclei to the bases of blastomeres was also demonstrated in couplets of 8-cell blastomeres examined after their formation by the division *in vitro* of cells isolated from 4-cell embryos. At increased times after cell division, the nuclei appeared closer to each other and to the region of intercellular contact (Fig. 3.12).

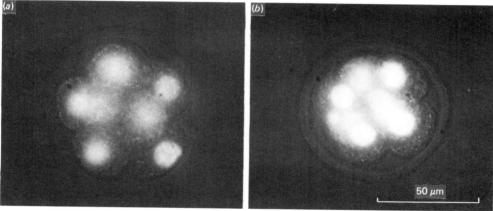

Fig. 3.10. (*a*) A precompact 8-cell embryo fixed and then stained with Hoechst 33258 has its nuclei located peripherally. (*b*) A decompacted late 8-cell embryo fixed and then stained with Hoechst 33258. The nuclei are clustered at the centre of the embryo.

It has been demonstrated by the pattern of surface-labelling with fluorescent ligand, the distribution of microvilli, the restricted localisation of HRP and the basal nuclear position that each blastomere of the 8-cell embryo becomes polarised axially, and that the embryo acquires a radial polarity. Does this polarity have significance for subsequent development?

THE 16-CELL EMBRYO: THE FIRST APPEARANCE OF INSIDE–OUTSIDE
DIFFERENCES

Surface features

The mouse 16-cell morula contains an inside and an outside population of cells. Previously, it had been estimated from serial reconstruction of sectioned material that there were rarely more than two inside cells at this stage (Barlow, Owen & Graham, 1972; Herbert & Graham, 1974). However, it has since been suggested that this number may be artefactually low due to shrinkage during fixation and sectioning procedures (Handyside, 1981). In a different approach, intact embryos were labelled with fluorescent ligand to mark their external surface, and then disaggregated to single cells. When all blastomeres of individual 16-cell embryos were examined, embryos contained on average ten cells that showed fluorescent labelling over part of their surface and six cells that were unlabelled. These unlabelled cells were interpreted as

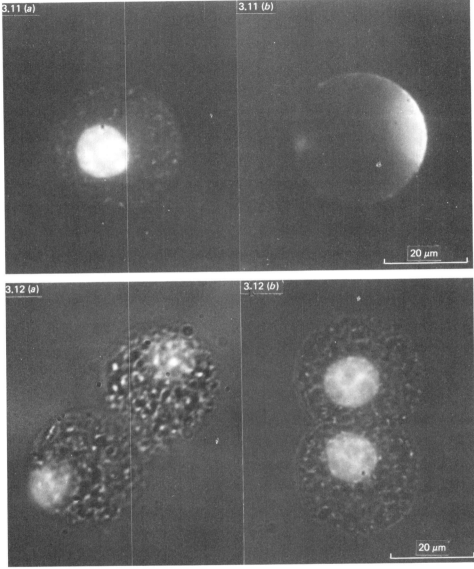

Figs. 3.11 and 3.12. An isolated 8-cell blastomere was surface-labelled with fluorescent ligand, and fixed before labelling of the nucleus with Hoechst 33258.

3.11(a) The fluorescent image of the nucleus was superimposed on a brief bright-field exposure of the cell. (b) Usually, the pole of ligand binding was located away from the nucleus. Couplets of 8-cell blastomeres formed by the division *in vitro* of cells isolated from 4-cell embryos were fixed and labelled with Hoechst 33258.

3.12(a) In newly formed couplets, the nuclei tend to be displaced maximally from the point of contact between the two blastomeres. (b) In late couplets (8–9 hours), the nuclei are closer than in early couplets.

being inside cells to which the antibodies in the labelling were denied access. In a subsequent experiment, 16-cell embryos were disaggregated to single cells that were then labelled with fluorescent ligand. Two populations of blastomeres were again identified: most cells showed intense binding of ligand over a small region of the cell surface; others were labelled uniformly. Later, these two procedures were combined

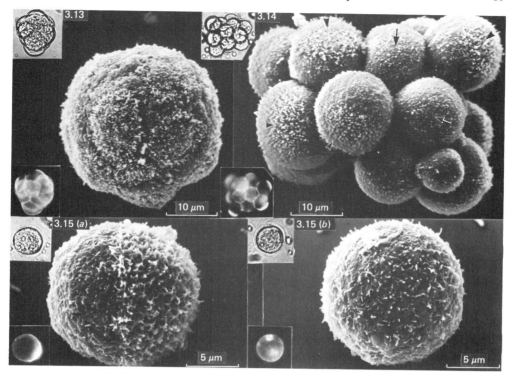

Figs. 3.13–3.15. Each figure includes a fluorescence photomicrograph with a bright-field comparison and a SEM photomicrograph.

3.13. A 16-cell embryo shows a uniform binding of fluorescent ligand over its surface, which is predominantly microvillous.

3.14. The outermost cells of a decompacted 16-cell embryo have apical regions of increased binding of fluorescent ligand, which correspond to poles of microvilli (▲) on the normally exposed surface. Cells with a uniform covering of sparse microvilli (▲) tend to be more internal.

3.15. Dissociated cells of 16-cell embryos show either (*a*) polarised distributions both of fluorescent-ligand binding and of microvilli or (*b*) uniform binding of fluorescent ligand and an overall population of sparse microvilli.

in a double-labelling experiment in which intact embryos were labelled to mark the outer aspects of cells, and then disaggregated to single cells that were labelled with a ligand conjugated to a different fluorochrome. The second fluorescent ligand labelled inside cells uniformly, whereas the outside cells had a concentration of ligand-binding sites in the region of cell surface that originally represented the external surface of the embryo. Use of these immunolabelling techniques has led to estimates of six to eight inside cells in 93% of 16-cell embryos (Handyside, 1981; Johnson, 1981; Johnson & Ziomek, 1981*b*).

The compact 16-cell embryo has a uniform covering of microvilli (Fig. 3.13), but following decompaction in calcium-depleted medium, both apolar and polar blastomeres (1/16 cells) can be identified (Fig. 3.14). In fact, the outside cells have microvillous poles, whereas inside cells have a uniform distribution of microvilli (Fig. 3.15).

At the compacted 8-cell stage no cells occupy an inside position and, after disaggregation, each blastomere has a pole of increased ligand binding. When these isolated 1/8 cells were allowed to divide *in vitro*, they each formed a pair of cells (2/16 couplet) in which the two blastomeres usually had different phenotypes (Johnson &

Ziomek, 1981*b*). After labelling with ligand, most couplets consisted of a larger cell that showed polar labelling and a smaller cell that labelled uniformly. These couplets appeared similar to the pairs of cells that remained attached when intact 16-cell embryos were disaggregated. Furthermore, the incidence of these polar and apolar patterns of labelling did not differ significantly for cells from intact 16-cell embryos and those isolated from couplets generated *in vitro*. In addition to their different patterns of labelling, these polar and apolar cells have also been demonstrated to show different properties (Ziomek & Johnson, 1981). Pairs of apolar cells are adhesive and aggregate faster than do pairs of polar cells. Furthermore, in most 2/16 couplets the polar cell eventually engulfs the apolar cell. This phenomenon does not occur when pairs of polar or apolar cells are aggregated, suggesting that it depends on the differences in properties of the two cell types. Thus, at the 16-cell stage, not only do differences in surface phenotype arise from the moment that the cells are formed, but behavioural differences are also detectable without the cells having occupied different positions within the intact embryo.

Cytoplasmic features

The patterns of distribution of ingested HRP, unlike the polar and apolar distributions of microvilli, are not diagnostic for the inside, apolar and outside, polar cell subpopulations in the 16-cell embryo, both of which show a range of patterns of HRP distribution (Reeve, 1981*b*). However, polar blastomeres did show a greater incidence than did apolar cells of HRP restricted to a single large aggregate in the cytoplasm. Furthermore, the restricted localisation of HRP always occurred on the same axis as, and underlay, the microvillous pole in each polar 1/16 cell (Fig. 3.16).

The differences in patterns of staining between polar and apolar 1/16 cells were evident in natural couplets formed in the embryo *in situ* and in 2/16 couplets generated *in vitro*. When examined soon after their formation, the two cells of a 2/16 couplet generated *in vitro* could have different cytoplasmic distributions of ingested HRP. Moreover, these differences occurred whether the 1/8 blastomere divided in HRP, or after restoration to control medium following culture in HRP for several hours. Thus, it is unlikely that the difference in distributions of HRP between the two cells of a couplet depends on a difference between blastomeres in microvillous distributions, which could be associated with a difference in rates of endocytosis. Instead, the data are consistent with the sister blastomeres of a mitotic division, from the 8-cell to the 16-cell stage, inheriting different cytoplasmic features.

Nuclear position may affect the generation of the two cell types

There is much evidence to support the notion that the apical half of each 1/8 cell contributes to an outer, polar 1/16 cell, whereas the basal half forms an inner, apolar 1/16 cell. First, 16-cell embryos tend to disaggregate into pairs of attached cells, each consisting of one polar and one apolar cell (Handyside, 1980; see Fig. 3.16). Second, the restricted localisation of HRP lies peripheral to the nucleus in each blastomere of the 8-cell embryo; in the 16-cell embryo, the outside cells show more localisation of HRP than do the inside cells. Third, isolated 1/8 cells divide *in vitro* to form couplets of cells that consist usually of a polar and an apolar cell (Johnson & Ziomek, 1981*b*). Fourth, in cells examined in transition between 1/8 and 2/16, the pole of microvilli becomes less demarcated, but is nevertheless conserved at division, and is inherited usually by just one of the two daughter cells (Johnson & Ziomek, 1981*b*). However, in a small number of cases, on average once out of eight divisions, the plane of cleavage

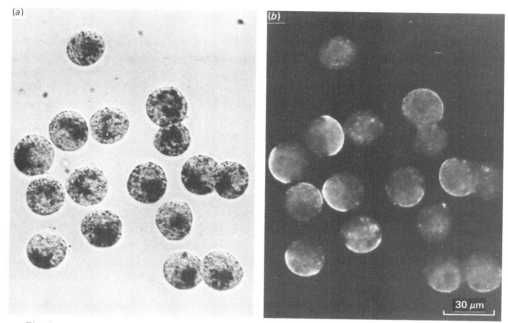

Fig. 3.16. All blastomeres of a 16-cell embryo were incubated in (*a*) HRP and (*b*) labelled with fluorescent ligand before embryo disaggregation. The isolated cells were then fixed and stained histochemically. The 11 outside cells tend to show greater localisation of HRP than the five inside cells, and this localisation underlies the pole of fluorescent labelling.

of a 1/8 cell bisects the microvillous pole, and generates two daughter cells with poles contiguous at the mid-body.

The mitotic apparatus, and especially the asters, acts as the stimulus for the position and orientation of the cleavage furrow (Wolpert, 1960; Rappaport, 1974). The cleavage furrow develops in the plane of the metaphase plate and usually bisects the metaphase spindle. Manipulation of the mitotic apparatus relative to the cell surface induces a new furrow in the surface adjacent to the asters in their new position. Eccentric division is indeed associated with the displacement of the mitotic apparatus from a central position and is typical of many embryos. For instance, the 16-cell eggs of echinoderms and molluscs contain 8 intermediate sized mesomeres, plus four macro- and four micromeres that are the unequal products of the division at the 8-cell stage. Likewise, the different sized cells present in yolky eggs, such as those of nematodes and amphibians, result initially from a gradient of yolk granules that displaces the nucleus from its central position in the egg. Finally, an extreme case of unequal division is illustrated by polar body formation in the mouse egg. However, when the maturation spindle is shifted by centrifugation from its eccentric position, the subsequent division can cause the polar body to be the same size as the egg.

The transition from an 8- to a 16-cell mouse embryo also involves the generation of two subpopulations of cells of different relative sizes (Johnson & Ziomek, 1981*b*). Generally, a polar 1/8 cell divides to form a larger, polar 1/16 cell and a smaller, apolar 1/16 cell, and this occurs whether division of cells is *in situ* or after isolation of 1/8 cells. The larger cells occupy an outer position in the morula and have properties that anticipate trophectoderm; the smaller cells occupy an inner position and are ICM-like (Handyside, 1981; Ziomek & Johnson, 1981). To what extent can the differences in size of 1/16 cells of each subpopulation be explained by the basal displacement of the nuclei in the polarised 1/8 cells?

The differences in sizes between the polar and apolar 1/16 cells can be explained on the basis of a random orientation of the cleavage plane passing through the eccentric position of the nucleus in each polar 1/8 cell, and not on the basis of a consistent, predictable orientation of the cleavage plane passing through the position of the nucleus (Reeve & Kelly, 1983). Moreover, there is a significant incidence (on average one out of eight divisions) of polar 1/8 cells dividing to form two polar 1/16 cells. Thus, the division of isolated 1/8 cells to 2/16 couplets does not appear to adhere to Hertwig's (1899) 'rule' that the metaphase plate becomes orientated at right angles to the long axis of the cell. It is, however, possible that a consistent, predictable plane of division, and hence the 'rule', applies to blastomeres of the 16-cell embryo and later developmental stages in which there is a tendency for the flattened outside cells to 'breed true' and produce only other outside cells (Ziomek & Johnson, 1982).

In conclusion, blastomeres of the 16-cell embryo are heterogeneous as shown by their different sizes, surface phenotypes and distributions of ingested HRP. Furthermore, this generation of distinct cell types by a process of differential inheritance depends on a dramatic cellular reorganisation or polarisation at the preceding 8-cell stage in which the basal migration of the nucleus in each cell is accompanied by the development of polarised distributions of microvilli and ingested HRP.

HOW DOES THE POLARISATION HYPOTHESIS ACCORD WITH ESTABLISHED NOTIONS?

The polarisation hypothesis suggests a novel mechanism for the generation of two distinct cell types in the pre-implantation mouse embryo. It proposes that individual cells of the 8-cell embryo develop an axial polarity, which is maintained through the succeeding cell division. The spherical cells of the intact precompact 8-cell embryo have a dispersed cytoplasmic distribution of organelles and bind fluorescent ligand uniformly over their surface. In contrast, the wedge-shaped blastomeres of the compacted 8-cell morula have their mitochondria and microtubules located near areas of intercellular apposition, and have microvilli concentrated at their external face, which has a high incidence of fluorescent-ligand binding sites. At division, the cleavage plane tends to bisect the axis of polarity within each cell, and thus ensures a differential inheritance by the two daughter 1/16 cells, most 2/16 couplets consisting of an apolar and a polar cell. These two cell types, although differing in their properties, are not yet committed to the ICM and trophectodermal lineages, respectively. Indeed, embryos consisting entirely of either 16 polar or 16 apolar cells will form normal blastocysts that are capable of forming foetuses (Ziomek, Johnson & Handyside, 1982a). However, the first differences between cells do arise by a process of differential inheritance, and subsequent interaction is thought to cause further differentiative divergence until the two types become committed eventually to different fates. The significance of the two distinct surface phenotypes *per se* is uncertain. The inheritance of these two forms may confer important differences upon cells at the 16-cell stage; alternatively, these differences in phenotype may represent merely an easily detected manifestation of a more complex underlying polarity.

Differences between the inside–outside and the polarisation hypotheses

The polarisation hypothesis proposes that cellular differences arise by a process of differential inheritance and, therefore, differs in an important aspect from the inside–outside or micro-environmental hypothesis (Tarkowski & Wroblewska, 1967), which proposes that initially all cells in the 16-cell embryo are identical and that differences are generated subsequently due to cells responding to their different relative positions within the morula. The distributions at division (from 1/8 to 2/16) of microvilli and ingested HRP vesicles demonstrate that some features, at least, can be inherited unequally by blastomeres of the 16-cell embryo. The difference in origins of cellular heterogeneity proposed by the two hypotheses has important implications for the mechanism of development of the ICM and trophectoderm. Tarkowski & Wroblewska (1967) postulated that an inside position was crucial to the formation of the ICM, and that reduction of cell numbers in the morula to a level at which no inside cells were present would result in 'blastocysts' comprised exclusively of trophectoderm. Thus, after the experimental removal of cells, the inhibition of cytokinesis or the impairment of normal cellular interactions, the micro-environmental hypothesis differs from the polarisation hypothesis in predicting the absence of inside markers. In contrast, under these conditions, the polarisation hypothesis predicts that while an overt ICM may or may not be present both ICM and trophectodermal characteristics will be. These contradictory predictions can be tested.

Culture of embryos in cytochalasin D for more than 15 hours irreversibly prevents cell division, whilst the continuing nuclear divisions result in each cell becoming polyploid (Surani, Barton & Burling, 1980; Pratt, Chakraborty & Surani, 1981). Cytochalasin D prevents compaction, but embryos that are restored to control medium can compact simultaneously with control embryos, and subsequently accumulate fluid to form 'blastocyst-like' vesicles. However, depending on the stage at which embryos were transferred to cytochalasin D, these vesicles may contain only two, four or eight cells, and consequently lack an overt ICM. Yet, whether the embryos are cultured continuously in cytochalasin D, or pulsed with the drug and then restored to control medium, they become indistinguishable in molecular terms from temporally equivalent 32- and 64-cell stage embryos. Thus, these arrested embryos become polarised, synthesise junctional proteins, gain sodium-dependent and ouabain-sensitive enzyme activities, develop mature mitochondrial, nucleolar and endoplasmic reticular morphologies, and have cholesterol biosynthetic patterns typical of control blastocysts. These features appear normally in cells of both the ICM and trophectoderm of control blastocysts. Consequently, their occurrence in arrested 2-cell embryos demonstrates maturation in molecular terms, but does not indicate whether the cells have differentiated solely as trophectoderm, or contain a combination of ICM and trophectodermal characteristics. Unfortunately, there is at present a shortage of markers that are restricted to the ICM. However, two pieces of evidence suggest that the arrested embryos do not become purely trophectodermal. First, the embryos stain positively for alkaline phosphatase activity, which is present in the ICM, but not in the trophectoderm, of control blastocysts. Second, they synthesise both ICM- and trophectoderm-specific proteins. A variant of the inside–outside hypothesis could postulate the development of inside (ICM) and outside (trophectoderm) characteristics in the corresponding regions in each blastomere of these 2-cell embryos. However, in its customary micro-environmental interpretation, the inside–outside hypothesis predicts that these embryos should be purely trophectodermal. The development of at least two ICM characteristics in the absence of an inside cell position provides important support for the polarisation hypothesis, which proposes that the basic ICM and trophectodermal characteristics are programmed temporally, and are segregated normally by cytokinesis.

The micro-environmental and polarisation hypotheses also predict different consequences if normal cellular interactions are manipulated, such that both compaction and subsequent blastocyst formation are prevented without interfering with cell division. When the cholesterol content of embryos is modified, or when embryos are cultured in antibody to embryonal carcinoma cells, low calcium or concanavalin A, cellular apposition and normal cellular relationships are both impaired; cells are not integrated properly into the embryo, and the eventual accumulation of fluid occurs in a disorganised, predominantly intracellular manner. The inside–outside hypothesis predicts that all cells should differentiate as trophectoderm since they are exposed to equivalent microenvironments. In fact, all these agents prevent the formation of zonular tight junctions, and prolonged periods of decompaction can be maintained without impairing the subsequent formation of blastocysts with overt ICMs. Moreover, embryos that were cultured in the antibody, at least, despite showing disorganised fluid accumulation, synthesised proteins characteristic of both ICM and trophectoderm (Johnson et al., 1979). Thus, although differentiation may require cellular perception of different relative positions within an aggregate of cells, distinct inside and outside micro-environments do not appear to be essential to the generation of ICM and trophectodermal characteristics.

Support for the importance of intercellular communication to the formation of the ICM has arisen from experiments in which morulae, either with or without zonae pellucidae, were injected into the blastocoel of a giant blastocyst (Pedersen & Spindle, 1980). A zona-enclosed morula, even though it was within the internal micro-environment, developed into a normal blastocyst. However, an injected zona-free morula formed cellular contacts with the cells lining the blastocoel and subsequently failed to form a blastocyst. Morphogenesis of the blastocyst appears to be governed more by intercellular communication than by the existence of distinct micro-environments. This regulation of cell fate through cellular interaction has indeed been stressed by the polarisation hypothesis, which emphasises the role of cellular interaction not only in generating the polarity at the 8-cell stage, but also in maintaining the distinct phenotypes at the 16- and 32-cell stages (Johnson, 1981; Johnson & Ziomek, 1982). Experimental manipulation that involves novel relative cell positions, such as after the injection of a zona-free morula into a blastocoel, alters the normal developmental fate. However, when left in situ the apolar and polar cells continue to interact, and show increasing divergence. How does this occur?

The polarisation hypothesis maintains that the first cellular differences are generated by a process of differential inheritance, and that these differences dictate the positions in the morula occupied by cells of different phenotypes. Thus, the microvillous poles and their associated cytocortex can be considered as analogous to the cytoplasmic determinants of other embryos. The few cytoplasmic determinants that have been identified morphologically stain heavily for RNA, and there is some evidence from other embryos that differential inheritance involves gene expression to generate fundamental differences between cells. However, the action of the morphogenetic determinants in the mouse embryo may be more straightforward. It is possible that the presence of a microvillous pole ensures merely that that cell always occupies an outside position with the pole directed outwards. The microvillous pole acts as a 'behavioural' determinant, and the subsequent perception of relative position relates causally to cell fate.

Recently, continuing interactions have been shown to influence the phenotypes of polar and apolar 1/16 cells and their progeny (Johnson & Ziomek, 1982). An increase in the degree of flattening of a polar cell on another blastomere is associated with an increase in the incidence of division through the microvillous pole. Furthermore, in a pair of apolar and polar 1/16 cells, the polar normally envelops the apolar, and each cell type breeds true (developing to trophectoderm and ICM, respectively). When envelopment fails to occur, or when 1/16 cells are isolated, the prospective fate may change. In this case, polar 1/16 cells show an increased incidence of division parallel to, rather than through, the microvillous pole. Instead of breeding true, the polar cell tends to undergo a 'differentiative division', generating both polar and apolar 1/32 cells. A corresponding change in prospective fate is also revealed by an isolated apolar 1/16 cell, which tends to polarise and generate a couplet consisting of either two polar cells or one polar and one apolar cell. An apolar 1/16 cell thus forms both apolar and polar cells by either the 32- or 64-cell stage.

The apolar and polar cells of the intact 16-cell embryo have the prospective cell fates of ICM and trophectoderm, respectively. Nonetheless, each type of 1/16 cell has also the developmental potency of the other cell type. The commitment of cells to either an ICM or trophectodermal lineage must occur after the late 16- or early 32-cell stage. Polar blastomeres are then no longer capable of differentiative division, and apolar cells cannot be cued to polarise.

Events of cleavage in relation to the polarisation hypothesis

Prior to polarisation and compaction, the asynchrony of division and the relative positions of cells in the early cleavage-stage embryo have been shown to affect the contribution of cells to the ICM (Graham & Deussen, 1978; Kelly, Mulnard & Graham, 1978; Graham & Lehtonen, 1979; Lehtonen, 1980). It has been demonstrated that the descendants of the first cell to divide at the 2-cell stage tend to divide ahead of those of the other 1/2 blastomere at all subsequent stages up to the blastocyst (Kelly *et al.*, 1978). Furthermore, at the 8-cell stage, the first cells to divide usually have more cell contacts (Graham & Deussen, 1978), due presumably to these cells having more microvilli with which to pull other cells around (Graham & Lehtonen, 1979). This was also observed when isolated cells were reaggregated, suggesting that continuous cellular interactions play a more important role in establishing relative cellular positions than do previous cytokinesis and morphogenetic movements. Moreover, the first cell to divide at the 4-cell stage contributed more descendants to the ICM than did the last cell to divide (Kelly *et al.*, 1978). Taking these results together, the progeny of the first cell to divide at the 2-cell stage tend to contribute a disproportionate number of inside cells and, thence, of cells to the ICM.

In contrast, the polarisation hypothesis proposes that the inside cells in the 16-cell embryo are the apolar cells generated at the division of polar 1/8 cells. Each polarised 1/8 cell divides, when the cleavage plane is at right angles to the axis of polarity, to form one polar and one apolar 1/16 cell. However, on average, one of the eight blastomeres in an embryo divides such that the cleavage plane bisects the microvillous pole, thus generating two polar 1/16 cells. A 16-cell embryo therefore contains more polar than apolar cells. In fact, six to eight apolar, inside cells are found in 93% of 16-cell embryos (Johnson, 1981). Whereas the polarisation hypothesis predicts the generation of the ICM from the apolar cells in the 16-cell embryo, Graham and his colleagues consider the early dividing cells to contribute disproportionately to the ICM. Can these two notions be reconciled? One explanation would be if division through the pole were more frequent among the late dividing than among the early dividing 1/8 cells. To test this possibility, 9- to 15-cell embryos can be examined for their numbers of polar and apolar cells to see if early dividing 1/8 cells tend to produce an apolar and a polar cell, whereas late dividing 1/8 cells produce two polar cells. This type of analysis does not support a relationship between order of division at the 8-cell stage and the plane of cleavage (Ziomek, Pratt & Johnson, 1982*b*). However, the same stage of embryo has not been examined both for the order of division of its blastomeres and for the planes of cleavage of these cells. Kelly *et al.* (1978) compared the respective contributions to the ICM made by the first and last cells to divide at the 4-cell stage. Since all the daughters of the early dividing cell at this stage may not always divide ahead of those derived from the late dividing cell, it is therefore necessary to relate the division order of cells at the stage labelled by Kelly *et al.* (1978) to the cleavage planes at division of 1/8 to 2/16 cells. This could be examined by marking the early dividing 1/2 or 1/4 cell and then, at the 16-cell stage, comparing its progeny with those of the equivalent late dividing cell. Perhaps more important, though, is the need to establish whether there are definite lineages between the apolar and polar cells at the 16-cell stage and the ICM and trophectoderm of the blastocyst. This is an important preliminary to the examination of the possible relationship between the order of division and the orientation of cleavage planes. Thus far, the data are consistent with the apolar cells of the 16-cell morula forming the ICM, whereas the polar cells form the trophectoderm of the blastocyst (Ziomek & Johnson, 1982).

CONCLUSION

A lineage-generated cell diversity relies normally on the inheritance by subpopulations of cells of different properties, associated with a high level of commitment of the different cell types to different lineages. Typically, embryonic developmental features two unique, distinct and quantal events: determination and differentiation. The event of determination (or commitment) is identified solely by the acquisition, by subpopulations of cells, of different restricted development potentials. Overt differentiation occurs subsequently (often much later) and is associated with the appearance of distinct differences between these subpopulations of cells.

The development of the pre-implantation mouse embryo appears to contradict these principles. Although differential inheritance generates two different cell types in the early 16-cell embryo, and guides these cells to particular positions in the morula *in situ*, its action can be overcome by the experimental manipulation of the embryo, a result which indicates that the two cell types are not committed to different fates. There is a mass of data to indicate that pre-implantation mouse embryos can regulate after the alteration of relative cellular position. When either blastomeres or intact embryos were placed in the centre of an aggregate of cells, their contribution to the ICM of the chimaeric blastocyst was increased significantly, whereas blastomeres on the outside differentiated as trophectoderm. The ability to regulate after the alteration of relative cell position arises from the totipotency of the two distinct cell types in the morula, and has been demonstrated perhaps most impressively by the aggregation of either 16 apolar or 16 polar 1/16 cells to form morulae that developed to blastocysts capable of forming foetuses (Ziomek *et al.*, 1982*a*). Thus, two distinct cell types exist normally in the morula, but cells of each type can independently form a complete embryo.

The crucial importance of cellular position in the morula to cell fate is, however, secondary to the mechanisms that dictate the positions that are occupied by particular cells. Apolar and polar cell types are not committed to different lineages, but their different phenotypes ensure they come to occupy different positions within the morula. In the morula *in situ*, the presence of a microvillous pole causes a blastomere to occupy an outside position, whereas apolar cells remain inside the cellular aggregate. Blastomeres with microvillous poles attempt to remain on the outside of the cellular aggregate, and therefore contribute to trophectoderm, whereas apolar cells are relegated to an inside position and differentiate as ICM (Ziomek & Johnson, 1982). Apolar and polar cells have been proposed as the respective precursors of ICM and trophectoderm, but the two subpopulations of cells are formed long before the commitment of blastomeres to either the ICM or trophectodermal lineages at about the $3\frac{1}{2}$ day, 32- to 64-cell blastocyst stage. In fact, a whole inventory exists of developmental changes that occur at different stages from the 2-cell onwards (Johnson *et al.*, 1977; Johnson, 1981). The differentiative processes reveal a series of changes throughout development, and a quantal differentiative event is absent.

In conclusion, the polarisation of cells serves two purposes. First, it may confer a necessary functional polarity. In this respect, the polarisation that occurs in the 8-cell mouse embryo bears close similarities to the generation of stable epithelia. A molecular heterogeneity has been identified in the cell surface of epithelial cells, but not yet in blastomeres. However, both cell types do become polarised as shown by an apical pole of microvilli and a basolateral surface of sparse microvilli. Moreover, though isolated cells of both types change shape and appear more rounded after isolation, they still retain these morphologically distinct surfaces. The morphological polarity appears to be more fundamental than does a molecular polarity since the molecular asymmetries do not persist in isolated epithelial cells, possibly due to the diffusion of molecules being allowed in the absence of tight junctions. It is possible that isolated blastomeres also lose their putative molecular asymmetries or, alternatively, these features of polarity may not appear until the development of zonular tight junctions, and epithelial integrity, at the 32-cell stage. Previous examinations of polarised epithelial cells have, in fact, provided little information on the induction of polarity, and have tended to involve the disruption of the established epithelium or the reversal of the polarity. In contrast, the development of the mouse embryo away from the influence of other cell types and the easy isolation of all its relatively large blastomeres offer considerable advantages in the study of cellular polarisation.

A second consequence of polarisation is that it enables the generation of cellular differences by a process of differential inheritance. The polarisation of individual blastomeres in the 8-cell mouse embryo is essential to the generation of the apolar and polar 1/16 cells, which differ from the time of their formation. The differential inheritance of determinants appears to guide cell fates by guiding cells to different positions, and position in the morula remains thereby causally related to lineage foundation. The placing of cells in different relative positions, and their retention there as a result of their inherited properties, ensures that cells continue to follow different differentiative pathways *in situ*. Nonetheless, the cell types retain their developmental lability and continued cellular interaction is required to ensure their increasing divergence. The differentiation of ICM and trophectoderm is not a single event; instead, the two cell types accumulate further differences until the phenotypic differentiation progresses beyond the point of reversal, when a state of commitment is reached.

I should like to thank Dr Martin Johnson for his advice and supervision during the progress of the above work submitted previously for a PhD; Drs Hester Pratt and Harry Goodall for stimulating discussion; Ian Edgar for photographic assistance. The work was supported by grants from the MRC and the CRC to Dr M. H. Johnson, and was conducted while the author was in receipt of an MRC Research Training Award and a grant from the Cambridge Philosophical Society.

REFERENCES

Barlow, P., Owen, D. A. J. & Graham, C. (1972). DNA synthesis in the pre-implantation mouse embryo. *Journal of Embryology and Experimental Morphology*, **27**, 431–45.
Calarco, P. G. & Epstein, C. J. (1973). Cell surface changes during pre-implantation development in the mouse. *Developmental Biology*, **32**, 208–13.
Dalcq, A. M. (1957). *Introduction to General Embryology*. London: Oxford University Press.
Davidson, E. H. (1976). *Gene Activity in Early Development*, 2nd edn. New York: Academic Press.
Ducibella, T. (1977). Surface changes of the developing trophoblast cell. In *Development in Mammals*, Vol. 1, ed. M. H. Johnson, pp. 5–30. Amsterdam: Elsevier/North-Holland.
Ducibella, T. (1980). Divalent antibodies to mouse embryonal carcinoma cells inhibit compaction in the mouse embryo. *Developmental Biology*, **79**, 356–66.
Ducibella, T., Albertini, D. F., Anderson, E. & Biggers, J. D. (1975). The preimplantation mammalian embryo: characterization of intercellular junctions and their appearance during development. *Developmental Biology*, **45**, 231–50.
Ducibella, T. & Anderson, E. (1975). Cell shape and membrane changes in the eight-cell mouse embryo: prerequisites for morphogenesis of the blastocyst. *Developmental Biology*, **47**, 45–58.
Ducibella, T., Ukena, T., Karnovsky, M. & Anderson, E. (1977). Changes in cell surface and cortical cytoplasmic organization during early embryogenesis in the preimplantation mouse embryo. *Journal of Cell Biology*, **74**, 153–67.
Goodall, H. & Johnson, M. H. (1982). The use of carboxyfluorescein diacetate to study the formation of permeable channels between mouse blastomeres. *Nature (London)*, **295**, 524–6.
Graham, C. F. (1971). The design of the mouse blastocyst. In *Control Mechanisms of Growth and Differentiation*, Society for Experimental Biology Symposium 25, ed. D. D. Davies & M. Balls, pp. 371–8. Cambridge University Press.
Graham, C. F. & Deussen, Z. A. (1978). Features of cell lineage in preimplantation mouse development. *Journal of Embryology and Experimental Morphology*, **48**, 53–72.
Graham, C. F. & Lehtonen, E. (1979). Formation and consequences of cell patterns in preimplantation mouse development. *Journal of Embryology and Experimental Morphology*, **49**, 277–94.
Graham, C. F. & Wareing, P. F. (1976). *The Developmental Biology of Plants and Animals*. Oxford: Blackwell Scientific Publications.
Handyside, A. H. (1980). Distribution of antibody- and lectin-binding sites on dissociated blastomeres from mouse morulae: evidence for polarization at compaction. *Journal of Embryology and Experimental Morphology*, **60**, 99–116.
Handyside, A. H. (1981). Immunofluorescence techniques for determining the numbers of inner and outer blastomeres in mouse morulae. *Journal of Reproductive Immunology*, **2**, 339–50.
Herbert, M. C. & Graham, C. F. (1974). Cell determination and biochemical differentiation of the early mammalian embryo. *Current Topics in Developmental Biology*, **8**, 151–78.
Hertwig, O. (1899). *Text-book of the Embryology of Man and Mammals*, translated from German by E. L. Mark. London: Swan Sonnenschein.
Hillman, N., Sherman, M. I. & Graham, C. (1972). The effect of spatial arrangement on cell determination during mouse development. *Journal of Embryology and Experimental Morphology*, **28**, 263–78.
Izquierdo, L. (1977). Cleavage and differentiation. In *Development in Mammals*, vol. 2, ed. M. H. Johnson, pp. 99–118. Amsterdam: North-Holland.
Johnson, M. H. (1979). Intrinsic and extrinsic factors in preimplantation development. *Journal of Reproduction and Fertility*, **55**, 255–65.
Johnson, M. H. (1981). Membrane events associated with the generation of a blastocyst. *International Reviews of Cytology*, Supplement **12**, 1–37.
Johnson, M. H., Chakraborty, J., Handyside, A. H., Willison, K. & Stern, P. (1979). The effect of prolonged decompaction on the development of the preimplantation mouse embryo. *Journal of Embryology and Experimental Morphology*, **54**, 241–61.

Johnson, M. H., Handyside, A. H. & Braude, P. R. (1977). Control mechanisms in early mammalian development. In *Development in Mammals*, Vol. 2, ed. M. H. Johnson, pp. 67–97. Amsterdam: North-Holland.

Johnson, M. H., Pratt, H. P. M. & Handyside, A. H. (1981). The generation and recognition of positional information in the preimplantation mouse embryo. In *Cellular and Molecular Aspects of Implantation*, ed. S. R. Glasser & D. W. Bullock, pp. 55–74. New York: Plenum Press.

Johnson, M. H. & Ziomek, C. A. (1981*a*). Induction of polarity in mouse 8-cell blastomeres: specificity, geometry and stability. *Journal of Cell Biology*, **91**, 303–8.

Johnson, M. H. & Ziomek, C. A. (1981*b*). The foundation of two distinct cell lineages within the mouse morula. *Cell*, **24**, 71–80.

Johnson, M. H. & Ziomek, C.A. (1982). Cell interactions influence the fate of mouse blastomeres undergoing the transition from the 16- to the 32-cell stage. *Developmental Biology*, **91**, 431–9.

Johnson, M. H., Ziomek, C. A., Reeve, W. J. D., Pratt, H. P. M., Goodall, H. & Handyside, A. H. (1983). The mosaic organisation of the preimplantation mouse embryo. In *Current Topics in Ultrastructure Research. Preimplantation Embryogenesis*, ed. J. Van Blerkom & P. Motta. The Hague: Martinus Nijhoff, in press.

Kelly, S. J. (1975). Studies of the potency of early cleavage blastomeres of the mouse. In *The Early Development of Mammals*, British Society for Developmental Biology Symposium 2, ed. M. Balls & A. E. Wild, pp. 97–105. Cambridge University Press.

Kelly, S. J. (1977). Studies of the developmental potential of 4- and 8-cell stage mouse blastomeres. *Journal of Experimental Zoology*, **200**, 365–76.

Kelly, S. J., Mulnard, J. G. & Graham, C. F. (1978). Cell division and cell allocation in early mouse development. *Journal of Embryology and Experimental Morphology*, **48**, 37–51.

Kemler, R., Babinet, C., Eisen, H. & Jacob, F. (1977). Surface antigen in early differentiation. *Proceedings of the National Academy of Sciences, USA*, **74**, 4449–52.

Lehtonen, E. (1980). Changes in cell dimensions and intercellular contacts during cleavage stage cell cycles in mouse embryonic cells. *Journal of Embryology and Experimental Morphology*, **58**, 231–49.

Lewis, W. H. & Wright, E. S. (1935). On the early development of the mouse egg. *Contributions to Embryology, Carnegie Institute*, **148**, 115–43.

Lo, C. W. (1980). Gap junctions and development. In *Development in Mammals*, Vol. 4, ed. M. H. Johnson, pp. 39–80. Amsterdam: Elsevier/North-Holland Biomedical Press.

McLaren, A. (1976). *Mammalian Chimaeras*. Cambridge University Press.

Magnuson, T., Demsey, A. & Stackpole, C. W. (1977). Characterization of intercellular junctions in the preimplantation mouse embryo by freeze–fracture and thin-section electron microscopy. *Developmental Biology*, **61**, 252–61.

Pedersen, R. A. & Spindle, A. I. (1980). Role of the blastocoele microenvironment in early mouse embryo differentiation. *Nature (London)*, **284**, 550–2.

Pratt, H. P. M., Chakraborty, J. & Surani, M. A. H. (1981). Molecular and morphological differentiation of the mouse blastocyst after manipulations of compaction with cytochalasin D. *Cell*, **26**, 279–92.

Pratt, H. P. M., Ziomek, C. A., Reeve, W. J. D. & Johnson, M. H. (1982). Compaction of the mouse embryo: an analysis of its components. *Journal of Embryology and Experimental Morphology*, **70**, 113–32.

Rappaport, R. (1974). Cleavage. In *Concepts of Development*, ed. J. Lash & J. R. Whittaker, pp. 76–100. Stamford, Connecticut: Sinauer Associates.

Reeve, W. J. D. (1981*a*). Cytoplasmic polarity develops at compaction in rat and mouse embryos. *Journal of Embryology and Experimental Morphology*, **62**, 351–67.

Reeve, W. J. D. (1981*b*). The distribution of ingested horseradish peroxidase in the 16-cell mouse embryo. *Journal of Embryology and Experimental Morphology*, **66**, 191–207.

Reeve, W. J. D. & Kelly, F. P. (1983). Nuclear position in the cells of the mouse early embryo. *Journal of Embryology and Experimental Morphology*, **75**, 117–39.

Reeve, W. J. D. & Ziomek, C. A. (1981). Distribution of microvilli on dissociated blastomeres from mouse embryos: evidence for surface polarization at compaction. *Journal of Embryology and Experimental Morphology*, **62**, 339–50.

Rossant, J. & Papaioannou, V. E. (1977). The biology of embryogenesis. In *Concepts in Mammalian Embryogenesis*, ed. M. I. Sherman, pp. 1–36. Cambridge, Massachusetts: MIT Press.

Seidel, F. (1960). Die Entwicklungsfähigkeiten isolierter Furchungszellen aus dem Ei des Kaninchens *Oryctolagus cuniculus*. *Wilhelm Roux' Archiv für Entwicklungsmechanik der Organismen*, **152**, 43–130.

Solter, D., Damjanov, I. & Skreb, N. (1973). Distribution of hydrolytic enzymes in early rat and mouse embryos – a reappraisal. *Zeitschrift für Anatomie und Entwicklungsgeschichte*, **139**, 119–26.

Surani, M. A. H., Barton, S. C. & Burling, A. (1980). Differentiation of 2-cell and 8-cell mouse embryos arrested by cytoskeletal inhibitors. *Experimental Cell Research*, **125**, 275–86.

Tarkowski, A. K. & Wroblewska, J. (1967). Development of blastomeres of mouse eggs isolated at the 4- and 8-cell stage. *Journal of Embryology and Experimental Morphology*, **18**, 155–80.

Wilson, E. B. (1925). *The Cell in Development and Heredity*, 3rd edn. New York: Macmillan.

Wolpert, L. (1960). The mechanics and mechanism of cleavage. *International Reviews of Cytology*, **10**, 163–216.

Ziomek, C. A. & Johnson, M. H. (1980). Cell surface interaction induces polarization of mouse 8-cell blastomeres at compaction. *Cell*, **21**, 935–42.

Ziomek, C. A. & Johnson, M. H. (1981). Properties of polar and apolar cells from the 16-cell mouse morula. *Wilhelm Roux's Archives of Developmental Biology*, **190**, 287–96.

Ziomek, C. A. & Johnson, M. H. (1982). The roles of phenotype and position in guiding the fate of 16-cell mouse blastomeres. *Developmental Biology*, **91**, 440–7.

Ziomek, C. A., Johnson, M. H. & Handyside, A. H. (1982a). The developmental potential of 16-cell mouse blastomeres. *Journal of Experimental Zoology*, **221**, 345–55.

Ziomek, C. A., Pratt, H. P. M. & Johnson, M. H. (1982b). The origins of cell diversity in the early mouse embryo. In *Functional Integration of Cells in Animal Tissues*, British Society for Cell Biology Symposium 5, ed. M. E. Finbow & J. D. Pitts, pp. 149–65. Cambridge University Press.

4 Stereology: progress in quantitative microscopical anatomy

T. M. MAYHEW

Department of Anatomy, University of Aberdeen, Aberdeen AB9 1AS, UK

INTRODUCTION

Anatomy is no longer the static study of structure by examination of dissected parts. Its progress has been marked by a willingness to apply new investigative techniques (light and electron microscopy, tissue culture, histochemistry, immunochemistry, autoradiography, tomography, etc.) which reveal not only the dynamism, intricacy and beauty of living organisms but also the intimate relation between biological structure and function and the artificiality of divisions between biomedical disciplines.

During the past two decades, research in microscopical anatomy has witnessed a resurgence of interest in morphometric, and particularly stereological, methods. Their continuing and expanding application is a reflection of many convictions: that all sciences rely on *exact* observation, that compartmentation of structure and subdivision of function are indissolubly linked and that living organisms are designed to perform in an economical manner so that 'no more structure is formed and maintained than is required to satisfy functional needs' (Taylor & Weibel, 1981).

In this chapter, there is no attempt to review the theory or derive the basic principles of stereology. These tasks have been undertaken by many others and the reader is referred to appropriate leading articles and books (DeHoff & Rhines, 1968; Dunnill, 1968; Weibel, 1969, 1979a, 1980; Underwood, 1970; Elias, Hennig & Schwartz, 1971; Weibel & Bolender, 1973; Miles & Davy, 1976; Williams, 1977; Mayhew, 1979a; Gundersen, 1980). Here, I wish to emphasise that the stereological approach can be at once simple, robust and efficient; to indicate the accidental and systematic errors which influence the validity, precision and efficiency of stereological estimates and to illustrate practical steps by which these sources of experimental uncertainty may be minimised or avoided. Practical problems and their solutions are illustrated further by a selection of experimental systems which, apart from their intrinsic biological significance, have involved the use of stereological techniques to quantify organ, tissue and cell composition. Due purely to lack of space, the examples are confined to lung, intestine, kidney and spinal cord.

THE STEREOLOGICAL APPROACH
The nature of stereology

Stereology involves the application of mathematical relationships to define three-dimensional structures from measurements performed on (ideally) two-dimensional images. In microscopical anatomy this usually means thin sections of tissue prepared for light and/or electron microscopy. The mathematical relationships are based on the reasonings of geometrical probability and statistics, but it is no more necessary to be able to derive the relationships in order to do good stereology than it is to be able to build an electron microscope in order to take good electron micrographs. All that is required is a little commonsense with an appreciation of the circumstances under which the relationships apply and of their advantages, limitations and weaknesses.

Measuring tissue sections

Measurements of structural components appearing on tissue sections can be made by superimposing a test lattice bearing a repeated pattern of areas, lines and points called test probes. By evaluating the *chance* encounters between test probes and the component(s) of interest, essentially planar morphometric information is obtainable. Since a single section is seldom representative of tissue composition, the information must be taken from sets of sections selected by a randomised sampling procedure.

Most of this information can be derived with comparatively little effort, by the simple expedient of reducing all 'measurements' to the counting of discrete events, e.g., the number of nuclear profiles (N), the number of intersections (I) between test lines and the contour of the nuclear envelope or the number of test points (P) falling on profiles of nuclei. Clearly, counting test points is not a very precise way of estimating the sectional area of an individual nuclear profile, just as counting intersections is a rather imprecise way of estimating the contour length of its envelope. However, it is important to appreciate at the outset that the resulting statistical uncertainty frequently pales into insignificance when set against that uncertainty which characterises most biological experiments: namely, 'biological variation' – the natural and irreducible variation between individual animals (Shay, 1975; Gundersen & Østerby, 1980, 1981; Gupta *et al.*, 1983). This has fundamental implications for the economical design of morphometrical experiments (see below).

The ease with which planar information may be obtained must be balanced against the fact that it can be misleading and, in consequence, can affect interpretations of its biological significance and relevance. For instance, the number of nuclear profiles per unit area of section is not always an accurate indicator of the number of nuclei in a volume of tissue. Its inaccuracy stems from the empirical observation that the number of nuclear profiles seen in a section depends not only on the real number of nuclei but also on section thickness, nuclear size and nuclear shape. More profiles tend to be seen in thicker sections and when nuclei are highly irregular (e.g., the nuclei of polymorphonuclear leukocytes). Furthermore, large nuclei have a greater chance of being sectioned than small ones.

To minimise problems of interpretation, it is preferable to convert planar data into more absolute structural quantities by applying appropriate stereological formulae (Weibel, 1979a, 1980). The majority, but by no means all, of these quantities are actually ratios or 'component densities'.

Component densities

Component densities relate the dimensions of a component (its volume V, surface area S, length L or number N) to a suitable reference (which can also be a volume, surface, length or number). In any stereological study, it is important to specify both the component and its reference. Thus, the ratio between the surface area of alveoli and lung volume is a component surface density in a volume, usually given the generic symbol S_V and having the units cm^2 cm^{-3} and dimensions cm^{-1}. However, this ratio would not have the same value as that between alveolar surface area and the volume of lung parenchyma (gas exchange regions). A synopsis of the basic component densities is given in Table 4.1 and principles for estimating them have been reviewed recently (Mayhew, 1979a; Weibel, 1979a).

Table 4.1. *List of fundamental component densities and their dimensions*

Component dimension	Reference dimension			
	Volume, V (cm^3)	Surface, S (cm^2)	Length, L (cm^1)	Number, N (cm^0)
Volume, V cm^3	V_V cm^0			
Surface, S cm^2	S_V cm^{-1}	S_S cm^0		
Length, L cm^1	L_V cm^{-2}	L_S cm^{-1}	L_L cm^0	
Number, N cm^0	N_V cm^{-3}	N_S cm^{-2}	N_L cm^{-1}	N_N cm^0

It is reassuring to note that reliable estimates of most component densities can be calculated without making any assumptions about the size, shape, spatial orientation or other properties of the individual structures. The only condition required is that the sample taken from each animal is random and independent in both orientation and location (Stuart, 1976; Weibel, 1979a; Gundersen, 1980). Failure to follow this fundamental rule-of-thumb usually requires the application of correction formulae to compensate for systematic errors, e.g., those introduced by deliberately restricting section planes to some favourable location and/or orientation (such as through the cell nucleus or perpendicular to an epithelial surface).

A notable exception to freedom from underlying assumptions is the estimation of component numerical densities: accurate estimates of particle numbers from random and independent sections can only be obtained when their size and shape are known (Weibel, 1979a, 1980; Cruz Orive, 1980a).

Volume, surface and length densities

Reliable information can be obtained for any arbitrary components appearing in random, independent sections. The robustness of these component densities is related to the fact that they characterise the sum total of all components of a given type present in a particular reference, e.g., the volume of all hepatocytes in liver volume, the surface area of all desmosomes on the surface of epithelial cells, the length of all seminiferous tubules in testicular volume. They are therefore densities which define aggregates rather than individuals within aggregates. As such, they are far easier to estimate than numerical densities and should, wherever possible, be selected in preference to numerical densities.

It is helpful to try to establish which component densities best suit the requirements of a particular investigation. For this it may be necessary to perform a preliminary (pilot) study on the experimental system. By analysing the results of such a study, it is often possible to focus on a few quantities which will permit one to pick up statistical differences between animals in different experimental groups and thereby reduce unwarranted effort. As we shall see, a pilot study also allows a rationalisation of future experimental designs in terms of the cost-effective division of sampling labour.

Numerical densities

Numerical densities differ from other component densities because they seek to characterise individual particles within populations. Unfortunately, numbers of

particles cannot be estimated solely from random, independent sections when the
particles are of arbitrary size, shape and orientation. In view of these difficulties, it is
advisable to give serious consideration to the question: 'Do I need to estimate the
number of particles?'

Generally speaking, number is a valuable structural index for correlating with
functional information in two main biological areas. These may be grouped conveniently under the headings of (a) communication and (b) genesis and transformation
(Mayhew et al., 1979; Gundersen, 1980). Thus, when investigating the phenomena of
intercellular communication (e.g., mediated by synapses and gap-junctions) and
morphogenesis (e.g., growth by hyperplasia as opposed to hypertrophy or accretion;
differentiation during normal and pathological conditions) estimates of particle
number can play an important part in our interpretation and understanding of cell and
tissue behaviour.

In other areas, number may be redundant information. Consider the case of
mitochondria: these are semi-autonomous organelles whose number, size and shape
may not be fixed but plastic, fluctuating as the chondriome as a whole fuses and
fragments. Under these circumstances, the number of organelles has little meaning
and, in terms of function, the overall energy requirements of the cell might be
described better by the surface density of inner mitochondrial membranes and the
volume density of the chondriome or its mitochondrial matrix (Mayhew et al., 1979;
Mathieu et al., 1981b). These component densities have the added advantage of being
size- and shape-independent.

If it is decided that estimates of number are required, the next step is to judge
whether it is reasonable to approximate the shapes of particles by some simple
geometric model such as a sphere, disc, cylinder or ellipsoid. Provided this can be
achieved, estimates of particle number suitable for comparative purposes at least can
be obtained (various methods are reviewed by Weibel, 1979a). If not, then it may be
necessary to resort to serial sectioning (Cruz Orive, 1980a). Studies on mitochondria
in lymphocytes (see Mayhew et al., 1979) have indicated the substantial systematic
errors which can be introduced by making erroneous assumptions about particle
shape.

Converting densities to absolute quantities

Component densities are merely ratios between the component and reference
dimensions, a fact which should not be disregarded. It is easy to make the mistake of
treating them as absolute values and this is another way in which erroneous
interpretations can be made. It is possible for a control population and an experimental population to have the *same* component density and yet have *vastly
different* absolute amounts of the component. Consider, for instance, a cell of volume
$200\,\mu m^3$ having a nucleus of volume $100\,\mu m^3$ and harbouring within its cytoplasm a
total of 600 primary lysosomes. Let us suppose that this cell hypertrophies as the result
of experimental treatment so as to occupy a volume of $400\,\mu m^3$ with a nuclear volume
of $200\,\mu m^3$ and a complement of 1200 lysosomes. Before and after treatment, this cell
would have a nuclear volume density of $0.5\,\mu m^3\,\mu m^{-3}$ and a numerical density of
3 lysosomes per μm^3. Clearly, the biological significance of the treatment would be
lost if stereological estimates were confined to these component densities.

Therefore, it behoves us to convert component densities into absolute quantities
where this is practicable. The way in which this is usually achieved is by estimating the
reference dimension in absolute terms. If the reference is cell volume, it may be

possible to estimate this directly (by measuring the cells themselves) or indirectly (by estimating nuclear volume and nuclear volume density). If the reference is organ volume, this might be estimated from its wet weight and specific gravity, by fluid displacement or by cutting parallel sections through it (see Dunnill, 1968; Weibel, 1979*a*).

Once absolute structural quantities have been obtained, it may be possible to explore allometric relationships, e.g., those between the surface area of pulmonary alveoli and body weight (Gehr, Bachofen & Weibel, 1978) or the volumes of skeletal muscle mitochondria, body weight and oxygen consumption (Mathieu *et al.*, 1981*b*).

Useful derived quantities

Component densities can be used to derive other quantities which are difficult to estimate directly from sections. A few examples will suffice. Blood capillaries in random thin sections present a variety of profile shapes which make it difficult to obtain estimates of their calibre diameter. However, their transverse sectional area can be estimated by calculating the ratio between capillary volume density and length density in the same reference volume. For a long, tubular structure, this ratio is equivalent to that between the volume and length of an open cylinder which is, of course, equivalent to its mean transectional area. In a study of blood capillaries in the rat spinal medulla (Mayhew & Momoh, 1974), these relationships were exploited and it was found that these vessels had a mean diameter of $6.4\,\mu$m. This roughly corresponds to the diameter of an erythrocyte.

Ratios between surface densities and volume densities have been used to derive estimates of the thickness of the alveolar air–blood barrier, a measure which cannot be obtained directly from thin sections (Weibel & Knight, 1964). The same ratios have been applied to estimate the surface area : volume relationships of particles and also their number (Weibel, 1979*a*). When comparing populations of particles, it is important to realise that the surface : volume ratio is determined by size *and* shape. This raises the question of how we might resolve the two in order to distinguish between populations having the same shape but different sizes and vice versa. In this context, it is useful to derive shape factors.

Particles having the same shape and the same or different sizes share the same shape factors. One shape factor, β, relates the volume of a particle to its mean sectional area and is employed widely to derive estimates of particle number. For spheres, the value is 1.382 and values are available for other simple geometric models (Weibel, 1979*a*). Another set of shape factors refers particle surface area to particle volume in the forms $S^{3/2}/V$ and $S/V^{2/3}$. Like β, these are dimensionless coefficients. For a sphere, the factor $S^{3/2}/V$ has the value 10.63 and $S/V^{2/3}$ has the value 4.85. Similar shape factors have been used to test for isomorphous growth of renal glomeruli during diabetes mellitus (Østerby & Gundersen, 1980) and of chorionic villi in human placentae during normal and abnormal pregnancies (Aherne & Dunnill, 1966).

SOURCES OF ERROR

Having established which quantities are to be calculated, the next step is to plan the biological experiment. In order to do so, it is wise to pay some attention to the sorts of error which are likely to be introduced, either wittingly or unwittingly. So far, I have spoken of the need to take random, independent samples and of stereological estimates being valid, precise and efficient. What do these terms signify and what can we do to ensure validity, precision and efficiency of our final estimates?

Accidental and systematic errors

In stereology, as in computing, the validity of our results (and hence of our biological interpretations) depends crucially on what we put into the system. Stereology relies on measurement and most measurements are liable to errors. In general, stereological errors are of two kinds: accidental (or random) and systematic.

Accidental errors arise because of variation in the biological material itself, in the way in which it is prepared for microscopical examination and in the way in which it is measured. Collectively, these errors influence the reliability or *precision* of the final estimate which we obtain for a group of animals. On the other hand, systematic error (bias) influences the validity or *accuracy* of the final estimate. It is a measure of the magnitude and direction of departure of this estimate from the 'true' value which, of course, is usually unknown. Precision and accuracy are synonymous only where there is no bias (Cochran, 1977).

It is intuitively clear that accidental errors also influence the efficiency of estimation. The efficiency of a final estimate is a measure of the precision it offers per unit of cost, precision being proportional to the reciprocal of variance and cost being expressed in whatever terms are deemed most appropriate or convenient. However, it is often easier to think of cost in terms of effort invested (working hours, time taken for measurement, etc.) rather than money spent – though one's head of department may disagree; both are appropriate ways of defining efficiency in stereological work, provided one is consistent in their use when comparing experimental groups and other sample items (tissue blocks, sections, micrographs and so on).

When designing stereological investigations, systematic error and efficiency can be balanced against each other so as to achieve an optimal design. The best design (and the best final estimate) is the one which gives the smallest systematic and accidental errors for a given cost (Stuart, 1976; Cochran, 1977). Occasionally, systematic errors can be introduced deliberately (Mayhew & Williams, 1971; Mayhew, 1979b) and biased estimates corrected by suitable formulae (Mayhew & Cruz Orive, 1973, 1975). Indeed, this route to obtaining a final estimate can improve overall efficiency.

Sources of accidental error

Variation between animals

Most biological experiments have to cater for natural differences between individual animals in a given group. When planning experiments, it is prudent to try to minimise this variation by selecting groups of animals matched for age, sex, body weight, genetic strain and so on. This is straightforward in many cases, but occasionally difficulties may arise and this is often true of pathological material. One of the characteristics of pathological change is an increase in variability between animals so that several heterogeneous disease stages are found concurrently. We may also attempt to reduce the contribution which inter-animal variation makes to the variance of a group mean by trying to ensure that adequate numbers of animals are investigated. It makes little statistical or biological sense to make lots of measurements on one or two animals. Indeed, if measurements are confined to one animal per experimental group there are *no* statistical grounds for detecting significant biological differences between groups and, in this sense, the effort is totally wasted.

Nested sampling designs

Much of quantitative microscopical anatomy is concerned with measurements made on tissue sections. This introduces further sources of error into the experimental scheme because the routine preparative steps for microscopical observation require that the animals (or parts thereof) be sampled at a series of successive levels. For example, each *animal* provides a set of tissue *blocks* and some of these are cut to obtain thin *sections* from which *fields* of view are selected for *measurement*.

Such hierarchical schemes are described as nested, cluster, multi-level or cascade sampling designs (Shay, 1975; Weibel, 1979a; Cruz Orive & Weibel, 1981). The need for these schemes partly reflects the requirement of good lateral resolution in the final image and partly the realisation that it is seldom practicable to examine all of the material which is present in a group of animals. A typical scheme is illustrated in Fig. 4.1.

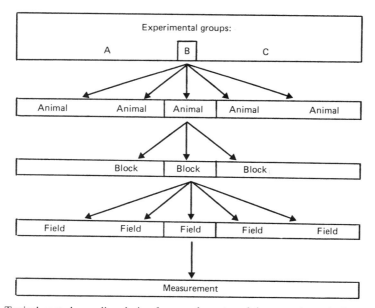

Fig. 4.1. Typical nested sampling design for morphometry of tissue sections. A single section is taken from each block so that, in this design, $(3 \times 5) = 15$ fields are analysed per animal.

It is easy to see that the final variation which we observe between animals in a particular group is really compounded of several sources of variation. These can be classified as inter-animal and intra-animal errors. The former includes the biological variation over which we have no absolute control but has superposed upon it the intra-animal errors ascribable to differences between blocks, between sections and between fields. Finally, there is the error determined by the inherent precision of the method of measurement. Over these intra-animal errors we can and should exercise control. We shall see how anon.

Sources of systematic error

The danger of introducing systematic errors unwittingly, stems from the likelihood that they may lead us to detect 'significant differences' where none exist or to detect 'no significant difference' where one actually exists (Shay, 1975). Moreover, once a sample of fields has been obtained and analysed, no amount of examination or manipulation of the results alone will disclose these errors (Stuart, 1976; Cochran, 1977). The best we can hope to say is that no systematic errors are apparent and this means that we must scrutinise carefully all those steps in the selection process at which errors of this sort might be introduced (Stuart, 1976).

In stereological studies, systematic errors arise in three main ways: (a) selection bias may be introduced into the sampling design, (b) technical bias may occur because of limitations of technique and (c) estimation bias may be introduced by applying inappropriate formulae when converting planar data to stereological data, component densities to absolute quantities and so on.

Selection bias

Randomised sampling at all levels is of decisive importance. Paradoxically, random sampling offers no guarantee that the final sample will be representative of each animal or organ being investigated (Stuart, 1976). It serves primarily to ease our conscience that we have not selected deliberately 'average' or 'typical' features. Therefore, random sampling is relevant not only to quantitative studies but also to investigations of qualitative morphology. Selecting 'average' or 'typical' micrographs implies that we know *a priori* what is average or typical and usually ensures only that we do not find either of them.

How then do we aim for a sample free from selection bias? The answer is simple: select animals (or organs), blocks, sections, fields and histological components regardless of their quality or content. Obviously, this must be tailored to suit the demands of a particular study. Often, we want to study only animals of a given age, strain, weight, etc.; sometimes, to facilitate identification of cell type, we may find it expedient to select fields which contain cell profiles sectioned across particular planes, such as those which pass through the nucleus or nucleolus (Mayhew & Williams, 1971; Mayhew & Cruz Orive, 1975). But even here, we must try to select cell profiles so that the only qualitative criterion is whether or not they contain a nucleus or nucleolus. Later, we may try to compensate for the specific bias towards nuclear/nucleolar planes of sectioning by applying mathematical correction procedures (Mayhew & Cruz Orive, 1973, 1975; Cruz Orive, 1976a,b).

When counting and sizing individual particle profiles appearing on thin sections, it often happens that a proportion of the profiles lie at the edges of the microscopical field of view. In such cases it is important to deal with those profiles which do not fall completely within the field of view by means of an unbiased selection rule. Several rules are available for circumventing so-called edge effects and are described in Gundersen (1977) and Miles (1978).

A convenient and efficient way of selecting sampling items at successive levels is systematic random sampling (Weibel, 1979a). The essence of this approach is that the position and orientation of the first item in the sample is decided purely by chance (e.g., by lottery, tables of random numbers) but that the position and orientation of all subsequent items are determined by those of the first. A practical example at the organ level would be to cut the organ into a series of slices, select the first slice at random and then select every fourth slice in the complete series. Test lattices may also be designed so that test points, intersections and areas are selected on a systematic random basis (various lattice designs are illustrated in Weibel, 1979a).

The virtues of systematic random sampling are illustrated here with a synthetic model. Imagine a cube of tissue T containing a histological component C which accounts for 50% of tissue volume (i.e. the volume density of C in T = 0.5) and arranged as shown in Fig. 4.2(*a*). Now let us cut the cube by section planes which, for ease of presentation, pass parallel to its front face so that we obtain a total of 10 slices. We propose to estimate the volume density of C in T by point counting methods (Weibel, 1979*a*).

We will begin by throwing a single random point on to each section in turn. It is easy to appreciate that this test point has an equal chance of falling inside or outside C but always hits the tissue T (Fig. 4.2*b*). Therefore, the probability that the point will hit C

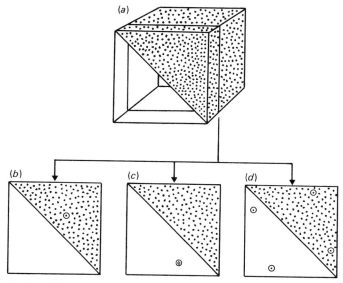

Fig. 4.2. Synthetic model to compare simple with systematic random sampling for point counting volumetry. The model (*a*) comprises a tissue cube T containing a component C (stippled) of volume density = 0.5. Ten sections are cut parallel to the front face of the cube and one such section plane is indicated. Each section is analysed with different test point arrangements: (*b*) a single random point (circled and hitting C); (*c*) a simple random set of 4 near-coincident points (circled and all hitting T but not C); (*d*) a systematic array of 4 points (each point circled, 2 hitting C and 4 hitting T). For further details, consult text and Table 4.2.

is equal to 0.5 which is equivalent to the volume density of C in T. The appropriate calculations will reveal that the expected variance between 10 sections is 0.2778 (Table 4.2) and that this estimate is achieved at a relative cost of 10 test points (one point per section). An index of efficiency for this simple random sampling scheme can be expressed as $1/(0.2778 \times 10)$ or roughly 0.36.

Now let us analyse the same sections with a set of four test points so close together as to be almost coincident but, again, positioned randomly on each section (Fig. 4.2*c*). Effectively, the fixed set of points now behaves as the single point used above and so we expect to obtain the same unbiased mean of 0.5 and the same variance between sections of 0.2778 (Table 4.2). However, the relative cost is now 40 test points (four per section) so the efficiency index now falls to $1/(0.2778 \times 40)$ which is roughly 0.09. We have obtained the *same* mean and variance for four times the effort!

Finally, we analyse the same sections with a systematic array of four test points (arranged, for instance, at the corners of an imaginary square) randomly positioned

Table 4.2. *Relative efficiencies of different test point arrangements for estimating the volume density of component C in tissue T (for model, see Fig. 4.2)*

Section number	Simple random 1 point		Simple random 4 points		Systematic random 4 points	
	P_C	P_T	P_C	P_T	P_C	P_T
1	0	1	0	4	2	4
2	0	1	4	4	2	4
3	1	1	4	4	1	4
4	0	1	4	4	2	4
5	1	1	0	4	2	4
6	1	1	0	4	2	4
7	1	1	4	4	2	4
8	1	1	0	4	3	4
9	0	1	4	4	2	4
10	0	1	0	4	2	4
Point totals	5	10	20	40	20	40
Means (P_C/P_T)	0.5		0.5		0.5	
Variance between sections	0.2778		0.2778		0.0139	
Cost in points	10		40		40	
Index of efficiency	0.36		0.09		1.80	

and orientated on each section in turn. If these points are sufficiently far apart, we can ensure that only one, two or three points can hit C on each section (Fig. 4.2d). On average, we anticipate that two out of four points will hit C and expect the same unbiased estimate of 0.5 for the volume density. Note, however, that the variation between sections falls dramatically. In the trial indicated in Table 4.2, the variance between sections is found to be 0.0139 for a relative cost of 40 test points. Therefore, the corresponding index of efficiency rises to 1/(0.0139 × 40) or 1.80, which is far higher than either of the indices for the two simple random sampling schemes.

This synthetic model emphasises several important practical considerations. First, all the randomised sampling schemes produce unbiased estimates of the volume density of C in T. Second, a dense packing of test points is less efficient than a widely dispersed arrangement. Third, a systematic random array is more efficient than a simple random array.

The superior efficiency of systematic random over simple random can be explained by the fact that, with the latter arrangement, two or more test points can come to lie very close together. Statistically speaking, the additional points convey no new information and are superfluous; they decrease efficiency because more points are counted to obtain the same information. In practice then, it is better to scatter test points systematically over as wide an area of section as possible.

These considerations apply equally well to other sampling levels. Thus, it is usually unnecessary to take more than one section from each block of tissue; taking more than one section effectively samples the same region and is unlikely to provide new information. Microscopical fields of view should be spread over as wide an area of this section as is practicable, preferably using a systematic random selection procedure (using, for instance, an eyepiece graticule or the x, y-axes of stage micrometers in the case of light microscopy; the squares of the supporting copper grid in the case of electron microscopy).

The principal caution in using systematic random sampling is to check for inherent periodicities in the biological specimen which may coincide with the periodicity of the systematic sampling design. If the patterns coincide, efficiency is likely to suffer (Weibel, 1979*a*).

Technical bias

Various systematic errors are influenced by technical limitations. It is impracticable to review all of these here, but mention will be made of the most common sources. These include tissue processing, image resolution, specimen contrast, section thickness and sectioning angle. More detailed discussions of these topics will be found elsewhere (see Reith, Barnard & Rohr, 1976; Williams, 1977; Weibel, 1979*a*).

Tissue processing (fixation, dehydration, embedding, sectioning) may alter the dimensions of the specimen by shrinkage, swelling and compression. For comparative studies, the resulting biases may not be important provided that they are similar in the different experimental groups. In this case, if you have a standardised procedure which provides reproducible results, stick to it! Where more absolute data are required (say for comparison with biochemical or physiological data), it is advisable to estimate pertinent shrinkage/swelling/compression factors. Remember, however, that if the shrinkage/swelling is concentric and uniform throughout the specimen, then estimates of component densities having the same dimensions in the component and reference (i.e. volume density V_V, surface density S_S, length density L_L and numerical density N_N – refer to Table 4.1) should not be affected. Other component densities will have to be corrected accordingly.

The amount of tissue shrinkage depends on the particular procedures employed. Paraffin embedding may incur substantial shrinkage but with epoxy resin embedding there is much less of a problem. The question of the effective osmolarity of buffered fixatives remains a moot one, though it appears that both the fixative concentration and buffer osmolarity determine the effective osmotic pressure of glutaraldehyde fixatives (see also Lee *et al.*, 1982).

In addition to the choice of fixative and buffer, it may be necessary to consider the method of fixation. With human material, one may be forced to take biopsies and immerse them in cold fixative. In other situations, it may be advantageous to fix tissues *in situ* by vascular perfusion at body temperature; in the case of lung, there may be advantages in doing this whilst air-inflating at various positive pressures rather than by instilling fixative into the respiratory passages (Gehr *et al.*, 1978; Weibel, 1979*a*).

Some stereological estimates seem to be especially sensitive to resolution effects. In particular, surface densities of pulmonary alveoli (Gehr *et al.*, 1978) and certain intracellular membranes (Paumgartner, Losa & Weibel, 1981) may be seriously underestimated at lower magnifications. In the case of mitochondrial and endoplasmic reticulum membranes, it is not yet clear to what extent the so-called resolution effect is influenced by the observer's criteria for identifying organelles and their membranes (Reith & Mayhew, 1980). Estimates of other structural quantities, such as organelle number (Mayhew & Williams, 1974), are also susceptible to magnification effects. Therefore, it is advisable to check that the magnification at the microscope is sufficient to ensure satisfactory lateral resolution of the structures under examination.

Specimen contrast also influences our ability to identify microscopical structures unambiguously. Generally speaking, insufficient contrast results in the underestimation of component densities. When this is due to the near-tangential sectioning of components, the systematic errors incurred can be appreciable. This is especially true of numerical density estimates where it is often necessary to compensate for resolution and contrast effects which lead to optically 'lost caps' (see Elias *et al.*, 1971; Weibel, 1979*a*).

A perennial bugbear in stereological work is section thickness. Most of the basic stereological principles are derived on the assumption that sections are true planes (i.e. have zero thickness). In fact, histological sections (and this includes ultrathin sections prepared for electron microscopy) have a positive thickness. Moreover, most sections are viewed by transmission (electron transmission or transmitted light) and, consequently, the images of components (especially contrasty components) are really projected through the section thickness.

This effect, the Holmes (or overprojection) effect, tends to overestimate component densities. The magnitude of the bias depends crucially on the relationship between section thickness (t) and particle mean projected height (H), the latter being determined by particle size, shape and spatial orientation. For spheres, H is equivalent to their mean diameter. Using this simple model and correction formulae reviewed elsewhere (Weibel, 1979*a*), the approximate magnitudes of these effects on estimates of V_V, S_V and N_V are illustrated in Fig. 4.3. Note that the graphs assume

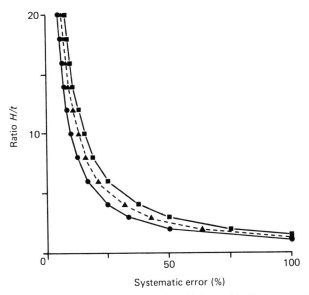

Fig. 4.3. Approximate systematic errors due to section thickness (t) effects on various component densities of spheres with mean diameter H. In practice, the errors may be smaller than indicated due to opposing contrast and resolution effects. Numerical density, N_V ●——● ; surface density, S_V ▲--▲; volume density, V_V ■——■ .

perfect specimen contrast and resolution so that the errors obtained in practice may be partially compensated by the underestimations due to these effects.

Overprojection can be ignored, provided that H is at least ten times t and that it does not have differential effects in different experimental groups. In other circumstances, it is desirable to try to estimate section thickness in order to compensate for overprojection. Various methods for doing so are available (see Williams, 1977; Weibel, 1979*a*). Correction procedures for component densities and particle shapes other than those used to construct Fig. 4.3 will be found in Gundersen (1979), Mayhew (1979*c*) and Weibel (1979*a*, 1980).

Finally, the angle of sectioning can lead to technical bias. Images of biological membranes prepared for inspection by transmission electron microscopy tend to disappear when tilted at too large an angle (beyond about 30°) within the section (Loud, 1967). To some extent, the magnitude of the membrane loss is influenced by the observer's criteria for recognising membrane images but it also depends on the class to which a particular organelle membrane belongs (Reith & Mayhew, 1980). Possible approaches to minimising these sources of error, which influence primarily estimates of membrane surface densities, are considered elsewhere (Reith *et al.*, 1976; Mall, Kayser & Rossner, 1977; Reith & Mayhew, 1980). In individual circumstances, it may be more appropriate to estimate the critical angle by goniometry rather than rely on angles and correction factors used by other investigators (T. M. Mayhew & A. Reith, unpublished observations).

Estimation bias

Systematic errors may be introduced inadvertently by applying inappropriate stereological and/or statistical formulae. Remember that certain stereological formulae only apply under particular conditions (e.g., that a membrane surface shows no preferred direction of orientation or that particles have a specific shape and ·size distribution).

An example of a statistical source of possible bias is offered in Mayhew & Cruz Orive (1974). More comprehensive treatments will be found in Miles & Davy (1977), Coleman (1979), Cruz Orive (1980*b*, 1982), Cruz Orive & Weibel (1981) and Jensen & Gundersen (1982).

When estimating the observed variance between animal means, straightforward statistical procedures can be followed in most cases (e.g., Bailey, 1972). However, when estimating variances between blocks and between fields of view it must be remembered that component densities are ratios, because more appropriate ways of estimating their means and variances may be required (Cochran, 1977; Gundersen, 1979; Mathieu *et al.*, 1981*a*; Mayhew, 1981). The procedures described in Shay (1975) are suitable for single variables, such as profile diameter measurements, but would not be applicable to estimates of component densities unless the reference area (or reference length) was the same on every field.

Therefore, it is important to apply correct statistical procedures when deriving and analysing stereological data. Whenever in doubt, consult a statistician but be sure to present the biological problem clearly as well as the statistical problem. The experience can be mutually rewarding.

ECONOMY OF EFFORT IN STEREOLOGY

An illustration of the efficiency of sampling

The accuracy, precision and cost-effectiveness which can be enjoyed by sampling histological components will be illustrated by results from a morphometric analysis of myelinated fibres in peripheral nerve trunks. A preliminary account of part of this work has been given elsewhere (Gupta *et al.*, 1983).

Biopsies of tibial nerves from four experimental diabetic rats were removed from a constant site, immersion-fixed in glutaraldehyde/paraformaldehyde, post-fixed in osmium tetroxide and embedded in Araldite. One block of tissue per animal was chosen by lottery and cut to provide a single, arbitrary transverse section. This was photographed to produce a montage of the complete nerve transection at a final print magnification of × 800.

This is a very useful experimental system because, with only 3000 myelinated fibres per montage, it is possible to measure the diameter of every fibre in each biopsy. By doing so, one obtains 'true' estimates of the mean diameter and variance for a group of animals virtually free of sampling errors due to variation between fibres and the precision of the method of measurement. Such estimates are used here as a yardstick for evaluating the accidental errors incurred by systematic random sampling.

To make these evaluations, we began by positioning and orienting a simple square lattice independently on each montage. All squares containing fibre centres were then assigned a number. This provided a basis for sampling groups of fibres with replacement. After first measuring every fibre on a digitising tablet and recording the time taken, we started a sampling trial by choosing one number (and hence one square) by lottery. The location of this square determined the positions of all subsequent squares because we decided beforehand to select every fourth square in 'vertical' and 'horizontal' directions (see Fig. 4.4). On average, this design succeeded in capturing about 6% of the 3000 fibres found on each montage.

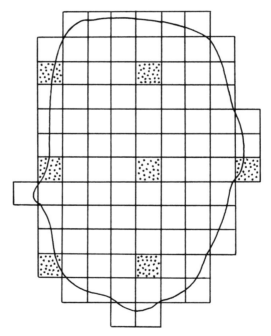

Fig. 4.4. Procedure for systematic random sampling of groups of nerve fibres. A test lattice of squares is positioned independently on a complete transverse section across a tibial nerve trunk (curved outline). Only lattice squares which contained fibre centres are illustrated. One square was selected by lottery and this determined the positions of all the other squares in the sample (stippled). Fibres whose centres lay within these squares were measured.

To avoid selection bias due to edge effects, we measured only those fibres whose centres lay within each square (Miles, 1978). We also noted the time taken to measure these fibres. Altogether, five sampling trials were undertaken. After each trial, we estimated the group mean fibre diameter from the individual animal means and the observed variance between the four rats.

Table 4.3. *Efficiency of systematic random sampling for estimating mean fibre diameter of tibial nerve biopsies from n = 4 rats. 'True' values were obtained by measuring every myelinated fibre in each complete nerve transection*

	'True' values	Sampling trials				
		1	2	3	4	5
Total fibre number	11 801	749	788	664	730	700
Measurement time (h)	19.5	1.2	1.3	1.1	1.2	1.2
Group mean fibre diameter (μm)	5.87	5.96	5.88	5.59	5.95	5.83
Observed variance between rats (μm^2)	0.306	0.320	0.533	0.630	0.409	0.340
Efficiency index	0.17	2.60	1.44	1.44	2.04	2.45

The results are summarised in Table 4.3. Measuring every fibre on each montage (a total of nearly 12 000 fibres) yielded a group mean diameter of 5.9 μm and an overall variance of 0.306 μm^2. This analysis took almost 20 hours, giving an efficiency index of 0.17. Note that the five sampling trials gave estimated group means which were all within 5% of the 'true' value. This range is a measure of the accidental error incurred by sampling and does *not* represent its systematic error. Therefore, the group estimates obtained by sampling were unbiased and highly reproducible. Their precision, reflected in the reciprocal of the observed variance between animals, was generally less than that achieved by measuring all fibres. Observed variances fell within the range 0.320–0.630 μm^2 and this serves to underline the point that estimated variances can be rather imprecise (Gundersen & Østerby, 1981). In this case, the imprecision is probably due mainly to the small number of animals studied and might be diminished in the final biological experiment by examining biopsies from more rats.

Despite the relative imprecision revealed by these results, we are comforted by the observation that the relative cost of sampling was only 1.1–1.3 hours. In consequence, it transpires that the indices of efficiency varied from 1.44 to 2.60 and this means that the sampling design was *at least* eight times more efficient than measuring every fibre! The time saved by sampling is more than enough to compensate for the increased number of animals that *may* be required to detect significant differences between experimental groups.

Designing cost-effective sampling schemes

The above example emphasises the fact that a particular sampling scheme can often be improved by analysing the results of a pilot study and identifying the sources of variation which contribute to the overall precision of the final morphometric estimate(s). With a multi-level sampling design, this means exploring variation at each sampling level. Assuming that prior consideration has been given to the question of what biological variable to measure, we will discuss sampling levels starting with the lowest level: the measurement of microscopical fields.

How many 'measurements'?

Under this heading, we can consider both the number and type of measurements. It has been stated already that all component densities can be estimated by counting events (numbers of profiles, test points and test intersections). Experience has shown that the concomitant loss of measuring precision is often of no consequence when compared with the variation between profiles, between fields, between blocks and between animals (Gundersen & Østerby, 1980, 1981; Mathieu *et al.*, 1981*a*; Gupta *et al.*, 1983). Even when specific dimensions are sought (e.g., the mean size and size distributions of nerve fibres, or of particle profiles in order to estimate numerical densities), it may not be necessary to measure every individual profile – it may suffice merely to classify them, with considerable saving of analysis time and little or no loss of overall precision (Gundersen, Seefeldt & Østerby, 1980; Gundersen, Boysen & Reith, 1981). The unifying theme then is 'classification' – is this profile a nucleus to be counted? Is this test point hitting the nuclear profile? Is this test line intersecting the nuclear envelope? Is this nuclear profile in size class 4, 5 or 6?

By now the reader may be unconvinced, even frankly incredulous. I therefore include a comparison of measurement versus classification based on analysis of the nerve fibres described above. As part of our pilot study, we wished to compare the precision of machine (digitiser) measurement with that of a simple classification procedure, i.e. the 'circle of best fit' method (Fernand & Young, 1951). For this purpose, estimates of fibre diameter were obtained by analysing the same systematic random samples of fibres from the four montages.

Fibres were measured first on the digitiser tablet and then classified with the aid of ten concentric circles varying in equal diameter increments equivalent to 1.5 μm on the specimens and reproduced onto a transparent overlay. For the size distributions based on digitisation, the class interval was slightly smaller than that of the concentric circles (1.48 μm versus 1.5 μm, a difference of less than 2%).

After each sample had been analysed, we calculated the mean fibre diameter for that animal together with its standard deviation (S.D.). We then calculated the group mean fibre diameter together with its standard error (S.E.M.).

The results are given in Table 4.4. Animal means for this sample of 749 fibres varied between 5.4 μm and 6.7 μm when individual fibre diameters were measured precisely

Table 4.4. *Measuring versus classifying nerve fibres. Results based on a systematic random sample of 749 myelinated fibres from 4 rats*

Animal		Fibre no.	Diameter (μm) mean ± S.D.
(a) Measuring			
	1	210	6.72 ± 2.35
	2	197	5.36 ± 2.00
	3	156	5.85 ± 2.27
	4	186	5.89 ± 2.03
		Group mean ± S.E.M.:	5.96 ± 0.28
(b) Classifying			
	1	210	6.69 ± 2.39
	2	197	5.36 ± 2.00
	3	156	5.87 ± 2.29
	4	186	5.81 ± 1.98
		Group mean ± S.E.M.:	5.94 ± 0.28

on the digitiser tablet. The group mean ± S.E.M. was 6.0 ± 0.28 μm. Within each animal the fibre-to-fibre variation was very similar, the S.D. being in the order of 34–39% of the individual animal mean.

Classifying the same fibres yielded a group mean ± S.E.M. of 5.9 ± 0.28 μm, the range of individual animal means being 5.4–6.7 μm. Moreover, the within-animal between-fibre variation was, again, 34–39%.

Thus, estimates of group mean fibre size and overall precision obtained by these extremes of measuring precision were not significantly different. Indeed, nor were the final fibre size-frequency distributions (T. M. Mayhew, A. K. Sharma & K. S. Bedi, unpublished observations).

It is also pertinent to note that the analysis times were 1.2 hours for digitisation and 1.0 hours for classification. Classifying fibres was slightly more efficient than measuring them.

These general conclusions are supported by results from several independent studies (Fraher, 1980; Mathieu *et al.*, 1981a; Gundersen *et al.*, 1981) which confirm that the precisions of different methods of 'measurement' are comparatively unimportant.

We now turn to the question of the requisite numbers of test points and test intersections to be counted in order to obtain reliable estimates of animal means, a recurrent question in morphometry. This can be tackled in several ways which vary in sophistication, depending on the determination of the individual investigator to achieve maximal economy of effort.

At the basic level, we can consider the design of the test lattice. We have seen already how spreading test points can improve overall precision and efficiency. Exactly analogous models could be used for test intersections and give similar conclusions. With point counting volumetry, the simplest precaution is to apply a test lattice of such a point density that the area of each square is no smaller than that of the largest profile in the population being evaluated (Weibel, 1979a). Alternatively, one may design a lattice so that no more than about 200 test points fall on the component and no more than 200 on the reference. These totals represent the limits on any given animal and the same limitations can be employed for intersection counts (Gundersen & Østerby, 1980, 1981). These suggestions emphasise the value of designing dual-purpose lattices bearing coarse points (lines) for evaluating the reference and fine points (lines) for the component (see Weibel, 1979a).

Where a more statistical approach is felt desirable, it is possible to estimate the minimal number of points and intersections required to attain an acceptable level of precision on a given set of fields taken from one animal. For example, the relative standard error approach has been employed to calculate test probe numbers for volume densities (Hally, 1964) and surface densities (Weibel, 1979a). By consulting nomograms relating test point number and test line length to relevant component densities and expected relative standard errors, more economical numbers of events can be counted for a given experimental design.

An alternative method involves the construction of cumulative or progressive mean plots which can be used to decide on the minimal numbers of profiles, points and intersections (Dunnill, 1968; Weibel, 1979a). The method involves analysing a pilot sample of fields and deriving the desired quantities for the component(s) of interest. The raw data are then used to compute cumulative mean estimates of these quantities for increasing numbers of fields (and, hence, increasing numbers of points, intersections, etc.). The number required to attain and remain within, say, ± 10% of the final cumulative mean is taken to be the minimal sample size for that particular quantity in that particular experimental group of animals. It is therefore sensible, as with the relative standard error approach, to analyse sets of fields from more than one animal in each pilot group so as to allow for inter-animal differences.

It is advisable to do this much at least in the search for economical sampling schemes. However, the methods just outlined have the disadvantage that whilst they permit us to estimate the numbers of events and fields they do not tell us the best way in which to divide those items amongst the blocks representing a given animal. Herein lies the practical benefit of studying variances at different sampling levels (Shay, 1975; Gundersen & Østerby, 1980, 1981).

The optimal sampling scheme (blocks and fields)

The biologist is rightly interested more in the biological problem than in fine details of technique such as how to design the optimal sampling regime for the material which he has available. After all, provided there are enough animals in each group there is no need to be worried unduly about the division of sampling labour within animals. Two factors influence this generalisation: firstly, additional constraints (e.g., the time taken to prepare and process material, ethical considerations) may make it difficult for us to select more animals or to add more animals to existing groups. This is particularly true for the pathologist working with human material and of quantitative electron microscopical autoradiography where exposures may take many months (Williams, 1977). Secondly, there are the increasing external demands for financial economies within research institutions. In this context, we are forced to be more conscious of the purchase and running costs of equipment and materials. Methods which allow experimental designs to be rationalised, by reducing numbers of blocks and micrographs, are of increasing concern to a growing number of research workers.

Procedures for providing cost-beneficial sampling schemes, suitable for multi-level designs, are founded on the well-established statistical device known as analysis of variance (e.g., see Sokal & Rohlf, 1969). A new, elegant and simple approach has been proposed as an alternative to multi-level sampling (Stringer, Wynford-Thomas & Williams, 1982). In this method, the natural architecture of the specimen is physically randomised *before* embedding, thereby minimising at an early stage the block-to-block and field-to-field differences built in to multi-level sampling regimes.

The idea behind analysis of variance is to balance the isolated variances at successive sampling levels against the costs of making additional observations at those levels. Clearly, it would be imprudent to analyse many micrographs per block if the micrographs were found to vary very little and/or were much more expensive than blocks.

In the typical nested scheme shown in Fig. 4.1, it can be seen that the total variation observed between animals, which we can denote as Os_a^2, is really a summation of four elements of variation: (a) s_a^2, the true variation between the animals, (b) s_b^2, the variation between tissue blocks selected from those animals, (c) s_f^2, the variation between fields selected from the tissue blocks (we suppose that only one section is cut from each block) and (d) s_m^2 variation due to the measuring precision. Since we now know that the last element is usually unimportant, we need not resolve the variances s_f^2 and s_m^2 and may instead use the composite term s_{fm}^2 to signify the sampling variance due to 'fields plus measurement'.

The relationships between these variances can be expressed as follows:

$$Os_a^2 = s_a^2 + s_b^2/n_b + s_{fm}^2/(n_b \times n_f)$$

(e.g., Gundersen & Østerby, 1981) where n_b is the mean number of independent tissue blocks per animal and n_f is the mean number of independent microscopical fields per tissue block.

By applying similar relationships to estimated variances from actual pilot experiments, it is possible to evaluate the contribution made by each sampling level to the overall variation observed between animals. In fact, there is a substantial body of experimental evidence to suggest that inter-animal variation often overshadows all sources of intra-animal variation which are present within nested sampling designs. In several tissue systems, differences between animals account for 53–86% of the total observed variation (Shay, 1975; Gundersen & Østerby, 1980, 1981; Gupta *et al.*, 1983). Such studies serve to emphasise that there is much to be gained by making relatively crude measurements on more animals rather than precise measurements on few animals. Increasing the number of individuals per experimental group often provides the most efficient division of effort for reducing the s.e.m. of a group of animals, the crucial statistic for comparing one group with another.

Inter-animal variation is not always the major contributor to total variance. There are plenty of examples in biology of individual animal means varying very little (e.g., blood pH in man is normally between 7.35 and 7.45; oral temperature is normally 35.8–37.7° C). Gundersen & Østerby (1980) have found that the total glomerular filtration surface of the rat kidney does not vary between subjects. Moreover, the widths of podocytic pedicels in the renal corpuscles of normal men and rats show remarkably little variation between subjects, the biological significance of which is, as yet, unknown (Gundersen *et al.*, 1980). We cannot doubt that it *is* significant (because small differences between individuals are indicative of rigid control being exercised over variables of major adaptive and functional import) but the model does offer an example of the way in which Nature cherishes her secrets – like Einstein's God, she is 'subtle but not malicious'.

A second caution to note is that the influence which inter-animal variation exerts on a sampling scheme is itself a product of that scheme. In a badly designed experiment, intra-animal differences can be so large that they reduce or even overwhelm the contribution to total variance made by inter-animal differences. This is another good reason for keeping a close scrutiny of all sources of variation.

Having isolated sampling variances, it is now possible to deal with costs and design the optimal sampling scheme. We have stated earlier that costs are most conveniently described in terms of time rather than money. Therefore, let us define C_a as being the cost (in minutes, working hours, etc.) of including one extra animal, C_b as the cost of trimming and cutting one additional block and C_f as the cost of recording and analysing one extra microscopical field. To predict the optimal number of fields per block (On_f) and the optimal number of blocks per animal (On_b), we can use the formulae:

$$On_f = [(s_{fm}^2/s_b^2)\,(C_b/C_f)]^{1/2} \text{ and}$$
$$On_b = [(s_b^2/s_a^2)\,(C_a/C_b)]^{1/2}$$

(Sokai & Rohlf, 1969; Shay, 1975). The resulting estimates should be treated as reasonable working approximations in view of the fact that the estimated sampling variances and costs may be rather imprecise (Gundersen & Østerby, 1981; but also refer to the sampling trials on tibial nerve fibres).

In order to test the reproducibility of the analysis of variance approach and to illustrate actual results, I have applied it to the tibial nerve samples described above. The reader will recall that each animal provided one block which was cut to furnish one complete transverse section from which a photographic montage was constructed. Each montage was used to select a systematic random sample of squares (each containing a set of fibre centres). The sampling design therefore adopted two principal sampling levels, animals and squares, each having a particular element of variance (s_a^2, s_s^2) and a particular cost (C_a, C_s) associated with it. On average, the cost of measuring one extra myelinated fibre was 6 seconds, so the cost of one additional square could be expressed in terms of the time taken to measure all of the fibres which the average square contained. In the five sampling trials, estimates of C_s varied from 2.5 to 3 minutes. The cost of including one extra animal ($C_a = 90$ minutes) could be divided as follows: roughly 20 minutes for taking the biopsy, 45 minutes for trimming and sectioning the tissue block and a further 25 minutes for photography and preparing the montage.

Table 4.5. *Predicting optimal schemes for sampling myelinated nerve fibres in biopsies from n = 4 rats. Estimates of optimal numbers based on systematic random samples evaluated by analysis of variance*

	Sampling trials				
	1	2	3	4	5
No. of squares sampled per rat (range)	5–8	6–9	4–10	5–8	6–9
No. of fibres captured per rat (range)	156–210	162–221	105–206	146–214	149–196
Observed variance between rats (μm^2)	0.320	0.533	0.630	0.409	0.340
Proportion due to animals (%)	81	82	91	79	69
Proportion due to squares (%)	19	18	9	21	31
Optimal no. of squares per rat (mean)	6.6	7.3	4.8	7.1	10.6
Optimal no. of fibres per rat (mean)	197	197	122	207	264

Results are summarised in Table 4.5. Despite the imprecision of estimated sampling variances, inter-animal differences in all trials accounted for the overwhelming proportion (69–91%) of the total variance observed between animals, supporting earlier conclusions regarding its importance. The predicted optimal number of squares per animal ranged from 5 to 11 and, when interpreted in terms of optimal numbers of fibres, this represented 122–264 fibres per animal. There is therefore a reasonable measure of agreement between sampling trials, illustrating the reproducibility of the design.

The results further suggest that, for future studies on these diabetic rats, the preliminary sampling scheme within animals is already near-optimal. It might be improved only slightly, i.e. by sampling about 7% of the total number of fibres per animal rather than the 6% sampled by the original design. In other words, this would mean selecting about 200 fibres rather than 180 per animal – a modest investment when compared with the effort involved in measuring all 3000 fibres in the average biopsy.

Methods for reducing intra-animal variability

An elementary precaution for reducing field-to-field variation is to ensure that the instrument magnification is the lowest which still permits satisfactory resolution of the histological/subcellular structures being analysed (Cruz Orive & Weibel, 1981).

Unnecessarily high magnifications only increase variability between fields and reduce sampling efficiency.

Another way of achieving smaller variation between fields relies on a sensible choice of the reference. Thus, when dealing with components associated with cell membranes (e.g., synapses, desmosomes, microvilli) it may be more efficient to estimate component densities on a surface in preference to densities in a volume. Studies on desmosomes in forearm skin from human patients have revealed that this can reduce electron micrograph requirements by about 50% with no loss in precision of the final estimate (Mayhew, 1981). In more general terms, when estimating component densities, try to choose the smallest reference which bears or contains the component of interest (Cruz Orive & Weibel, 1981).

Occasionally, it pays to transform raw data into an alternative form: for instance, take the logarithm, sine, square root or reciprocal of a particular variable. Transformations of this sort have proved extremely valuable for dealing with microscopical structures whose dimensions vary greatly: for instance, glomerular basement membrane thickness and pedicel width (Gundersen, 1980; Gundersen *et al.*, 1980).

For small organs, such as the rat thyroid gland, considerable savings in sectioning can be effected by dicing the tissue and randomly embedding the pieces in one block (Stringer *et al.*, 1982). This method has been shown to yield very efficient estimates of component volume densities, even when thyroid architecture is rendered more heterogeneous by goitrogen-induced alterations.

How many animals?

Since inter-animal variation is often the decisive factor and the only variation over which we have no absolute control, it is natural to enquire: 'How many animals do I need in a given experimental group?'

Whilst it might seem prudent to investigate as many subjects as possible or to aim to achieve an s.e.m. of, say, ± 5% of the group mean, it is worth pausing to consider that the number of animals you require does not depend solely on the observed group variation. It also depends on the magnitude of the between-group difference you wish to detect as being statistically significant and on the statistical confidence with which you wish to detect it. Clearly, it is easier to detect significant group differences when the groups display little inter-animal variation and the group means differ greatly. Relatively few animals will be needed in such circumstances. Differences are harder to detect when the group means are very similar and when animals within those groups exhibit large differences. A pilot study will usually indicate the sort of investment that is required to suit particular circumstances.

Having performed a pilot study and analysed the within- and between-group variations, numbers of animals can be estimated by methods such as those described by Shay (1975) and Gundersen (1980).

Of machines and men

Many measuring devices are currently available commercially for quantifying microscopical components. These vary from the relatively simple and inexpensive planimeters and opisometers to the relatively sophisticated and expensive semi-automatic and automatic image analysing systems.

So far, we have seen how unbiased estimates of group means can be derived by applying a simple test lattice to carefully sampled sets of microscopical fields; how the precision of the group estimate depends crucially on the variation between animals and how precision of measurement on an individual profile or on a single field frequently introduces little uncertainty into the estimate of a group mean. At all levels of sampling, efficiency can be improved by balancing variation against cost.

Undoubtedly, the semi-automatic and automatic devices measure extremely precisely. But what of their efficiency? Do they speed up the measuring process so that more blocks and animals can be studied in a unit time? What is their financial cost when compared with the cost of manual methods? Do they introduce machine bias? These are the questions which define their value to the potential user interested in microscopical morphometry.

Analyses of tibial nerve fibres have shown that classification is slightly more efficient than digitisation in the sense that it provided essentially the same observed variance between animals in a shorter analysis time. Independent studies on other experimental and synthetic models (Gundersen et al., 1981; Mathieu et al., 1981a) have shown that semi-automatic digitiser systems and automatic image analysis are, at best, only as efficient as event counting and classification. A digitiser-based system measured structures accurately but at the expense of analysis time; an automatic image analyser failed to recognise different structures of similar grey level densities in specimens of skeletal muscle but was as efficient as point counting when employed to evaluate a synthetic model possessing sufficient contrast.

The real advantage of simple classification methods is best appreciated by comparing financial costs. A test lattice has a price which can be expressed in pence; the cost of a digitiser system currently varies from hundreds to thousands of pounds and the cost of an automatic device must be expressed in tens of thousands of pounds. 'Due to the lack of any obvious benefit of digitisers for the bulk of morphometric studies in biology, the choice of device is in favour of manual procedures' (Gundersen et al., 1981).

This is not to say that (semi-)automatic devices have no place in morphometry. It merely expresses the opinion that with most variables, especially component densities, manual methods are entirely satisfactory. This is an opinion with which I must concur. Certainly, I would not recommend purchasing a digitiser system expressly to estimate component densities or even particle (e.g., nerve fibre) size-frequency distributions. However, if one is available already, there appears to be no great disadvantage in employing it to measure selected nerve fibres at least (see above). Indeed, for certain sizing schemes it may be beneficial to do so. One advantage of such systems is that they allow several variables to be measured simultaneously. Fraher (1980) has found that digitisation yielded simultaneous estimates of axon area and circumference in about one-sixth of the time taken by making successive measurements. There is an obvious advantage here for studies requiring multiple measurements on the same structure and for pilot studies which seek to establish those variables which are suitable for detecting significant differences between populations.

Two final remarks about bias and cost: first, Fraher (1980) has concluded that alternative methods of measurement can engender small, but statistically significant degrees of bias. In consequence, one should be wary about comparing 'absolute' values published by different investigators employing different methods to estimate the same variable. The problem should be less important when a comparative study of experimental groups adopts the same method throughout, but it is wise to check that this is so.

Second, some digitiser systems are cheaper and more flexible than others. In those systems which interface the tablet to a dedicated computer, access to the computer as a general-purpose aid is extremely limited. It is far better to interface a digitiser-tablet to a non-dedicated computer which can be used for other purposes. The cost of digitisation then reduces to the price of the tablet alone. The most valuable piece of machinery for most morphometric purposes is the flexible computer, programmable to handle the raw data and subject them to statistical evaluation.

BIOLOGICAL EXAMPLES

The following applications of stereology in microscopical anatomy have been chosen to illustrate its power and potential and to offer examples of solutions to some of the practical problems mentioned in the preceding text. The selection is entirely personal; it is not intended to be exhaustive or to reflect on the quality of the numerous other applications which are to be found in the literature.

Anatomy and physiology of the lung

Pioneering studies by E. R. Weibel and his co-workers have indicated (*a*) the extent to which stereology has helped to interpret the microscopical anatomy and physiological performance of the mammalian lung and (*b*) the experimental precautions required to validate such correlations of structure and function. References to original articles can be found in recent reviews (Weibel, 1979*b*,*c*, 1982). The most recent investigations (see the special issue of *Respiration Physiology*, vol. 44, 1981) have dealt with the overall design and oxygen flow of the mammalian respiratory system from the pulmonary alveolus to skeletal muscle mitochondria.

Although the lung has many functions, its principal role is in respiration. Exchange of gases between the alveolus and blood is mediated by diffusion across the alveolar–capillary membrane or 'air–blood barrier'. Actually, this membrane comprises several barriers arranged in series.

The rate at which oxygen (O_2) diffuses across these barriers depends on the prevailing pressure gradient and on lung conductance. Physiologists express the latter in terms of the O_2 diffusion capacity, D_L, but this can also be estimated from a combination of morphometric and physical attributes of the diffusion pathway. It is proportional to the surface area between air and blood, to the permeability coefficients of tissue and plasma for O_2 and to the rate of O_2 binding to whole blood. It is also inversely proportional to the thickness of the air–blood barrier.

In the morphometric model proposed by Weibel, the O_2 diffusion route is divided into three parts: the tissue barrier, the blood plasma and the erythrocyte. For each component, a conductance is calculated from stereological data and from available physiological constants. In this way, a morphometric estimate of D_L is derived and can be compared with values obtained by physiological means.

Results for the 'healthy' human lung (see also Gehr *et al.*, 1978) have demonstrated that its exchange surface is less well-developed and substantially thicker than in many other mammals. Estimates of average alveolar surface area are extremely sensitive to technical bias from resolution effects and the value derived using electron microscopy (roughly $145\,m^2$) is considerably higher than that obtainable by light microscopy (about $80\,m^2$). On the basis of this improved value and other structural quantities, the morphometric D_L was calculated to be $125-265\,ml\ O_2\,min^{-1}\ (mm\,Hg)^{-1}$ the range reflecting discrepancies in published figures of the pertinent physical constants.

It was noted that the morphometric D_L is far higher than standard physiological estimates of $20-30\,ml\ O_2\,min^{-1}\ (mm\,Hg)^{-1}$. However, this range is based on measurements made under *basal* metabolic conditions, when O_2 uptake is minimal. Physiological measurements made under conditions of *maximal* workload give values of 80–100 ml O_2 min^{-1} (mm Hg)$^{-1}$.

The residual discrepancy could be partly explained by technical biases introduced by the method of fixation. The human lungs were fixed *in situ* by instilling glutaraldehyde into the airways *post mortem*. This has the tendency to wash away the alveolar surface lining, producing systematic overestimates of alveolar surface area and morphometric D_L values. Studies on air-inflated rat lungs fixed by vascular perfusion suggested that the bias was in the order of 25–50%. The revised morphometric D_L estimates fell in the range 60–190 ml O_2 min^{-1} (mm Hg)$^{-1}$ and were more in accord with the physiological estimates obtained under conditions of work.

Future technical improvements (Weibel, 1982) may lead to more refined estimates of morphometric D_L but, already, these investigations have provided a remarkable example of the mutual dependence of biological structure and function.

Similar studies may be performed on other respiratory exchange surfaces, such as the placenta (Laga, Driscoll & Munro, 1974). Indeed, for the human placenta, morphometry seems to offer at present the only way of assessing respiratory potential at full term.

Anisotropy and the intestinal villous surface

A recurring problem in stereological analysis of biological structures is anisotropy or preferential orientation. For a detailed discussion of this general problem, the reader is referred to Weibel (1980). Examples of highly anisotropic structures are skeletal muscle, kidney and stratified squamous epithelium. When sectioning such tissues, the planar data which are obtained will vary according to the position and/or orientation of the section plane. Therefore, stereological information may be biased if it is decided to restrict sectioning to some specific plane. It will be necessary to compensate for any imposed selection bias by correcting the final estimate. Alternatively, modified stereological formulae may be used (e.g., Whitehouse, 1974; Mall *et al.*, 1977). This possibility is illustrated by reference to the villi of the rat small intestine.

The ability of small intestine to digest and absorb food materials depends, amongst other things, on its surface area. The primary mucosal surface (defined, for convenience, as the imaginary boundary between bases of villi and openings of crypts) forms a long and much folded tube. In the rat, this surface is enlarged in two main ways: by villi and by microvilli. Amplification factors for these projections can be treated as component surface densities on a surface and estimated by intersection counting (Mayhew, 1979a).

For dealing with villous amplification factors, the basic stereological principle of value is $S_S = I_I$ (Mayhew, 1979a,b; Weibel, 1979a) where S_S represents the ratio between the villous and primary mucosal surfaces and I_I represents the ratio of intersection counts between these surfaces and independently positioned test line probes. However, the principle only holds for arbitrary section planes when both surfaces share the same orientation characteristics (Mayhew, 1981). It would only hold for transverse and longitudinal sections through an anisotropic tube, like the small intestine, if villi shared the same orientation characteristics as the near-cylindrical primary mucosa.

Mere inspection of intestine, by light or scanning electron microscopy, demonstrates that these conditions are not met. Quantitative studies, using transverse and longitudinal sections prepared for light microscopy, have confirmed subjective impressions and indicate that the intersection ratio I_I is always larger when estimated using longitudinal sections of proximal small intestine from the rat (Stenling & Helander, 1981). Significantly, longitudinal sectioning produced an intersection ratio which was, on average, 1.58 times larger than that obtained from transverse sections. This observation suggests that the overall villous surface is isotropic (i.e. shows no preferred orientation). In fact, geometrical reasoning predicts, that, for an isotropic surface arising from the internal surface of a circular cylinder, the factor linking intersection ratios on longitudinal and transverse sections is $\pi/2$ which is roughly 1.57 (unpublished results). Though the surface of an individual villus is patently anisotropic, the collective isotropy of villi may possibly be explained by the empirical observation that their long (height) axes tend to be arranged radially.

These considerations allow us to construct a geometric model of the rat small intestine which can be used to derive correction factors to substitute into a more suitable stereological principle, $S_S = kI_I$, where k is a constant determined by the sectioning approach. It transpires that $k = 4/\pi$ in the case of transverse sections and $8/\pi^2$ in the case of longitudinal sections. Moreover, systematic errors due to departures from villous isotropy should not exceed 10% provided that the factor linking longitudinal and transverse sections does not differ from 1.57 by more than about ± 0.15 (T. M. Mayhew, unpublished results).

Stenling & Helander (1981) estimated villous amplification factors by taking the mean of intersection ratios derived from longitudinal and transverse sections. This method tends to furnish estimates which are less sensitive to departures from isotropy but it may also be less efficient in view of the extra work involved. Unfortunately, it is not known to what extent these considerations influence amplification factors derived from biopsies of human material where the anatomy is complicated by plicae circulares. It is possible that systematic errors alter when the geometry of the villus/mucosa interface changes, as it does for instance during malabsorption syndromes (see e.g., Meinhard, Wadbrook & Risdon, 1975).

At present, we are using transverse sections to analyse regional differences in villous amplification factors along the rat small intestine (C. Middleton & T. M. Mayhew, unpublished results). Preliminary studies indicate that the amplification is larger in proximal regions (about seven-fold) and smaller in distal ileum (about three-fold). The findings are entirely in accord with the functional importance of proximal sites as the principal regions for digestion and absorption.

Regional variations in villous shape

Villi alter their relative and absolute dimensions in different regions of the small intestine. Though it is possible to estimate the dimensions of villous *profiles* seen in histological thin sections, there have been very few attempts to convert these data into values which quantitatively define variations in villous shape independent of their size. In this example, a stereological solution to this problem is described.

The method makes use of the shape factor $S^{3/2}/V$ as described in Østerby & Gundersen (1980). The studies were based on light microscopical morphometry of transverse sections taken from five different sites along the small intestines of rats (C. Middleton & T. M. Mayhew, unpublished results). At each site, estimates of villous surface area were derived from amplification factors (*see above*) and estimates of the circumference of the primary mucosa (determined by intersection counting). From these quantities, we calculated the surface area of all villi associated with an intestinal segment of length 1 cm. Estimates of the volume of all villi in the same length were obtained by point counting. Methods for counting the number of villi per unit length are described in Forrester (1972).

From these simple counts, we estimated the surface area (S) and volume (V) of the average villus at each site. Shape factors were calculated on the basis of these estimates. Regional differences in shape were tested in a group of nine animals.

The results indicate that there is no significant change in villous shape as one passes from the duodenum (site 1) to the first quarter of the jejunum and ileum (site 2, see Table 4.6). In both regions, the shape factor for the average villus was 15. Passing

Table 4.6. *Regional differences in the shapes of villi at five sites along the small intestine of n = 9 rats. Each shape factor is given as mean ± S.E.M.*

Shape factor	Site 1	Site 2	Site 3	Site 4	Site 5
$S^{3/2}/V$	15.2 ± 0.6	15.1 ± 0.6	12.4 ± 0.6	9.2 ± 0.5	8.3 ± 0.6

Site 1, duodenum; site 2, proximal jejunum; site 3, second quarter of jejunum + ileum; site 4, third quarter; site 5, terminal ileum.

from the first to second and from the second to third quarters of jejunum and ileum, shape factors dropped steadily and significantly to about 9. From this region to the terminal ileum, the apparent decrease was not significant. The results further indicate a progressive increase in variation between animals at more distal sites. This was evident when each S.E.M. was expressed as a percentage of its corresponding mean and may be another manifestation of the greater functional significance of proximal regions.

These quantitative findings are consistent with studies on intact villi made by scanning electron microscopy. Villi in more proximal regions (duodenum, proximal jejunum) tend to be rather broad and tall and have been described as leaf- and tongue-shaped. In contrast, villi in the ileum tend to be short and finger-like (e.g., Kessel & Kardon, 1979). Interestingly, our results suggest that villi in the terminal ileum possess a shape factor which is similar to that of a cylinder with a length : diameter ratio of about 2 : 3.

Shape factors offer a convenient way of defining the shapes of irregular villi such as those which appear to be incompletely fused or become damaged as a consequence of irradiation (Clarke, 1970; Carr, Hamlet & Watt, 1981).

Stereology in pathology : diabetic glomerulopathy

By applying stereological techniques to compare normal and diseased tissues, the experimental pathologist relies less upon subjective impressions and can define more exactly those morphological changes which might improve diagnosis and prognosis. They can also play an important part in assessing the efficacy of drugs and other forms of control. Though many examples could be offered, I have chosen to illustrate stereology in pathology by reference to diabetes mellitus.

Two manifestations of this disease, neuropathy and angiopathy, continue to attract especial morphometric attention. Much of this attention has been directed towards the microangiopathy which affects the renal glomeruli of human diabetics and experimental diabetic animals, though angiopathy affects most, if not all, of the organs in long-term diabetics. Studies by Ruth Østerby and her colleagues have helped to elucidate several aspects of glomerular microangiopathy and the following includes a summary of some of their findings. Additional references may be found in Østerby (1975), Rasch (1979), Steffes *et al.* (1979), Gundersen (1980) and Østerby & Gundersen (1980).

Glomerular changes are remarkably similar in human and animal models. Ultrastructural investigations on human patients and rats have established that the thickness of the glomerular capillary basement membrane (a component of the ultrafiltration barrier) provides a very reliable and sensitive indicator of the progressive development of the abnormality. Two measures of this thickness are of biological interest: its arithmetic mean thickness and its harmonic mean thickness (see also Weibel & Knight, 1964). The former offers a measure of membrane mass and has been employed to detect changes in basement membrane thickness at early stages of diabetes; the latter is directly proportional to the resistance which the membrane presents to ultrafiltration. Both variables may be estimated by simple classification procedures.

In the case of harmonic mean thickness, attention has been directed towards solving the question of the efficiency and bias of different methods for its estimation. It has been shown that transformations of the reciprocal type serve to normalise distributions of membrane thickness, increase overall efficiency and reduce estimation bias.

During the natural course of glomerular microangiopathy, basement membrane thickness increases significantly over a period of less than two years and the same phenomenon has been quantified in rats with long-term experimental diabetes. Indeed, there is a substantial thickening in rats after only four days of induced diabetes. Up to this point, the membrane thickening represents an increase in both the volume and surface area of glomeruli but thereafter it is due entirely to an increase in surface area, an observation which correlates well with the augmentation of glomerular filtration rate.

More recent studies (e.g., Rasch, 1979) have demonstrated that experimental diabetic glomerulopathy can be controlled by insulin treatment, indicating that good control of blood glucose can preserve normal basement membrane thickness. Transplanting pancreatic islets into diabetic animals has failed to preserve normal thickness (Steffes *et al.*, 1979), but this may be due to failure to achieve normal insulin levels in recipients.

Though these studies provide further evidence of good correlation between structure and function, one fundamental question remains unanswered – the causative factor(s) responsible for diabetes mellitus. It remains to be seen what role, if any, stereology can play in solving this mystery.

Particle number (counting synapses)

Counting synapses in thin sections illustrates the general problem of estimating particle number. Alternative methods for counting synapses in ultrathin sections are reviewed in Mayhew (1979c).

From its inception, the concept of a synapse has been at once functional and structural. Physiological transmission from one neuron to another has a morphological substrate which can be visualised by light and/or electron microscopy. With the electron microscope, three principal components of this substrate can be counted and each may give a different estimate of the number of 'synapses'. Clearly, it is important to specify the counting unit so that independent investigators can draw realistic comparisons but the choice of unit will also influence the extent of biases introduced into the experimental design. For instance, numbers of boutons may be underestimated if unequivocal identification depends on favourable planes of sectioning.

In recent years, there has been a tendency to count synaptic apposition zones or membrane thickenings rather than boutons. The tendency partly reflects advances in staining techniques but is also a recognition that these components tend to be easier to describe geometrically, e.g. as circular discs. Serial sectioning has demonstrated that, in some cases at least, the assumption of circularity is reasonable. Consequently, biases due to erroneous assumptions about particle size and shape can be minimised in these instances.

It is also advisable to consider the most suitable reference when estimating component numerical densities. Estimating number of synapses per reference surface may be more efficient than estimating number per reference volume (see a study on desmosomes – an analogous counting problem – in Mayhew, 1981). With axosomatic synapses at least, estimating numbers per soma surface can be combined with light microscopical determinations of soma surface area to provide estimates of absolute number per soma (Momoh & Mayhew, 1982). Another alternative is to relate the numerical density of synapses to the numerical density of neurons in the same reference volume and derive estimates of synapse : neuron ratios (see Thomas et al., 1979). This component density is preferable to others because it helps to minimise the range of biological interpretations which can be made on results from comparative studies. Thus, one can often assume that neuron number will not increase with age, disease or experimental manipulation.

To illustrate a method for obtaining estimates of absolute numbers per neuron, I will refer to calculations based on studies of rat spinal motoneurons performed in collaboration with the late C. K. Momoh. Part of this investigation analysed postnatal changes in synaptic predominance on the soma surface of cells in the cervical spinal medulla. Preparative and sampling details may be found in Mayhew & Momoh (1974) and Momoh & Mayhew (1982). Present results are confined to rats aged 1, 10, 30, 60 and 120 days post partum.

Light micrographs were used to estimate the surface area of the average motoneuron soma. Electron micrographs were recorded in order to estimate numbers of synapses per unit area of soma surface. Four morphological classes of synapse – designated S, F, C and M – were identified using established criteria (e.g., Bodian, 1972). The counting unit was the synaptic apposition zone which was treated as a flat circular disc. All numerical densities were corrected for technical bias due to section thickness effects (Mayhew, 1979c).

Results for S and F synapses are summarised in Table 4.7. Estimates of the numbers of C and M synapses are excluded because these types are uncommon. In newborn rats, there was an overwhelming preponderance of S synapses (roughly 83% of all

Table 4.7. *Postnatal changes in synaptic predominance on motoneurons in the rat cervical spinal medulla. Each value is the mean ± s.e.m. for n = 9 animals*

No. of synapses per soma	Days *post partum*				
	1	10	30	60	120
All types	316 ± 20	968 ± 38	800 ± 22	817 ± 31	731 ± 38
S synapses	263 ± 20	492 ± 25	302 ± 7	325 ± 18	307 ± 20
F synapses	51 ± 4	440 ± 28	479 ± 21	481 ± 25	416 ± 31

axosomatic synapses). By day 10, there had been a significant net increase in the total number of S synapses per average soma but, owing to a preferred increase in the number of F synapses, they now accounted for only 51% of all somatic input.

By day 30, F synapses predominated and this was due exclusively to a net loss of S synapses from the soma. This predominance of F synapses persisted without significant change until day 120.

The mechanism responsible for the differential loss of S synapses is uncertain, though similar studies on cat motoneurons suggest that there may be spontaneous phagocytosis of synapses by glial cells (Ronnevi, 1977). At least in the rat, the net loss of synapses seems to affect S synapses in preference to F synapses. The synapses could be phagocytosed but their displacement to other parts of the neuronal surface cannot be ruled out at present.

These postnatal changes at the motoneuron surface coincide with a period of great physiological development with respect to dominance of inhibition versus excitation. In this regard, it is interesting to note that S synapses are putative excitatory synapses whereas F synapses employ glycine as neurotransmitter and are expected to be inhibitory. The present stereological results may represent the morphological substrate for the shift towards inhibition which occurs postnatally.

These studies offer one last proof of the value of stereology in quantitative microscopical anatomy. Though similar information could be obtained by reconstruction using serial sections, this approach is technically demanding and severely limits the amount of material which can be examined. Nevertheless, it occasionally happens that synapses are so irregular in shape that serial sectioning is presently the only way to obtain accurate estimates of their number. This is true of the so-called perforated synapses found, for instance, in the rat hippocampus (Didima de Groot, personal communication).

SUMMARY

Stereology is a body of geometrico-statistical principles suitable for quantifying microscopical images in thin sections. Provided that careful attention is paid to all aspects of experimental design, these principles can provide valid and efficient estimates of structural quantities. In most situations, no expensive measuring equipment is required: relevant quantities can be obtained simply by classifying events and counting them. Many examples attest to the power of stereology in helping to bridge the artificial divide between biological structure and function and to identify objectively structural changes which occur with age, disease and experimental treatment.

This chapter is dedicated to the memory of Christopher Kunaye Momoh for whom the cartographer's wheel was the best way of measuring and, like the stone of Sisyphus, must roll forever. As a friend and foil he is missed greatly.

I am grateful to many colleagues who have contributed to this review in thought or deed. In particular, I would like to thank all students and co-teachers who have attended the annual Scandinavian Course in Morphometry and Stereology. Finally, I am indebted to Professor E. J. Clegg, Dr K. S. Bedi and Dr M. J. Moore for their many suggestions for improving the original manuscript.

REFERENCES

Aherne, W. & Dunnill, M. S. (1966). Quantitative aspects of placental structure. *Journal of Pathology and Bacteriology*, **91**, 123–39.

Bailey, N. T. J. (1972). *Statistical Methods in Biology.* London: The English Universities Press.

Bodian, D. (1972). Synaptic diversity and characterisation by electron microscopy, In *Structure and Function of Synapses*, ed. G. D. Pappas & D. P. Purpura, pp. 45–65. New York: Raven Press.

Carr, K. E., Hamlet, R. & Watt, C. (1981). Scanning electron microscopy, autolysis and irradiation as techniques for studying small intestinal morphology. *Journal of Microscopy*, **123**, 161–8.

Clarke, R. M. (1970). Mucosal architecture and epithelial cell production rate in the small intestine of the albino rat. *Journal of Anatomy*, **107**, 519–29.

Cochran, W. G. (1977). *Sampling Techniques*, 3rd edn. London: John Wiley.

Coleman, R. (1979). *An Introduction to Mathematical Stereology.* Institute of Mathematics, University of Aarhus, Denmark.

Cruz Orive, L.-M. (1976a). Correction of stereological parameters from biased samples on nucleated particle phases. I. Nuclear volume fraction. *Journal of Microscopy*, **106**, 1–18.

Cruz Orive, L.-M. (1976b). Correction of stereological parameters from biased samples on nucleated particle phases. II. Specific surface area. *Journal of Microscopy*, **106**, 19–32.

Cruz Orive, L.-M. (1980a). On the estimation of particle number. *Journal of Microscopy*, **120**, 15–27.

Cruz Orive, L.-M. (1980b). Best linear unbiased estimators for stereology. *Biometrics*, **36**, 595–605.

Cruz Orive, L.-M. (1982). The use of quadrats and test systems in stereology, including magnification corrections. *Journal of Microscopy*, **125**, 89–102.

Cruz Orive, L.-M. & Weibel, E. R. (1981). Sampling designs for stereology. *Journal of Microscopy*, **122**, 235–57.

DeHoff, R. T. & Rhines, F. N. (1968). *Quantitative Microscopy.* New York: McGraw-Hill.

Dunnill, M. S. (1968). Quantitative methods in histology. In *Recent Advances in Clinical Pathology*, Series V, ed. S. C. Dyke, pp. 401–16. London: Churchill.

Elias, H., Hennig, A. & Schwartz, D. E. (1971). Stereology: applications to biomedical research. *Physiological Reviews*, **51**, 158–200.

Fernand, V. S. & Young, J. Z. (1951). The sizes of the nerve fibres of muscle nerves. *Proceedings of the Royal Society of London, series B*, **139**, 38–58.

Forrester, J. M. (1972). The number of villi in rat's jejunum and ileum: effect of normal growth, partial enterectomy and tube feeding. *Journal of Anatomy*, **111**, 283–91.

Fraher, J. P. (1980). On methods of measuring nerve fibres. *Journal of Anatomy*, **130**, 139–51.

Gehr, P., Bachofen, M. & Weibel, E. R. (1978). The normal human lung: ultrastructure and morphometric estimation of diffusion capacity. *Respiration Physiology*, **32**, 121–40.

Gundersen, H. J. G. (1977). Notes on the estimation of the numerical density of arbitrary profiles: the edge effect. *Journal of Microscopy*, **111**, 219–23.

Gundersen, H. J. G. (1979). Estimation of tubule or cylinder L_V, S_V and V_V on thick sections. *Journal of Microscopy*, **117**, 333–45.

Gundersen, H. J. G. (1980). Stereology – or how figures for spatial shape and content are obtained by observation of structures in sections. *Microscopica Acta*, **83**, 409–26.

Gundersen, H. J. G., Boysen, M. & Reith, A. (1981). Comparison of semiautomatic digitizer-tablet and simple point counting performance in morphometry. *Virchows Archiv B (Cell Pathology)*, **37**, 317–25.

Gundersen, H. J. G. & Østerby, R. (1980). Sampling efficiency and biological variation in stereology. Special Supplement, *Mikroskopie (Wien)*, **37**, 143–8.

Gundersen, H. J. G. & Østerby, R. (1981). Optimizing sampling efficiency of stereological studies in biology: or 'Do more less well!' *Journal of Microscopy*, **121**, 65–73.

Gundersen, H. J. G., Seefeldt, T. & Østerby, R. (1980). Glomerular epithelial foot processes in normal man and rats. Distribution of true width and its intra- and inter-individual variation. *Cell and Tissue Research*, **205**, 147–55.

Gupta, M., Mayhew, T. M., Bedi, K. S., Sharma, A. K. & White, F. H. (1983). Inter-animal variation and its influence on the overall precision of morphometric estimates based on nested sampling designs. *Journal of Microscopy*, in press.

Hally, A. D. (1964). A counting method for measuring the volumes of tissue components in microscopical sections. *Quarterly Journal of Microscopical Science*, **105**, 503–17.

Jensen, E. B. & Gundersen, H. J. G. (1982). Stereological ratio estimation based on counts from integral test systems. *Journal of Microscopy*, **125**, 51–66.

Kessel, R. G. & Kardon, R. H. (1979). *Tissues and Organs: A Text-Atlas of Scanning Electron Microscopy.* San Francisco: W. H. Freeman.

Laga, E. M., Driscoll, S. G. & Munro, H. N. (1974). Human placental structure: relationship to fetal nutrition. In *Problems of Human Reproduction*, vol. 2, ed. J. B. Josimovich, M. Reynolds & E. Cobo, pp. 143–81. London: John Wiley.

Lee, R. M. K. W., McKenzie, R., Kobayashi, K., Garfield, R. E., Forrest, J. B. & Daniel, E. E. (1982). Effects of glutaraldehyde fixative osmolarities on smooth muscle cell volume, and osmotic reactivity of the cells after fixation. *Journal of Microscopy*, **125**, 77–88.

Loud, A. V. (1967). Quantitative estimation of the loss of membrane images resulting from oblique sectioning of biological membranes. In *Proceedings of the 25th Anniversary Meeting of the Electron Microscopy Society of America*, ed. C. J. Arceneaux, pp. 144–6. Baton Rouge: Claitor's Book Store.

Mall, G., Kayser, K. & Rossner, J. A. (1977). The loss of membrane images from oblique sectioning of biological membranes and the availability of morphometric principles – demonstrated by the examination of heart muscle mitochondria. *Mikroskopie (Wien)*, **33**, 246–54.

Mathieu, O., Cruz Orive, L.-M., Hoppeler, H. & Weibel, E. R. (1981*a*). Measuring error and sampling variation in stereology: comparison of the efficiency of various methods for planar image analysis. *Journal of Microscopy*, **121**, 75–88.

Mathieu, O., Krauer, R., Hoppeler, H., Gehr, P., Lindstedt, S. L., McNeill Alexander, R., Taylor, C. R. & Weibel, E. R. (1981*b*). Design of the mammalian respiratory system. VII. Scaling mitochondrial volume in skeletal muscle to body mass. *Respiration Physiology*, **44**, 113–28.

Mayhew, T. M. (1979*a*). Basic stereological relationships for quantitative microscopical anatomy – a simple systematic approach. *Journal of Anatomy*, **129**, 95–105.

Mayhew, T. M. (1979*b*). Isolated peritoneal macrophages: component-biased sampling. In *Stereological Methods*, vol. 1, *Practical Methods for Biological Morphometry*, ed. E. R. Weibel, pp. 331–7. London: Academic Press.

Mayhew, T. M. (1979*c*). Stereological approach to the study of synapse morphometry with particular regard to estimating number in a volume and on a surface. *Journal of Neurocytology*, **8**, 121–38.

Mayhew, T. M. (1981). On the relative efficiencies of alternative ratio estimators for morphometric analysis of cell membrane surface features. *Journal of Microscopy*, **122**, 7–14.

Mayhew, T. M., Burgess, A. J., Gregory, C. D. & Atkinson, M. E. (1979). On the problem of counting and sizing mitochondria: a general reappraisal based on ultrastructural studies of mammalian lymphocytes. *Cell and Tissue Research*, **204**, 297–303.

Mayhew, T. M. & Cruz Orive, L.-M. (1973). Stereological correction procedures for estimating true volume proportions from biased samples. *Journal of Microscopy*, **99**, 287–99.

Mayhew, T. M. & Cruz Orive, L.-M. (1974). Caveat on the use of the Delesse principle of areal analysis for estimating component volume densities. *Journal of Microscopy*, **102**, 195–207.

Mayhew, T. M. & Cruz Orive, L.-M. (1975). Some stereological correction formulae with particular applications in quantitative neurohistology. *Journal of Neurological Sciences*, **26**, 503–9.

Mayhew, T. M. & Momoh, C. K. (1974). Stereological description of the anterior horn cervical cord of the adult rat. A quantitative study using the optical microscope. *Journal of Comparative Neurology*, **156**, 107–22.

Mayhew, T. M. & Williams, M. A. (1971). A comparison of two sampling procedures for stereological analysis of cell pellets. *Journal of Microscopy*, **94**, 195–204.

Mayhew, T. M. & Williams, M. A. (1974). A quantitative morphological analysis of macrophage stimulation. II. Changes in granule number, size and size distributions. *Cell and Tissue Research*, **150**, 529–43.

Meinhard, E. A., Wadbrook, D. G. & Risdon, R. A. (1975). Computer card morphometry of jejunal biopsies in childhood coeliac disease. *Journal of Clinical Pathology*, **28**, 85–93.

Miles, R. E. (1978). The sampling, by quadrats, of planar aggregates. *Journal of Microscopy*, **113**, 257–67.

Miles, R. E. & Davy, P. J. (1976). Precise and general conditions for the validity of a comprehensive set of stereological fundamental formulae. *Journal of Microscopy*, **107**, 211–26.

Miles, R. E. & Davy, P. (1977). On the choice of quadrats in stereology. *Journal of Microscopy*, **110**, 27–44.

Momoh, C. K. & Mayhew, T. M. (1982). A stereological evaluation of synaptic diversity on spinal motoneurons in the rat. *Experientia*, **38**, 694–5.

Østerby, R. (1975). Early phases in the development of diabetic glomerulopathy. A quantitative electron microscopic study. *Acta Medica Scandinavica*, Supplement 574.

Østerby, R. & Gundersen, H. J. G. (1980). Fast accumulation of basement membrane material and the rate of morphological changes in acute experimental diabetic glomerular hypertrophy. *Diabetologia*, **18**, 493–500.

Paumgartner, D., Losa, G. & Weibel, E. R. (1981). Resolution effect on the stereological estimation of surface and volume and its interpretation in terms of fractal dimensions. *Journal of Microscopy*, **121**, 51–63.

Rasch, R. (1979). Prevention of diabetic glomerulopathy in streptozotocin diabetic rats by insulin treatment. *Diabetologia*, **16**, 319–24.

Reith, A., Barnard, T. & Rohr, H. (1976). Stereology of cellular reaction patterns. In *Critical Reviews in Toxicology*, vol. 4, ed. L. Goldberg, pp. 219–69. Cleveland, Ohio: CRC Press.

Reith, A. & Mayhew, T. M. (1980). Caveat bei der morphometrisch–stereologischen Bestimmung von Biomembranen. *Gegenbaurs Morphologische Jahrbuch (Leipzig)*, **126**, 206–15.

Ronnevi, L.-O. (1977). Spontaneous phagocytosis of boutons on spinal motoneurons during early postnatal development. An electron microscopical study in the cat. *Journal of Neurocytology*, **6**, 487–504.

Shay, J. (1975). Economy of effort in electron microscope morphometry. *American Journal of Pathology*, **81**, 503–12.

Sokal, R. R. & Rohlf, F. J. (1969). *Biometry. The Principles and Practice of Statistics in Biological Research*. San Francisco: W. H. Freeman.

Steffes, M. W., Brown, D. M., Basgen, J. M., Matas, A. J. & Mauer, S. M. (1979). Glomerular basement membrane thickness following islet transplantation in the diabetic rat. *Laboratory Investigation*, **41**, 116–18.

Stenling, R. & Helander, H. F. (1981). Stereologic studies on the small intestinal epithelium of the rat. 1. The absorptive cells of the normal duodenum and jejunum. *Cell and Tissue Research*, **217**, 11–21.

Stringer, B. M. J., Wynford-Thomas, D. & Williams, E. D. (1982). Physical randomisation of tissue architecture: an alternative to systematic sampling. *Journal of Microscopy*, **126**, 179–82.

Stuart, A. (1976). *Basic Ideas of Scientific Sampling*, 2nd edn. London: Charles Griffin.

Taylor, C. R. & Weibel, E. R. (1981). Design of the mammalian respiratory system. I. Problem and strategy. *Respiration Physiology*, **44**, 1–10.

Thomas, Y. M., Bedi, K. S., Davies, C. A. & Dobbing, J. (1979). A stereological analysis of the neuronal and synaptic content of the frontal and cerebellar cortex of weanling rats undernourished from birth. *Early Human Development*, **3**, 109–26.

Underwood, E. E. (1970). *Quantitative Stereology*. Reading, Massachussetts: Addison-Wesley.

Weibel, E. R. (1969). Stereological principles for morphometry in electron microscopic cytology. *International Review of Cytology*, **26**, 235–302.

Weibel, E. R. (1979a). *Stereological Methods*, vol. 1, *Practical Methods for Biological Morphometry*. London: Academic Press.

Weibel, E. R. (1979b). Morphometry of the human lung: the state of the art after two decades. *Extrait du bulletin européen de physiopathologie respiratoire*, **15**, 999–1013.

Weibel, E. R. (1979c). Oxygen demand and the size of respiratory structures in mammals. In *Evolution of Respiratory Processes*, vol. 13, ed. S. C. Wood & C. Lenfant, pp. 289–346. New York & Basle: Marcel Dekker.

Weibel, E. R. (1980). *Stereological Methods*, vol. 2, *Theoretical Foundations*. London: Academic Press.

Weibel, E. R. (1982). Stereology – a bridge between morphology and physiology. *Acta Stereologica*, **1**, 23–33.

Weibel, E. R. & Bolender, R. P. (1973). Stereological techniques for electron microscopic morphometry. In *Principles and Techniques of Electron Microscopy*, vol. 3, ed. M. A. Hayat, pp. 237–96. New York: Van Nostrand Reinhold.

Weibel, E. R. & Knight, B. W. (1964). A morphometric study on the thickness of the pulmonary air–blood barrier. *Journal of Cell Biology*, **21**, 367–84.

Whitehouse, W. J. (1974). A stereological method for calculating internal surface areas in structures which have become anisotropic as the result of linear expansions or contractions. *Journal of Microscopy*, **101**, 169–76.

Williams, M. A. (1977). *Quantitative Methods in Biology*. Oxford: North-Holland.

5 Anatomical, biomolecular and morphometric views of the primates

CHARLES E. OXNARD

The Departments of Anatomy and Cell Biology, and Biological Sciences, School of Medicine, University of Southern California, Los Angeles, California 90033, USA

INTRODUCTION

There are especially exciting stages in the development of sciences when separate types of investigations and different lines of evidence start to impinge upon common problems. Such a time has come in the development of our understanding of the evolutionary relationships between the primates.

Many decades, nay many centuries, of study of the evolution of the primates have come about through the activities of classical morphologists. This work involves time-consuming, painstaking and infinitely careful investigation of the detailed structure of the body together with growing knowledge of the function of its various component organs and organ systems, and indeed of whole organisms and populations of organisms themselves. These findings have been capped during the present century by the investigations of individuals such as D. G. Elliot (1913), F. Wood Jones (1929), A. H. Schultz (1936), S. Zuckerman (1932, 1933) and W. E. Le Gros Clark (1934). Their contributions stand, in turn, upon those of a host of earlier investigators such as St G. Mivart (1867, 1873), T. H. Huxley (1872) and R. Owen (1866) among many others. In recent years these organismal relationships have been summarised in compendia such as those of G. G. Simpson (1945), W. C. Osman Hill (1953–1970), and P. Hershkovitz (1977).

Within the last two decades, in contrast, the work of an increasing number of individuals in the area of molecular evolutionary biology, broadly defined, has started to supply new types of information about the relationships between the various primates. This work involves studying the similarities of and differences between the primates through increasing understanding of the subcellular, biochemical, and molecular structures to be found in these animals. Yet, though we now have a not inconsiderable bulk of such data from the studies of individuals such as E. H. Y. Chu (e.g. Chu & Bender, 1961), N. A. Barnicott (e.g. Barnicott, 1969), W. M. Fitch (e.g. Fitch & Langley, 1976; Fitch, 1977), M. Goodman (e.g. Dene, Goodman & Prychodko, 1976a), V. Sarich, J. E. Cronin and A. C. Wilson (e.g. Sarich & Cronin, 1976, 1977, 1980; Sarich & Wilson, 1967, 1973), F. J. Ayala (e.g. Bruce & Ayala, 1978, 1979), A. E. Romero-Herrera and K. A. Joysey (e.g. Romero-Herrera *et al.*, 1976, 1978; Romero-Herrera *et al.*, 1979), it is also fitting to remember that the concept of studies such as these is actually quite old. Zuckerman (1933) understood very clearly how such information might tell us about the relationships between the primates. Perhaps the earliest definitive work (but not of large enough bulk to provide any overall picture) stems from the turn of the century (e.g. Friedenthal, 1900; Nuttall, 1904). The writings of Darwin himself, half a century earlier, make it quite clear that he had glimpsed the possibility of molecular evolution.

The present time is an especially pertinent period to attempt to draw together results obtained by classical morphology and molecular evolutionary biology. Although studies in the biomolecular area are now quite old, it is only now that a large enough bulk of molecular information has become available to allow us to compare the results of the two technologies. Indeed, even the present time is still somewhat early for such a synthesis because, though primate anatomists have long known of the detailed structures of every primate (even such rarities as the aye aye were studied over a century ago: e.g. Owen, 1862), by no means has every living species of primate been investigated using the various biomolecular tools.

ORGANISMS AND MOLECULES

Classical organismal studies

As we come to look at the entire Order Primates, it would seem that organismal techniques define a pattern for the major divisions of the primates that is agreed by almost all. Whether we study the structures of primate hands and feet, hips and shoulders, trunks, heads, brains, reproductive structures, developmental patterns, growth series, or any other parameter, the living primates can be described as a relatively linear series with prosimians at the one extreme, then New World monkeys, then Old World monkeys, then apes with humans at the other, opposite, end (e.g. see the overall volumes of Simpson, 1945; Le Gros Clark, 1959; Hershkovitz, 1977; summary in Oxnard, 1983a).

Molecular biology

Likewise, whether we study immunogenetic distances, foetal gamma haemoglobins, maps of beta globin clusters, primate karyologies, protein sequencing methods or DNA–DNA hybridisations we see, broadly speaking, the same approximately linearly related groups: prosimians, New World monkeys, Old World monkeys, and apes and humans (e.g. see the edited volumes of Goodman & Tashian, 1976; Chivers & Joysey, 1978; Ciochon & Chiarelli, 1980; summary in Oxnard, 1983a).

Morphometrics

The concordance between the organismal and biomolecular approaches to primate relationships is most satisfying. It is, therefore, of some interest that yet another form of investigation (classical in the sense that it studies relationships at the organ/organismal level, of recent origin in that it examines them through a type of quantification and analysis not readily available before the development of computers: Oxnard, 1978b) has also started to provide some understanding of the overall relationships of the primates. Perhaps 10–20% of the papers in most journals dealing with the primates now encompass such 'morphometric' studies, yet, in fact, these studies are even less extensive than are those of the molecular biologists. Very recent investigations, however, have started to supply enough data so that a 'morphometric view' of the entire primate order can be entertained.

These morphometric views of the primates vary depending upon whether the objects of study are individual anatomical regions or whether attempts are made to meld many individual anatomical regions into the morphometrics of entire organisms. The studies have mostly been carried out in a fairly standard way. The form of the individual anatomical regions or of the overall proportions of entire specimens is characterised by measurement. Suites of such measurements taken upon samples of specimens, grouped into species or genera depending upon availability of materials, are then analysed using appropriate multivariate statistical techniques. The arrangements of the various primate groups according to the results of such statistical analyses are then studied in the light of independent information about the animals (such as function, behaviour, evolution, taxonomy, and so on).

In simple studies these arrangements are usually conveniently summarised by two- or three-dimensional plots based upon the first two or three canonical or factor axes derived from the multivariate statistical studies. But in more complex investigations in which there are bigger suites of variables and greater numbers of animal groups, more axes may be necessary to describe the arrangements. In such cases, the results may need to be displayed using minimum spanning trees (Gower & Ross, 1969) derived from the complete matrix of generalised distances, or using high-dimensional displays (Andrews, 1972, 1973) based upon large numbers of canonical or factor axes.

Although many of these studies are from the laboratories of Oxnard and Ashton and their various colleagues (for summaries, see Oxnard, 1973*a*, 1975, 1977), a number of other laboratories have also used such methods and have produced confirming results (e.g. Feldesman, 1976; Corruccini & Ciochon, 1976; Day & Wood, 1968; McHenry & Corrucini, 1975; see corroborative comparisons in Oxnard, 1983*b*). The type of information which results from such studies varies according to whether individual anatomical regions are the object of study, or whether attempts are being made to investigate the overall anatomy of entire animals.

Upper limbs

Thus, it now seems clear that morphometric examination of individual anatomical regions provides information mainly about the functional adaptations of those regions during the life cycle of different primates. Many morphometric studies of upper limb structure (of shoulders, arms, forearms, upper limbs as a whole, summarised in Oxnard, 1981*a*, 1983*a*) demonstrate that the primary arrangement of the various genera is into a band-shaped spectrum that is most closely associated with the different functions of upper limbs in the life styles of the different species (Fig. 5.1).

At one end of this spectrum lie species displaying life habits that involve using upper limbs in raised positions and bearing tension. Examples include orang-utans and spider monkeys. At the other end of the spectrum lie species that mainly use the upper limbs in lowered positions and bearing primarily compressive forces. Examples include baboons, patas monkeys, tarsiers and bushbabies. More centrally located within the spectrum are a variety of species whose life habits are such that their upper limbs are involved in raised positions and bearing tension to degrees intermediate between the others. Examples here are woolly and proboscis monkeys, sifakas and pottos. Humans are unique in not lying in the band-shaped spectrum; and even this finding is associated with the unique functions of the human upper limb (Fig. 5.1).

Lower limbs

Likewise, several morphometric studies of lower limb structures (of hips and thighs, of ankles and feet, of lower limbs as a whole, summarised in Oxnard, 1981*a*, 1983*a*) show that the primary arrangement of the various genera is into a star-shaped spectrum that is most closely aligned with the different functions of lower limbs in the life styles of the different species (Fig. 5.2).

In this case, all of the generalised quadrupedal species of all taxonomic groups, are centrally located within the nucleus of the star. Examples include Diana monkeys,

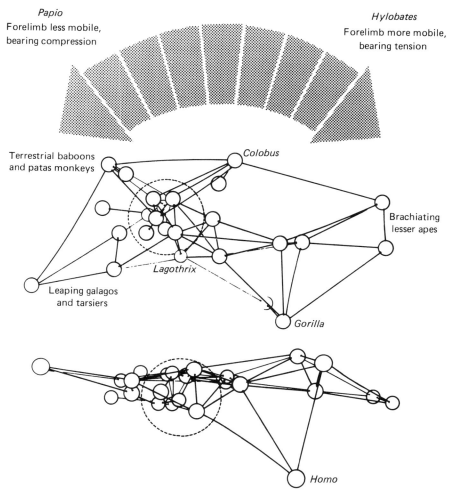

Fig. 5.1. Multivariate statistical analysis of Schultz's nine dimensions of the upper limb arranges the primates in a broad band-shaped spectrum (middle frame) that fits well with their arrangement according to the degree to which the upper limb bears compressive or tensile forces in lowered or raised positions during major locomotor activities (upper frame). Rotation of the multivariate statistical model along its long axis (lower frame) reveals the uniquely offset position of the genus *Homo*. Similar pictures are seen in analyses of other data taken from the various parts of the upper limb (Oxnard, 1982*a*).

The multivariate morphometric model has been constructed from the matrix of generalised distances that separate the various genera. Only a few genera are named in this figure, but the entire data are given in the original studies.

The general scale of the diagram is some 25 standard deviation units but a marker cannot be provided because the model is three-dimensional. Some of the connections between the genera are slightly curved; this is because they actually exist in a space of dimensionality higher than three.

squirrel monkeys and lemurs. The species with more specialised locomotion are located within separate peripheral rays of the star, again in ways which bear no relationship to taxonomy but are closely related to lower limb function. An example is the juxtaposition of bushbabies and tarsiers in one ray of small leaping forms; another is the inclusion of spider and woolly spider monkeys together with the gibbons and siamangs in an arboreal acrobatic ray. A third example is the grouping of patas

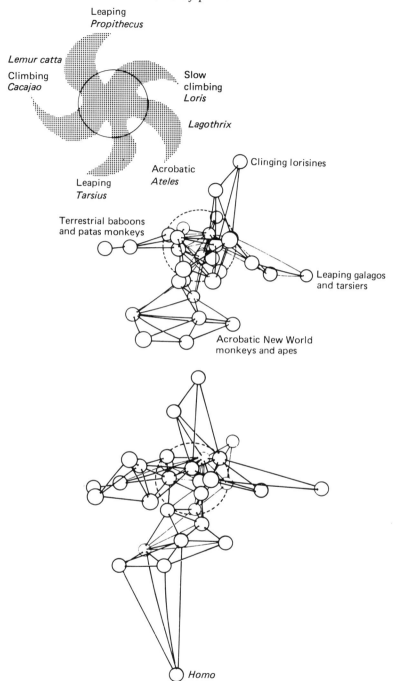

Fig. 5.2. Multivariate statistical analysis of Schultz's seven dimensions of the lower limb arranges the primates in the form of a star-shaped spectrum (middle frame) that fits well with their arrangement according to the degree to which the lower limb is involved in a variety of quite different forces during major activities (upper frame). Rotation of the star-like model reveals a unique position for the genus *Homo*. Similar pictures are seen in analyses of other data taken from various parts of the lower limb.

The conventions and caveats for the morphometric model are as in Fig. 5.1. The general scale of the model is some 30 standard deviation units.

monkeys, baboons and *Cercopithecus aethiops* in a mainly terrestrial ray. Many other examples of such functional parallels exist. Again, humans do not lie within this star-shaped spectrum, and this too associates well with the unique functions of the human lower limb (Fig. 5.2).

Upper and lower limbs combined

One particular morphometric study of upper and lower limbs combined arranges the primates into a 'signet-ring-shaped' spectrum that seems to reflect, more than any other feature, the balance between the weightbearing usages of the upper and lower limbs in locomotion (Oxnard, 1981a, 1983a, and Fig. 5.3).

Most of the species fall in the 'seal' of the signet ring. The only feature that these forms have in common is that, irrespective of taxonomic group and irrespective of the precise form of their locomotion, they all share locomotor forces approximately equally between the upper and lower limbs. This is so whether they move on the ground (baboons) or in the trees (Diana monkeys), above the branches (cercopitheques) or below the branches (pottos), by scurrying (marmosets) or bounding (squirrel monkeys), by relatively slow cautious quadrupedal movement (douroucoulis) or acrobatic quadrupedal climbing (uakari monkeys), and so on.

Species in the rest of the left-hand part of the signet ring show a different parallel. Whatever their taxonomic group or mode of locomotion, they are all heavily upper limb dependent (orang-utans as a result of acrobatic climbing; gibbons and siamangs as a result of brachiation; spider monkeys and woolly monkeys as a result of acrobatic tail-assisted climbing and swinging; and, to peculiar degrees, chimpanzees and gorillas which, though terrestrial, are also accomplished arboreal acrobats). Species in the rest of the right-hand part of the signet ring show a third parallel in that, whatever their taxonomic group, they are heavily lower limb dependent (avahis, sifakas, bushbabies and tarsiers, presumably as a result of powerful leaping; and, again, to peculiar degrees and presumably as a result of a unique form of bipedalism, humans).

Overall morphometrics of primates

The various regional anatomical arrangements of the primates, described above, do not follow the simple pattern of overall primate relationships such as we have seen emanate from classical organismal studies or from the newer biomolecular investigations. When, however, such regional morphometric studies are organised in such a way that some coverage of the entire organism is obtained, then the functional, adaptive result disappears and a result which mirrors primate evolutionary relationships emerges.

Thus, first, study of the overall proportions of the primates as taken by Adolph Schultz during a long and vigorous lifetime (summarised in Schultz, 1929, 1969) and analysed using multivariate statistical methods involving minimum spanning trees of generalised distances (Oxnard, 1981a, 1983a, and see Fig. 5.4) provides a picture of the major primate subgroups in a linear relationship from prosimians, New World monkeys, Old World Monkeys, and apes to humans. And second, studies of the morphometric structures of more detailed anatomical regions by similar methods have begun to supply, when summed in an overall manner by even newer techniques (Andrews' high-dimensional method, 1972, 1973, as used by Oxnard, 1983a, and see Fig. 5.5), a picture of the same array of primate groups.

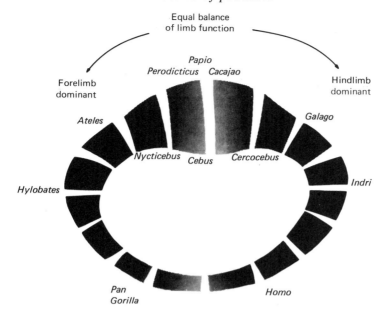

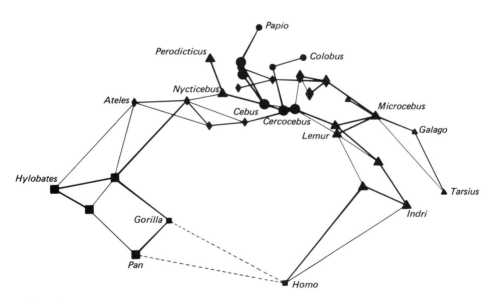

Fig. 5.3. Multivariate statistical analysis of Schultz's fifteen dimensions of upper and lower limbs combined arranges the primates in the form of a ring-shaped or doughnut-shaped spectrum (lower frame). Though this places species together that are vastly different from one another in their overall locomotor patterns (see text), it does arrange the primates according to the degree to which their major activities are upper-limb- or lower-limb-dominant, or use both limbs to approximately equal degrees (upper frame).

The conventions are again as in Fig. 5.1. The general scale of this model is some 35 standard deviation units. Squares, hominoids; circles, Old World monkeys; diamonds, New World monkeys; triangles, prosimians.

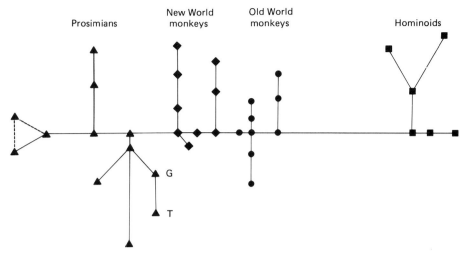

Fig. 5.4. The analysis of Schultz's twenty-three dimensions of the entire body. In this case the analysis is so complex that a three-dimensional model cannot be constructed; a large percentage of the information is contained within discriminant axes higher than three. The generalised distance connections between the genera have been laid out as a linear minimum spanning tree from one end to the other. The symbols are the same as in Fig. 5.3, and this indicates clearly that the result follows the linear set of relationships of the primates from prosimians, through New World monkeys, then Old World monkeys, to apes and finally humans.

The length of the minimum spanning tree is some 45 standard deviation units but because of the limitations of this display, the only distances in the diagram which are correct are those joining the genera. Any distances in the diagram not connected are unlikely to be correct. Dashed lines indicate neighbour relationships which are not minimum but are very close to minimum. *This constraint about lengths in the diagram is essential to its understanding.*

Comparisons among the three lines of investigation

Important though it may be that three such different technologies (classical study of organisms, molecular biology and morphometrics) give the same basic result, we may be pardoned for thinking that this result (clusters of prosimians, New World monkeys, Old World monkeys, apes and humans) is so self evident that it is scarcely of interest. Yet it turns out that this is not the case. Notwithstanding the broad consensus just described, the moment we turn our attention to the details of primate relationships at intermediate levels, we are faced with many areas of controversy and many disagreements between the results of the different methods. For instance it is not totally clear what are, or are not, primates. The notion that tree shrews are primates was emphasised by Le Gros Clark as long ago as 1926 and adopted by many workers since (e.g. Simpson, 1945). However, as a result of the activity of workers in the last decade (e.g. Martin, 1975), it would seem that most evidence now removes tree shrews from the Order Primates.

The basic split between prosimians and anthropoids is, likewise, by no means as obvious as indicated by the broad view. The prevailing theory in this century has been that tarsiers are prosimians and this is still held by many investigators (e.g. Simpson, 1945; Napier & Napier, 1967). More and more, however, we are seeing new evidence coming forward to support a much earlier view, that these little creatures (though far removed from any living primate) are more closely allied to the Anthropoidea than the Prosimii (e.g. Cave, 1973; Luckett, 1974; Minkoff, 1974; McKenna, 1975; Szalay, 1975*a,b*; Oxnard, 1978*a*).

Disagreements can be discerned at many other levels within the primates. Those studying organismal features tend to demonstrate disagreements about the levels of grouping that they discern: compare the very 'split' clusterings of the New World monkeys, as provided by Hershkovitz (1977) who recognises 12 groups, with the 'lumped' clusters of Simpson (1945) who sees only seven groups. Those studying biomolecular phenomena tend to disagree about distances between the groups that they see: compare the studies of the separations of various hominoids by Sarich & Cronin (1977) who view relationships between African and Asian apes as more distant, and by Dene, Goodman & Prychodko (1976a) who see this same relationship as being considerably closer.

However, the above disagreements *within* each classical organismal and biomolecular group of investigators are merely those that we might well expect, given different bases of judgment or opinions about matters such as clusterings of groups (i.e. differences of judgment between 'lumpers' and 'splitters') or distances between groups (i.e. differences of judgment between 'linear' as opposed to 'non-linear' biomolecular clocks). In contrast, far greater differences of opinion are now becoming evident *between* most of the classical organismal biologists on the one hand, and most of the molecular biologists on the other. These differences involve the more detailed relationships of the various primates as seen by each set of methods, and can perhaps be most easily noted by studying each individual group of primates separately. The most controversial of such differences is evident in the relationships between humans and apes in the Hominoidea. This is the group, therefore, that it is most provident to describe first.

HUMANS AND APES

Classical organismal studies have long seen the relationships among the hominoids as a tripartite clustering into lesser apes (gibbons and siamangs), great apes (orang-utans, gorillas and chimpanzees), and humans. (Indeed, it is this clustering that is responsible for the further, derivative, work of the primate taxonomists classifying the hominoids in the way that they do. And it is this view of these higher primates that conflicts most with the recent fossil evidence.) This tripartite clustering of the hominoids depends upon the voluminous data of many centuries (see Simpson, 1945), and it continues to be the picture provided by even very recent investigations of primate morphology such as those of Tuttle (1975, 1977).

In complete contrast (and with only a few exceptions: e.g. Bruce & Ayala, 1979), molecular biologists find relationships among the hominoids to comprise a primary split between humans, chimpanzees and gorillas on the one hand, and the various Asian apes on the other (Kohne, 1975; Dene *et al.*, 1976b; Goodman, 1976; Sarich & Cronin, 1976; Benveniste & Todaro, 1976; Romero-Herrera *et al.*, 1976; and a host of other workers since). Sometimes, it is true, these results also split the Asian apes themselves into (a) lesser apes (gibbons and siamangs), and (b) Asian great apes (orang-utans). The findings, however we study these relationships (on the basis of immunological comparisons, electrophoretic data, primate karyology, protein sequencing information, and so on), all concur.

It is of considerable interest that the very small number of multivariate morphometric studies that have been brought to bear upon this question, also place gorillas and chimpanzees close to humans, and gibbons and siamangs closer to orang-utans. This is shown in multivariate morphometric studies of the overall proportions (upper limb, lower limb, trunk, head and neck) of the entire body (the data of Schultz studied

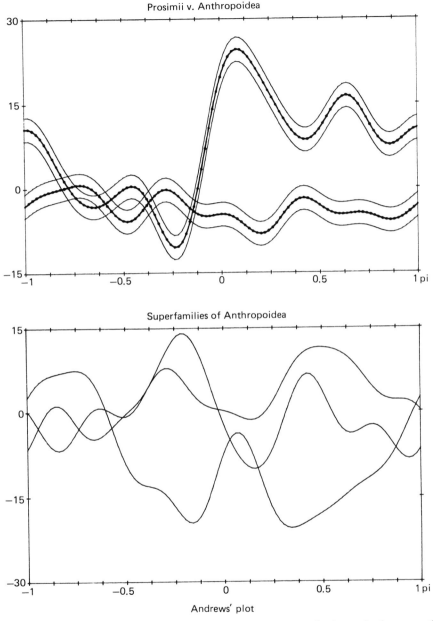

Fig. 5.5. This demonstrates the separations between major groups of primates in the summation by Oxnard (1983a) of separate regional analyses of shoulder, arm, forearm, forelimb as a whole, hip, foot, hindlimb as a whole, trunk, and head and neck using the data of Ashton, Oxnard and colleagues, and of Schultz. This has been done using Andrews' (1972, 1973) method of high-dimensional analysis.

This method of display, described non-mathematically in Oxnard (1975), indicates differences between groups even when the number of discriminant axes is too large to permit easy visualisation with two-dimensional plots or three-dimensional models. The mean positions of any given group are indicated by the curved plots extending from −pi to +pi. Similarity of groups is indicated by similarity in the curvatures of the plots; difference between groups is indicated by differences in curvature; a precise measure of difference is given by the area between plots (this is the squared generalised distance between the groups).

by canonical analysis and minimum spanning trees of generalised distances by Oxnard, 1981*a*). It is confirmed when we look at the summation, by high-dimensional studies, of detailed measurements of smaller bodily regions such as the shoulder girdle, arm, forearm, upper limb, pelvic girdle, foot, lower limb, trunk and head and neck (data of Ashton, Oxnard and many colleagues, summated by Oxnard, 1983*a*, and Fig. 5.6).

It is thus possible to compare and contrast the clusterings produced by these three approaches (Fig. 5.7). It is evident that the results of morphometric studies are most consistent with the biomolecular data.

OLD WORLD MONKEYS

In a similar way, there is a difference between the classical organismal view of the Old World monkeys and the biomolecular view. The former recognises a bipartite division into cercopithecines and colobines but with other differences between Old World monkeys being rather minor (the comparative uniformity of the Cercopithecoidea is well noted by Schultz, 1970; see also Thorington & Groves, 1970). The latter recognises an approximately equal tripartite division (e.g. Goodman, 1975; Hewett-Emmett, Cook & Barnicot, 1976; Sarich & Cronin, 1976) into a *Cercopithecus*-like species group, a macaque–baboon–mangabey species group, and a colobine group which is slightly more distant than the other two.

It is, therefore, again of interest that the arrangements of the Old World monkeys produced by morphometric studies using multivariate statistical analyses of overall bodily proportions (the data of Schultz studied by Oxnard, 1981*a*) and high-dimensional analyses of detailed measures of more localised anatomical regions also provide generally tripartite arrangements of these monkeys (the data of Ashton, Oxnard and colleagues as studied by Oxnard, 1983*a*, and Fig. 5.8). It is thus, again, possible to compare and contrast these three approaches (Fig. 5.9) from which it is evident, also again, that it is with the biomolecular studies that the morphometric results are most concordant.

NEW WORLD MONKEYS

In a similar way there is a difference between the classical organismal view of the clusterings of the New World monkeys and the biomolecular view. The former recognises a bipartite division into callithricids and cebids (e.g. Hershkovitz, 1977). The latter generally recognises a tripartite division into a special prehensile- and semiprehensile-tailed species group, an intermediate saki–uakari–*Chiropotes* species group, and a more generalised group combining callithricids and the remaining cebids (e.g. Dene *et al.*, 1976*a*; Baba, Darga & Goodman, 1979).

It is, therefore, again of interest that the arrangements of the New World monkeys produced by morphometric studies using multivariate statistical analyses of overall

The upper frame indicates that this method of summation easily separates prosimians from anthropoids. (Plots that are three standard deviation units away from each group have been drawn to give some notice of the scale of these separations, which are very large indeed.) The lower frame indicates that similarly large differences exist between the three superfamilies: Hominoidea, Cercopithecoidea and Ceboidea. The two frames taken together indicate that these morphometric data, when summarised in this way, show the same major groupings of the primates as are obtained from overall views of classical morphological and biomolecular data.

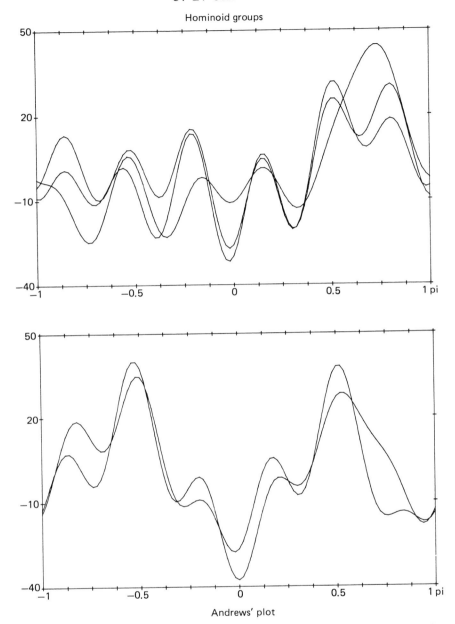

Fig. 5.6. Study of the summation of the several anatomical regions (as in Fig. 5.5) using Andrews' high-dimensional technique.

The upper frame demonstrates Andrews' plots for African great apes and for humans, the lower frame Andrews' plots for Asian apes (orang-utans and gibbons). Although each genus is different, two overall groups are clearly demonstrated, one in each frame. The differences between these two groups do not depend upon a single canonical axis or even two or three, but upon the pattern of difference within many canonical axes; hence they are most easily displayed by a medium such as Andrews' high-dimensional method.

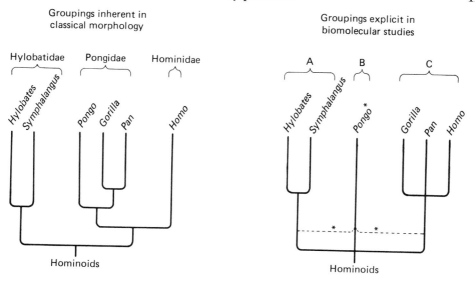

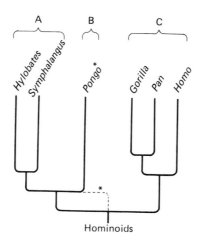

Fig. 5.7. Differences in the grouping patterns within hominoids as shown by the consensus of classical morphologists (upper left), the consensus of biomolecular studies (upper right), and the detailed morphometric result (lower). Asterisks indicate cluster links that are almost equally as likely in the various studies. The similarity between the biomolecular and morphometric results is quite marked.

bodily proportions (the data of Schultz studied by Oxnard, 1981*a*), and high-dimensional analyses of detailed measures of more localised anatomical regions (the data of Ashton, Oxnard and colleagues studied by Oxnard, 1983*a*, and Fig. 5.10) also provide a generally similar tripartite arrangement of these monkeys.

For a third time it is possible to compare and contrast these three techniques (Fig. 5.11). And for a third time it is clear that it is with the biomolecular studies that the morphometric results are most concordant.

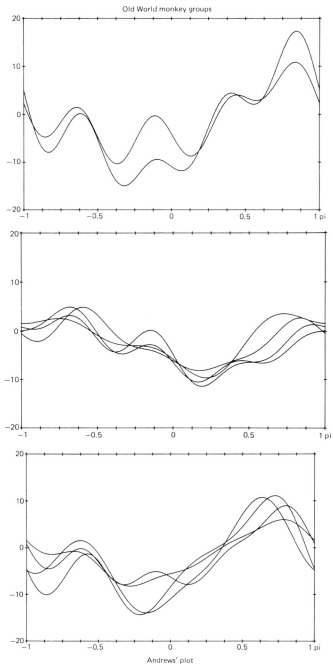

Fig. 5.8. Study of the summation of the several anatomical regions (as in Fig. 5.5) using Andrews' high-dimensional technique.

The upper frame demonstrates Andrews' plots for various colobine genera, the middle frame Andrews' plots for the combined group of genera (*Allenopithecus*, *Cercopithecus*, *Miopithecus* and *Erythrocebus*), the lower frame Andrews' plots for the combined group of genera (*Macaca*, *Cercocebus*, *Papio*, and *Mandrillus*).

The separation of these three overall groups from one another is marked. The lower plot shows within itself two pairs of plots, a separation of lesser degree, between macaques and mangabeys on the one hand, and baboons and mandrills on the other.

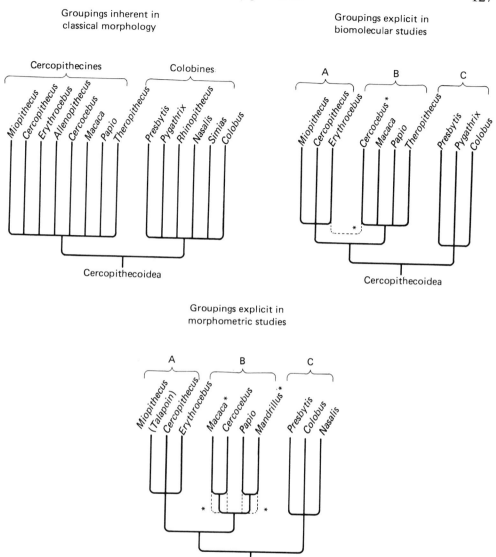

Fig. 5.9. Differences in the grouping patterns within Old World monkeys as shown by the consensus of classical morphologists (upper left), the consensus of biomolecular studies (upper right) and the detailed morphometric result (lower). Asterisks indicate cluster links that are almost equally as likely in the various studies. The similarity between the biomolecular and morphometric results is quite marked.

PROSIMIANS

It is considerably more difficult to discuss the operation of these three different methods as regards the various prosimian species. In part this is because these forms are remarkably more different from one another having been separated, presumably, for far longer periods of evolutionary time. In the main, however, the problem is that the biomolecular and morphometric techniques have not been applied to the full

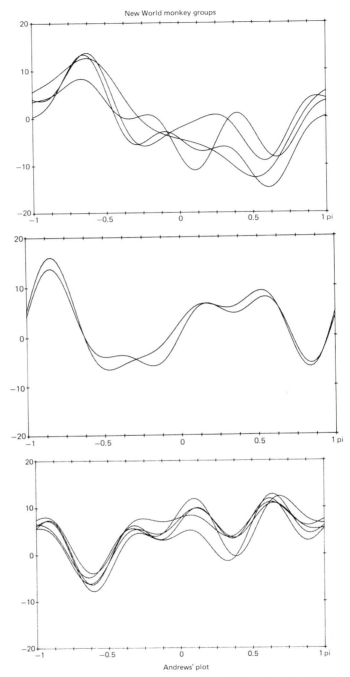

New World monkey groups

Andrews' plot

Fig. 5.10. Study of the summation of the several anatomical regions (as in Fig. 5.5.) using Andrews' high-dimensional technique.

The three frames demonstrate Andrews' plots for the various groups of New World monkeys. The first frame illustrates the prehensile-tailed and semiprehensile-tailed genera, including *Cebus*. The second plot includes only *Pithecia* and *Cacajao*. The third frame includes all the remaining cebid genera together with all the callithricid genera.

The reality of these groupings is clearly evident from the patterns of Andrews' plots, even though examination of individual canonical axes does not reveal marked separations.

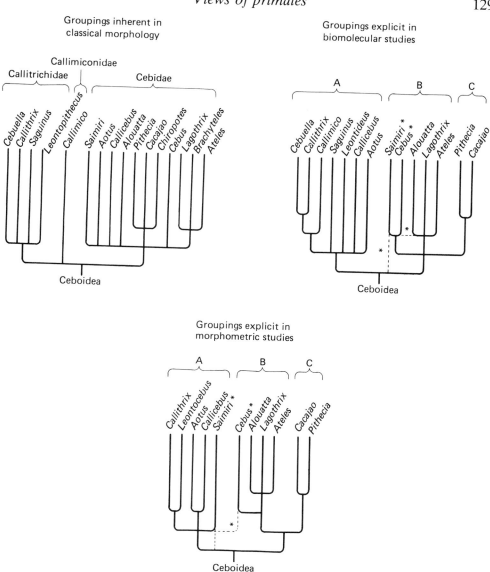

Fig. 5.11. Differences in the grouping patterns within New World monkeys as shown by the consensus of classical morphologists (upper left), the consensus of biomolecular studies (upper right) and the detailed morphometric result (lower). Asterisks indicate cluster links that are almost as equally likely in the various studies. The similarity between the biomolecular and morphometric results is quite marked.

range of species. Most of these animals are small and rare, and materials are not easily made available. But the classical studies, though somewhat limited in the same way, have the advantage of having been carried out over centuries rather than decades, and for that reason large quantities of data have been culled. Even so, however, we should be aware that some species (e.g. *Daubentonia* spp.) are quite rare, even in the collections of the oldest museums. Bearing these caveats in mind, we therefore note that classical organismal studies have long seen the living prosimians as divided into three: Lemuriformes (including tree shrews and aye-ayes), Lorisiformes and Tarsiiformes (e.g. Simpson, 1945; Le Gros Clark, 1959; Napier & Napier, 1967).

Those few biomolecular studies that have included sufficient prosimian species suggest a somewhat different picture (e.g. Beard, Barnicott & Hewett-Emmett, 1976; Beard & Goodman, 1976; Sarich & Wilson, 1967; Dene et al., 1976b). The grouping into Lemuriformes and Lorisiformes is generally fairly well recognised although the representation of genera is sparse. Such studies contrast, however, with classical ones in two ways. First, they do not place *Daubentonia* as close to Lemuriformes (at least some classical investigators would place this genus even within the indriids, a subgroup of the Lemuriformes). The new biomolecular studies locate *Daubentonia* as far distant from any extant species. Second, they do not place *Tarsius* with prosimians at all (as did Le Gros Clark, 1924, and many investigators since), but as more closely linked with anthropoids or, at the very least, intermediate between prosimians and anthropoids (which, if correct, would be a return to an earlier view).

Morphometric investigations once again mirror the biomolecular researches. Morphometric studies on the overall proportion of prosimians place both *Daubentonia* and *Tarsius* as being very far distant from each other and from the two main groups of lemuriform and lorisiform prosimians (Oxnard, 1973b; Jouffroy, Oxnard & German, 1982). When such studies also include anthropoids, then *Daubentonia* is further confirmed as being unique among primates (Oxnard, 1981b), and *Tarsius* is suggested as being closer to anthropoids than prosimians (Oxnard, 1978a, 1981a). The most recent studies of all (Oxnard, 1983b, and see Fig. 5.12) on high-dimensional investigations of summated detailed anatomical regions of these small animals also concur in defining two main groups of prosimians: Lemuriformes and Lorisiformes (each of which shows subgroups: cheirogaleines, lemurs and indriids in the former and lorisines and galagines in the latter), with *Daubentonia* and *Tarsius* each being markedly different from each other and from all the rest.

To conclude, it is possible to compare and contrast these three techniques (Fig. 5.13) and it is clear that it is with the biomolecular studies that the morphometric results are most concordant.

DISCUSSION

In summary, a similar picture of overall primate relationships (prosimians, New World and Old World monkeys, apes and humans) is presented by study of classical organismal biology and molecular biology. Though regional multivariate morphometric results reflect primarily the functions of individual anatomical regions, overall multivariate morphometric results concord with this same overall relationship of the animals, as found by study of both organisms and molecules.

There are, however, many detailed differences between the pictures presented by classical organismal and biomolecular ways of comparing the animals. These are most obvious within the hominoids but exist to greater or lesser degrees in each of the other major groups. The morphometric relationships mirror, in their details, the groupings which result from biomolecular studies rather than those resulting from classical organismal biology. The close relationships between humans and African apes, and their complete separation as a group from the other apes, is the most obvious part of this picture.

The classical approach is usually thought to provide the better picture of primate relationships because it depends upon such a huge volume of very different investiga-

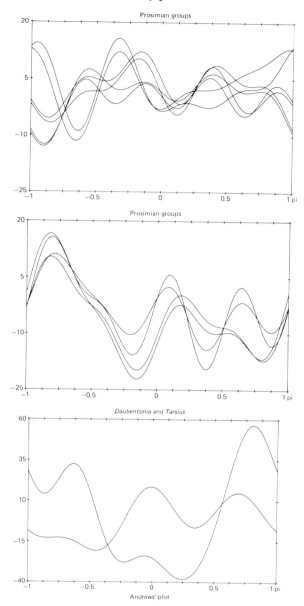

Fig. 5.12. Study of the summation of several anatomical regions (as in Fig. 5.5) using Andrews' high-dimensional technique.

The three frames demonstrate Andrews' plots for the various groups of prosimians. The first frame includes all genera currently described as Lemuriformes, except for *Daubentonia*. The second frame includes all genera currently described as Lorisiformes. These two frames demonstrate, notwithstanding the existence of appropriate subgroups within each, that these two major groups do indeed form coherent wholes. The third frame demonstrates the single individual plots for *Daubentonia* and *Tarsius*. These last two genera are, of course, totally different from each other; but they are also each totally different from any of the other prosimian genera. The reality of these groupings is clearly evident from the patterns of Andrews' plots, though examination of individual canonical axes does not reveal marked separations of this type.

It is of considerable interest that even within each of the major groups, Lemuriformes and Lorisiformes, similarities of high-dimensional plots indicate subgroups of each: galagines and lorisines for the Lorisiformes, lemurs, cheirogaleines and indriids for the Lemuriformes.

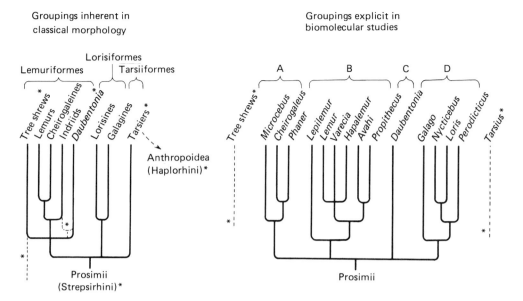

Groupings inherent in
classical morphology

Groupings explicit in
biomolecular studies

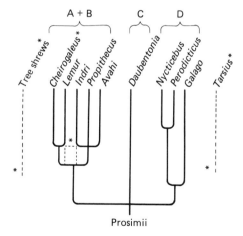

Groupings explicit in
morphometric studies

Fig. 5.13. Differences in the grouping patterns within prosimians as shown by the majority of classical morphologists (upper left), the consensus of biomolecular studies (upper right) and the detailed morphometric result (lower). Asterisks indicate cluster links that are equivocal or under dispute in various studies. For example, in the upper left frame, some investigators would not have tree shrews in the primates at all, some would link *Daubentonia* much more closely with the Indriidae, some would remove *Tarsius* from the prosimians. In other parts of the diagram asterisks indicate cluster links that are also at issue, or almost equally as likely in the various studies. Because of limitations explained in the text, these diagrams for prosimians are much less robust than those for anthropoids. Yet the similarity between the biomolecular and morphometric results is still quite marked.

tions carried out by many workers over the years, indeed over the centuries. On this count, the limited data stemming from the biomolecular studies can scarcely compare. In contrast, however, the biomolecular approach is believed by some to be better because it deals more directly with the basic materials of evolution. Its results are thought to be somewhat less diluted by non-genetic, developmental, biotic, environmental and other factors than are those of classical organismal biologists.

The new morphometric studies provide some individual findings that may provide insight into the differences between the classical organismal and biomolecular approaches.

Functional parts, evolutionary wholes

A first finding exists within the various morphometric studies themselves. A sufficient number of the regional anatomical investigations have now been carried out and it is not in doubt that the pictures they supply relate primarily to functional adaptation. Comparison of the results from a number of different laboratories provides the confirmation (e.g. the talus: Day & Wood, 1968; the arm and forearm: Feldesman, 1976; the pelvis: McHenry & Corruccini, 1975; the shoulder: Corruccini & Ciochon, 1976; all compared with studies of the same anatomical regions resulting from the collaborations of Oxnard and colleagues, confirmation supplied in Oxnard, 1983*b*).

Yet when the various anatomical regions are summated, either in a mode that carries out a single analysis on the overall proportions of all parts of the body (Oxnard, 1981*a*), or in a manner that adds together the results of separate analyses on each of the individual anatomical regions (Oxnard, 1983*a*), the overall results mirror primate relationships, not function. How can this be?

One possible explanation may be the following. The information that stems from each anatomical region is truly heavily functional. The addition of many such functional regions helps to mimic the addition of many different characters such as is normally attempted in studies of animal relationships. Though we may think, superficially, that only a single biological entity, the skeleton, is being examined, in fact, measurements of bones which comprise the primary data here must also be reflecting many other aspects of the morphology of the primates. As well as bone these include, of course, various soft tissues such as muscles, fasciae, ligaments and joints: i.e. the structure of the entire locomotor system is actually being sampled. Thus, these structural measurements must be reflecting the functions of those same locomotor tissues. And again, in addition to the biomechanical function of locomotion, these measurements must also be including some information about other systems such as the motor and sensory aspects of the nervous system, and even about environmental, ecological and behavioural aspects of the organisms. This widespread biological representation of these measurements follows simply because locomotion is such an all-pervasive activity of most primates. We can thus readily understand why suites of measurements apparently only from the skeleton add up to being very widely representative of the totality of the organism. It is, in fact, possible that these morphometric data summarise the entire organism better than the data of classical morphology, for these latter tend to be heavily biased towards skulls and teeth, and to ignore most other aspects of organisms.

There is, however, a second possible explanation why functional parts summate to evolutionary wholes. This resides in the fact that, though the structures of the anatomical regions reflect mainly the functions of those regions, some information about animal relationships is also contained within them. One example, for instance, is the structure of the shoulder. Though this anatomical region, when rendered morphometrically, seems to reflect mainly the function of the shoulder, some separations that coincide with overall primate relationships can be distinguished (e.g. a major division between prosimians and anthropoids by a second canonical axis: Ashton *et al.*, 1971). A second instance stems from the architecture of the arm and forearm. Though this reflects mainly the function of the upper limb, it is also possible to distinguish clusters that seem to indicate the overall relationships between the primates (e.g. separation between prosimians and anthropoids is partially effected by a second canonical axis: Ashton *et al.*, 1976). A third illustration can be seen in the pelvis. Though its chief features when rendered morphometrically mirror the functions of the pelvis, most especially in recognising the unique human pelvis, some clusterings reflecting primate relationships can be discerned (e.g. once again, a partial separation of prosimians and anthropoids can be discerned within several canonical axes combined: Zuckerman *et al.*, 1973; and especially Ashton *et al.*, 1981).

None of this is surprising; for though these morphological regions are extremely sensitive to function, there is no doubt at all that they must also reflect, to some degree or other, hereditary features other than functional ones. Thus, when we add several such anatomical regions together (something that can only be done when they have been rendered quantitatively), the following may occur. Functional components do not reinforce each other because the functions of the various parts are different. Components reflecting overall primate relationships do reinforce one another, gradually summating, because each (though statistically relatively independent) points in the same biological direction as the others.

A third type of finding emphasises the differences between morphometric analyses of anatomical regions as compared with morphometric surveys of whole organisms. Thus, though the usual flavour of these investigations has been to determine the clusterings of the animals, it is also possible to determine the clusterings of the anatomical variables (Oxnard, 1983*a*). Such studies reveal that clusters of variables in the regional anatomical investigations make most sense when viewed functionally. For example, clusters of variables in the shoulder studies are arranged around overall morphological features to do with function of the shoulder: its craniolateral torsion as related to the degree of rotation as in arm-raising and hanging, its mediolateral extent as related to degrees of terrestrial or arboreal quadrupedal movement (Oxnard, 1973*a*). Clusters of variables in the studies of the arm and forearm are arranged around morphological features to do with the function of the arm and forearm: e.g. a cluster of variables around the elbow related to its flexion and extension, a cluster of variables around the wrist related to both flexion and extension of the wrist and its ulnar and radial deviation, and a special cluster of variables from both elbow and wrist that relate to pronation and supination of the radio-ulnar joint (see Oxnard, 1983*a* and Table 5.1).

In contrast, clusters of variables in the morphometric studies of entire organisms present differently. Though it is not easy to see functional meaning in such clusters, meaning that may be related to a combination of developmental and evolutionary phenomena is discernible. Thus in the analyses by Oxnard (1983*a*) of the data on overall proportions of primates taken by Schultz, and on limb proportions of prosimians supplied by Jouffroy & Lessertisseur (see acknowledgements at end of this paper), the clusters of variables are into groups representing: (*a*) proximo-distal features of the limbs, (*b*) mediolateral arrays across limbs, (*c*) serially homologous

Table 5.1. *Example of functional clusters of variables: factor analysis of data on arm and forearm*

Clusters of variables	Anatomical features	Overall description
Shared factor pattern	Facet on humerus for ulna Facet on ulna for humerus Projection epicondyles Position radial tuberosity Insertion of triceps	Measures at elbow
Factor axis two	Projection of ulnar styloid Relative sizes, both styloids Projection of radial styloid Widths, radius, ulna	Measures at wrist
Shared factor pattern	Distal insertion of pronator Distal insertion of biceps Lateral bowing of radius Angle of interosseous ridge Maximum bowing of radius	Measures relating to pronation and supination

Table 5.2. *Evolutionary and developmental clusters of variables: factor analysis of data on proportions of prosimians*

Clusters of variables	Anatomical features	Overall description
Factor one	Eighteen variables: Four upper limb lengths Four lower limb lengths Five hand lengths Five foot lengths	Proximo-distal dimensions of the limb
Factor two	Length of fourth metacarpal Lengths of fourth phalanges Length of fourth digit	Variables pertaining to digit four
Factor four	Lengths of middle metacarpals Lengths of middle metatarsals Middle phalanges of hand Middle phalanges of foot	Pre-axial to post-axial in hand and foot
Factor three	Length of forearm Length of leg (shin) Length of hand Length of foot	Mirror image serial elements (see factor five)
Factor five	Length of upper arm Length of thigh Length of hand Length of foot	Mirror image serial elements (see factor three)

combinations of elements of limbs, and even (*d*) a special cluster relating to the fourth manual digit, a curious finding until we remember that the structure of the hand in prosimians differs from that in anthropoids through its organisation around the fourth digit (e.g. Oxnard, 1983*a* and Table 5.2).

Probably there is some truth in all these suggestions. We must, then, not be overly surprised to find that overall organismal relationships emerge when localised anatomical regions are summated morphometrically.

The difference between classical organismal studies and morphometrics

A second finding of the morphometric investigations relates to the difference from the results obtained by classical organismal investigations. Both depend purely upon assessments at organ and organismal levels. Why should the mere addition, to morphology, of measurement and analysis produce an answer different from that obtained by visual assessment?

There is one immediate way in which the morphometric method differs from the classical. Though the creative mind of the classical investigator is able to take account of a great deal of interesting detail in the complex forms and patterns that are studied, that mind is not able to cope so easily with quantitative relationships, and scarcely at all with associations in the data such as stem from statistical properties such as variance and covariance, autocorrelation and cross-correlation. It is not that these statistical relationships do not exist within classical data; they surely do. It is merely that the methods applied in classical studies have not been capable of identifying and allowing for them. The various methods (quantification and analysis) used in multivariate statistical approaches to studying these same structures are exactly designed to take account of such phenomena. This is the simple major difference between the classical morphological and multivariate morphometric approaches and it presumably accounts for the considerable difference in results.

The similarity between biomolecular studies and morphometrics

Let us move, then, to a third matter: why should the morphometric result resemble closely the general trend evident among the various biomolecular investigations? Why should the morphometric result contradict that of classical morphology in this particular direction? It cannot be because the initial data of the morphometric studies are as close to evolution as the biomolecules; being organismal, whether quantitative or not, these data are presumably as far from the genetic materials as are the classical organismal data themselves.

The classical organismal data display correlations (in addition to those that are accidental) for a multitude of causal reasons. Especially obvious examples are the correlations that are due to mechanisms of inheritance, to patterns of development and to processes of ontogenetic adaptation. The technology of classical studies does not remove any but the most obvious of such correlations, and hence, there is great redundancy in the information that it presents. In biomolecular studies many fewer 'characters' are examined and summated. However, because of the way in which molecular phenomena have been discovered and studied, because of our still very restricted understanding of the biomolecular picture of whole organisms, and because the coverage of biomolecular phenomena is extremely spotty, it is highly unlikely that there will be any very large intercorrelations among the various biomolecular items. There will, of course, be some correlations but these are likely to be little more than those necessarily resulting from the almost random selection of these data. There is, therefore, little correlation in the data and they can be thought of as being the equivalent of data with correlation removed. In biomolecular investigations, therefore, most of the information is new; there is probably only a small amount of redundancy.

I do not wish to imply that correlation does not exist in biomolecular data; clearly, it does. There must be DNA sequences that relate to (say) specific RNA formations, and particular RNA formations associated with (say) particular enzymes; these in turn must be linked with specific biochemical functions of (say) the blood; and these, finally, may have important repercussions on (say) the anatomy or physiology of some anatomical part. Such functional links will result in marked intercorrelations among biomolecular data but it is not at all common, in choosing characters of the biomolecular type in evolutionary studies, for investigators deliberately to select such obviously linked systems. Indeed, such linked systems are, so far, poorly known save in a few special experimental laboratory species. In general, those data that are chosen for biomolecular evolutionary studies are much *less* likely to be correlated (for reasons other than accidental) than are any of the data used in organismal studies. The molecular data, indeed, are rather likely to be almost totally independent from one another (although this will become less the case as we learn more about the molecular biology of whole organisms). Of course, once we do know a great deal about molecular biology, we will undoubtedly find many linkages; but at the moment we do not have many biomolecular examples, and it is rather likely that they are somewhat isolated from one another.

For organismal features, however, such an independence is very seldom the case. Though we might think, superficially, that there will be little correlation (except for that accidentally present) between, for instance, the form in humans of the head and the shape of the little finger, or between the structure of the human eye and the lengths of the digits, the existence of phenomena such as Down's syndrome and Marfan's disease reminds us immediately that even such apparently remote anatomical areas can be most closely linked. Though these particular examples do not operate, presumably, in normal individuals, many other equivalent and perhaps more subtle examples undoubtedly do.

We can now see that the morphometric method (morphological dimensions treated by multivariate statistical methods that eliminate correlation) may (for that reason) mimic the biomolecular results. Both of the more modern approaches depend, in a sense, upon the absence of redundant information; one through redundancy being accidentally missing, the other through redundancy being deliberately removed. Both may thus produce similar arrangements of the primates. Presumably, if we weighted classical morphological data to allow for the intercorrelations that are present among them, we would also obtain this result.

FUTURE POSSIBILITIES

Perhaps the most exciting part of all of these results is that they have been obtained using methods which seem capable of improvement in the future, for the morphometric results depend at present upon only two separate lines of investigation, one using overall bodily proportions and the second using summations of independent statistical studies of individual anatomical regions. Each has limitations.

In the case of the first (overall bodily proportions), it must be acknowledged that Schultz's data have limitations. They constitute a unique body of information and are more extensive than can be found in any other single study representing, as they do, the work of a single individual over a lifetime. However, they do not define the shapes of primates as well as do more detailed studies of all anatomical regions. They are generally restricted to indices embodying trunk length in the denominator and are less accurate measures of primate carcasses rather than more accurate measures of the skeleton. Moreover, they are defined purely as measures of overall proportions, rather than as succinct measures of detailed skeletal form. Finally, samples are very small for ten of the genera.

In the case of the second (summation of individual anatomical regions), it must again be acknowledged that the method of summation has its drawbacks. Though the data from the individual anatomical regions are accurate and detailed, the fact that the summation had to be carried out by adding separate analyses, rather than making one gigantic analysis of the entire data set, means that some information (the interactions between the individual anatomical regions) has been lost. This missing information may not be large because we already know that the intercorrelations between major anatomical regions tend to be small, but we do not actually know exactly what has been lost.

We can therefore expect that a series of future morphometric studies, employing discriminating measures for all the various bodily regions, using methods which are able to treat the data as a single universe and with a greater number of much larger samples, will provide information about primate relationships that will be much more sensitive than those which have been previously demonstrated. We may expect that such new studies will show (even more so than the above) both the view of humans as uniquely separated from non-human primates due to functional reflections of structure in individual anatomical regions, and the similarities of humans with certain non-human primates (African apes) based upon overall relationships.

In the same way, however, we can expect major advances in the area of biomolecular studies of primate relationships. These will probably involve at least two major features. One may relate to the development of techniques to eliminate redundant information, as these studies grow in volume so that they start to provide duplicate data. Whether this will be achieved by precise statistical estimators such as those currently applied in morphometrics, or whether this will be achieved by using cladistic methods (which allow, crudely, for correlation and thus attempt to remove redundant information), will probably depend upon the precise nature of the studies and the interests of the particular investigators (e.g. Henning, 1966; Funk & Brooks, 1981).

A second will probably relate to the methodology of new biomolecular studies. Thus the discovery of DNA–DNA hybridisation techniques provides the possibility of doing studies that (like the morphometric investigations) allow the researcher to see all the data at one time, in a grand averaged manner as it were (see, for example, the studies on various groups of birds by Sibley & Ahlquist, 1980, 1981). Such studies produce a distance resulting from the average across the entire genome (an enormous number of nucleotides). This 'grand average distance' differs from the individual distances that are produced by studies of each individual protein moiety, or each individual set of immunogenetic measures, or each individual group of chromosome comparisons (earlier forms of biomolecular studies). Such a distance is much more reminiscent of the 'generalised distance' of morphometric investigations that represents the distances of species from one another when a very large range of items is included.

It is of further interest that such 'distances' can be applied to 'rates of change' in a way that mutes the criticisms of methods of estimating biomolecular rates of change. At present, for instance, it is appropriate to criticise the idea of the molecular clock upon the basis that no one 'clock' model is especially useful for dating purposes: why should change in any one set of proteins have been especially stable or linear? Change in the 'grand average distance' provided by all nucleotides in the genome, such as stems from the DNA–DNA hybridisation method, though not necessarily totally linear or totally constant, will, simply because it is a grand average, be able to provide far better estimates of 'average rates' and hence of dating. This, too, is an exciting prospect.

Can we expect major improvements in classical organismal studies? Indeed, we can and I believe that the clue exists in the last paragraph. Though the methods of cladistics currently used are far from perfect, the general effect of cladistics is to take classical data, in all their many forms, some meristic, some quasi-continuous, even some genuinely continuous (even if currently only expressible in a non-continuous fashion) and, in a somewhat crude but nevertheless useful way, apply to them a method which has the equivalent effect of allowing for some correlation and of removing some redundant information. We can therefore expect that even classical studies, when utilising the cladistic method, will converge gradually upon the picture provided by biomolecular and morphometric investigations. We can also expect that removal of correlation in classical data by appropriate statistical methods will gradually come to be applied. This should give the best result of all.

All kinds of organismal studies have the advantage over the biomolecular in that, save for rare and special types of preservations, only they can be applied to fossils. This last is a most exciting conclusion when used with the new morphometric views in mind. For the new views allow us to obtain results about the relationships between humans and other primates that concur with the biomolecular approaches even when biomolecular studies themselves cannot be carried out. For many investigators this means the ability to assess rare specimens of which preserved or skeletal materials are available in museums but of which fresh biological materials do not exist or cannot easily be obtained. For palaeontologists, this especially means abilities to evaluate the more complete fossils, especially those possibly related to the human lineage.

It is true that for some types of fossils, materials are available that can be assessed by biomolecular methods. At present these are limited to uncommon examples: the examination of actual bodily tissues from the frozen carcasses of mammoths extinct for a relatively short period, the study of materials in which some of the original molecules (perhaps changed only slightly) still exist because of phenomena such as mummification or preservation within a matrix (the tar of the La Brea species, or the amber of certain insect remains). However, in the majority of cases the information that is available for extinct creatures is about form and pattern. These can only be studied by methods that assess organismal morphology; and though in the past this has mainly meant classical morphology, it now includes morphometric evaluations which may, if the above findings are not too far awry, better mirror the biomolecular assessment, the underlying stuff of evolution.

This paper has depended upon the willingness of the late Professor A. H. Schultz to make available his lifetime's collection of original data on the overall proportions of primates. Dr Françoise-K. Jouffroy and the late Dr Jacques Lessertisseur also made available their extensive data on the overall proportions of prosimians.

The paper includes a discussion of results and ideas stemming from collaborative studies carried out with Professor Lord Zuckerman of the Zoological Society of London and the University of East Anglia, with Professor F. P. Lisowski at the University of Hong Kong, with Professor E. H. Ashton, Dr R. M. Flinn and Mr T. F. Spence of the University of Birmingham, with Professor W. J. Moore of the University of Leeds, with Professor G. H. Albrecht of the University of Southern California, with Dr J. E. McArdle of the Laboratory of Applied Zoology, Illinois, and with Miss Rebecca Z. German of Harvard University.

Thanks are due to Miss Joan Hives, Mesdames Marsha Greaves and Eleanor Craycraft, and Messrs Hugh and David Oxnard for computational, secretarial and drafting work. The studies have been supported by NSF grants GS 30508 and DEB 81939, and by research funds from the University of Southern California.

REFERENCES

Andrews, D. F. (1972). Plots of high dimensional data. *Biometrics*, **28**, 125–36.

Andrews, D. F. (1973). Graphical techniques for high dimensional data. In *Discriminant Analysis and Application*, ed. T. Cacoullos. pp. 37–59. New York: Academic Press.

Ashton, E. H., Flinn, R. M., Moore, J. W., Oxnard, C. E. & Spence, T. F. (1981). Further quantitative studies of form and function in the primate pelvis with special reference to *Australopithecus*. *Transactions of the Zoological Society of London*, **86**, 1–98.

Ashton, E. H., Flinn, R. M., Oxnard, C. E. & Spence, T. F. (1971). The functional and classificatory significance of combined metrical features of the primate shoulder girdle. *Journal of Zoology*, **163**, 319–50.

Ashton, E. H., Flinn, R. M., Oxnard, C. E. & Spence, T. F. (1976). The adaptive and classificatory significance of certain quantitative features of the forelimb in primates. *Journal of Zoology*, **179**, 515–56.

Baba, M. L., Darga, L. L. & Goodman, M. (1979). Immunodiffusion systematics of the primates. The platyrrhini. *Folia Primatologica*, **32**, 207–38.

Barnicott, N. A. (1969). Some biochemical and serological aspects of primate evolution. *Science Progress* (*Oxford*), **57**, 459–93.

Beard, J. M., Barnicott, N. A. & Hewett-Emmet, D. (1976). Alpha and beta chains of the major haemoglobin and a note on the minor component of *Tarsius*. *Nature* (*London*), **259**, 338–41.

Beard, J. M & Goodman, M. (1976). The hemoglobins of *Tarsius bancanus*. In *Molecular Anthropology*, ed. M. Goodman & R. E. Tashian, pp. 239–55. New York: Plenum.

Benveniste, R. A. & Todaro, T. G. (1976). Evolution of type C viral genes: evidence for an Asian origin of man. *Nature* (*London*), **26**, 101–8.

Bruce, E. J. & Ayala, F. J. (1978). Humans and apes are genetically very similar. *Nature* (*London*), **276**, 264–5.

Bruce, E. J. & Ayala, F. J. (1979). Phylogenetic relationships between man and the apes: electrophoretic evidence. *Evolution*, **33**, 1040–56.

Cave, A. J. E. (1973). The primate nasal fossa. *Journal of the Linnean Society* (*Zoology*), **5**, 377–87.

Chivers, D. J. & Joysey, K. A. (1978). *Recent Advances in Primatology*. London: Academic Press.

Chu, E. H. Y. & Bender M. A. (1961). Chromosome cytology and evolution in primates. *Science*, **133**, 1399–405.

Ciochon, R. L. & Chiarelli, A. B. (1980). *Evolutionary Biology of New World Monkeys and Continental Drift*. New York: Plenum.

Clark, W. E. Le Gros. (1924). Notes on the living tarsier (*Tarsius spectrum*). *Proceedings of the Zoological Society of London*, **1924**, 217–23.

Clark, W. E. Le Gros. (1926). The anatomy of the pen-tailed tree shrew (*Ptilocercus lowii*). *Proceedings of the Zoological Society of London*, **1926**, 461–501.

Clark, W. E. Le Gros. (1934). *Early Forerunners of Man; a Morphological Study of the Evolutionary Origin of the Primates*. London: Baillière, Tindall & Cox.

Clark, W. E. Le Gros. (1959). *The Antecedents of Man*. Edinburgh University Press.

Corruccini, R. S. & Ciochon, R. L. (1976). Morphometric affinities of the human shoulder. *American Journal of Physical Anthropology*, **45**, 19–38.

Day, M. H. & Wood, B. A. (1968). Functional affinities of the Olduvai hominid 8 talus. *Man*, **3**, 440–55.

Dene, H. M., Goodman, M. & Prychodko, W. (1976a) Immunodiffusion evidence on the phylogeny of the primates. In *Molecular Anthropology*, ed. M. Goodman & R. E. Tashian, pp. 171–95. New York: Plenum.

Dene, H. M., Goodman, M., Prychodko, W. & Moore, G. W. (1976b). Immunodiffusion systematics of the Primates. *Folia Primatologica*, **25**, 35–61.

Elliot, D. G. (1913). *A Review of the Primates*. New York: Monographs of the American Museum of Natural History.

Feldesman, M. (1976). The primate forelimb: a morphometric study of locomotor diversity. *University of Oregon Anthropological Papers*, **10**, 1–154.

Fitch, W. M. (1977). The phyletic interpretation of macromolecular sequence information: simple methods. In *Molecular Anthropology*, ed. M. Goodman & R. E. Tashian, pp. 211–48. New York: Plenum.

Fitch, W. M. & Langley, C. H. (1976). Evolutionary rates in proteins: neutral mutations and the molecular clock. In *Molecular Anthropology*, ed. M. Goodman & R. E. Tashian, pp. 197–219. New York: Plenum.

Friedenthal, H. (1900). Ueber einen experimentellen Nachweis von Blutsverwandtschaft. *Archiv für Anatomie und Physiologie Leipzig, Physiologische Abteil*, 494–508.

Funk, V. A. & Brooks, D. R. (1981). *Advances in Cladistics*. New York: New York Botanical Gardens.

Goodman, M. (1975). Protein sequence and immunological specificity: their role in phylogenetic studies of primates. In *Phylogeny of the Primates*, ed W. P. Luckett & F. S. Szalay, pp. 219–48. New York: Academic Press.

Goodman, M. (1976). Towards a genealogical description of the Primates. In *Molecular Anthropology*, ed. M. Goodman & R. E. Tashian, pp. 321–53. New York: Plenum.

Goodman, M. & Tashian, R. E. (1976). *Molecular Anthropology*. New York: Plenum.

Gower, J. C. & Ross, G. J. S. (1969). Minimum spanning trees and single linkage cluster analysis. *Applied Statistics*, **180**, 54–64.

Hennig, W. (1966). *Phylogenetic Systematics*. Urbana: University of Illinois Press.

Hershkovitz, P. (1977). *Living New World Monkeys (Platyrrhini)*. University of Chicago Press.

Hewett-Emmett, D., Cook, C. N. & Barnicott, R. A. (1976). Old World monkey haemoglobins: deciphering phylogeny from complex patterns of molecular evolution. In *Molecular Anthropology*, ed. M. Goodman & R. E. Tashian, pp. 257–76. New York: Plenum.

Hill, W. C. O. (1953–1970). *Primates. Comparative Anatomy and Taxonomy*. Edinburgh University Press.

Huxley, T. H. (1872). *A Manual of the Anatomy of Vertebrated Animals*. New York: Appleton.

Jouffroy, F.-K., Oxnard, C. E. & German, R. Z. (1982). Interprétation phylogénétique des proportions des membres des tarsiers, par comparaison avec les autres prosimiens sauteurs. Analyse multivariée. *Comptes rendus hébdomadaires des séances de l'Académie des sciences, Paris*, **295**, 315–20.

Kohne, D. E. (1975). DNA evolution data and its relevance to mammalian phylogeny. In *Phylogeny of the Primates*, ed. W. P. Luckett & F. S. Szalay, pp. 249–61. New York: Plenum.

Luckett, W. P. (1974). Comparative development and evolution of the placenta in primates. *Contributions to Primatology*, **3**, 142–234.

McHenry, H. M. & Corruccini, R. S. (1975). Multivariate analysis of early hominid pelvic bones. *American Journal of Physical Anthropology*, **43**, 263–70.

McKenna, M. C. (1975). Towards a phylogenetic classification of the mammalia. In *Phylogeny of the Primates*, ed. W. P. Luckett & F. S. Szalay, pp. 21–41. New York: Plenum.

Martin, R. D. (1975). The bearing of reproductive behavior and ontogeny on strepsirhine phylogeny. In *Phylogeny of the Primates*, ed. W. P. Luckett & F. S. Szalay, pp. 265–98. New York: Plenum.

Minkoff, E. C. (1974). The direction of lower primate evolution: an old hypothesis revived. *American Naturalist*, **108**, 519–32.

Mivart, G. (1867). Additional notes on the osteology of the *Lemuridae*. *Proceedings of the Zoological Society of London*, 960–75.

Mivart, G. (1873). On *Lepilemur* and *Cheirogaleus*, and the zoological rank of the *Lemuroidea*. *Proceedings of the Zoological Society of London*, 484–510.

Napier, J. R. & Napier, P. H. (1967). *A Handbook of the Living Primates*. New York: Academic Press.

Nuttall, G. H. F. (1904). *Blood Immunity and Blood Relationships*. Cambridge University Press.

Owen, R. (1862). On the aye-aye (*Chiromys*, Cuvier; *Chiromys madagascariensis*, Gmel., Sonnerat; *Lemur psilodactylus*, Schreber, Shaw). *Transactions of the Zoological Society of London*, **5**, 33–101.

Owen, R. (1866). *On the Anatomy of Vertebrates*. London: Longman, Green & Co.

Oxnard, C. E. (1973a). *Form and Pattern in Human Evolution: Some Mathematical, Physical and Engineering Approaches*. University of Chicago Press.

Oxnard, C. E. (1973b). Some locomotor features of the pelvic girdle in primates. *Symposia of the Zoological Society of London*, **33**, 71–165.

Oxnard, C. E. (1975). *Uniqueness and Diversity in Human Evolution: Morphometric Studies of Australopithecines*. University of Chicago Press.

Oxnard, C. E. (1977). Human fossils: the new revolution. In *The Great Ideas Today*, ed. J. Van Doren. Chicago: Britannica Press.

Oxnard, C. E. (1978a). The problem of convergence and the place of *Tarsius* in primate phylogeny. In *Recent Advances in Primatology*, vol. 3, *Evolution*, ed. D. J. Chivers & K. A. Joysey, pp. 239–47. London: Academic Press.

Oxnard, C. E. (1978b). One biologist's view of morphometrics. *Annual Review of Ecology and Systematics*, **9**, 219–41.

Oxnard, C. E. (1981a). The place of man among the primates: anatomical, molecular and morphometric evidence. *Homo*, **32**, 149–76.

Oxnard, C. E. (1981b). The uniqueness of *Daubentonia*. *American Journal of Physical Anthropology*, **54**, 1–22.

Oxnard, C. E. (1983a). *The Order of Man: a Biomathematical Anatomy of the Primates*. University of Hong Kong Press.

Oxnard, C. E. (1983b). Multivariate statistics in physical anthropology: testing and interpretation. *Zeitschrift für Morphologie und Anthropologie*, **73**, 237–78.

Romero-Herrera, A. E., Lehmann, H., Joysey, K. A. & Friday, A. E. (1976). Evolution of myoglobin amino acid sequences in Primates and other vertebrates. In *Molecular Anthropology*, ed. M. Goodman & R. E. Tashian, pp. 289–300. New York: Plenum.

Romero-Herrera, A. E., Lehmann, H., Joysey, K. A. & Friday, A. E. (1978). On the evolution of myoglobin. *Philosophical Transactions of the Royal Society*, **283**, 61–163.

Romero-Herrera, A. E., Lieska, N., Goodman, M. & Simons, E. L. (1979). The use of amino-acid sequence analysis in assessing evolution. *Biochemie*, **61**, 767–79.

Sarich, V. M. & Cronin, J. E. (1976). Molecular systematics of the primates. In *Molecular Anthropology*, ed. M. Goodman & R. E. Tashian, pp. 141–70. New York: Plenum.

Sarich, V. M. & Cronin, J. E. (1977). Generation length and rates of hominoid molecular evolution. *Nature (London)*, **269**, 354–5.

Sarich, V. M. & Cronin, J. E. (1980). South American mammal molecular systematics, evolutionary clocks and continental drift. In *Evolutionary Biology of New World Monkeys and Continental Drift* ed. R. L. Ciochon & A. B. Chiarelli, pp. 399–421. New York: Plenum.

Sarich, V. M & Wilson, A. C. (1967). Immunological time scale for hominid evolution. *Science*, **158**, 1200–4.

Sarich, V. M. & Wilson, A. C. (1973). Generation time and genomic evolution in primates. *Science*, **179**, 1144–7.

Schultz, A. H. (1929). The technique of measuring the outer body of human foetuses and of primates in general. *Contributions to Embryology*, 213–57.

Schultz, A. H. (1936). Characters common to higher primates and characters specific for man. *Quarterly Review of Biology*, **11**, 259–83.

Schultz, A. H. (1969). *The Life of Primates*. New York: Universe Books.

Schultz, A. H. (1970). The comparative uniformity of the Cercopithecidae. In *Old World Monkeys*, ed. J. R. Napier & P. Napier, pp. 39–52. New York: Academic Press.

Sibley, C. G. & Ahlquist, J. E. (1980). The relationships of the 'primitive insect eaters' (Aves: Passeriformes) as indicated by DNA–DNA hybridization. *Proceedings of the International Ornithological Congress*, **17**, 1215–20.

Sibley, C. G. & Ahlquist, J. E. (1981). The relationships of the accentors (Prunella) as indicated by DNA–DNA hybridization. *Journal of Ornithology*, **122**, 369–78.

Simpson, G. G. (1945). The principles of classification and a classification of mammals. *Bulletin of the American Museum of Natural History*, **85**, 1–350.

Szalay, F. S. (1975a). Phylogeny, adaptations and dispersal of the tarsiiforme primates. In *Phylogeny of the Primates*, ed. W. P. Luckett & F. S. Szalay, pp. 357–404. New York: Plenum.

Szalay, F. S. (1975b). Phylogeny of primate higher taxa. The basicranial evidence. In *Phylogeny of the Primates*, ed. W. P. Luckett & F. S. Szalay, pp. 91–125. New York: Plenum.

Thorington, R. W. Jr. & Groves, C. P. (1970). An annotated classification of the Cercopithecoidea. In *Old World Monkeys: Evolution Systematics and Behavior*, ed. J. R. Napier & P. H. Napier, pp. 629–47. New York: Academic Press.

Tuttle, R. H. (1975). Parallelism, brachiation and hominoid phylogeny. In *Phylogeny of the Primates*, ed. W. P. Luckett & F. S. Szalay, pp. 447–80. New York: Plenum.

Tuttle, R. H. (1977). Naturalistic positional behavior of apes and models of hominid evolution, 1929–76. In *Progress in Ape Research*, ed. G. H. Bourne, pp. 277–96. New York: Academic Press.

Wood Jones, F. (1929). *Man's Place Among the Mammals*. London: Edward Arnold.

Zuckerman, S. (1932). *Social Life of Monkeys and Apes*. London: Kegan Paul.

Zuckerman, S. (1933). *Functional Affinities of Man, Monkeys and Apes*. London: Kegan Paul.

Zuckerman, S., Ashton, E. H., Flinn, R. M., Oxnard, C. E. & Spence, T. F. (1973). Some locomotor features of the pelvic girdle in primates. *Symposia of the Zoological Society of London*, **33**, 71–165.

6 The pattern of evolution within the genus *Homo*

ALAN BILSBOROUGH

Department of Physical Anthropology, University of Cambridge, Downing Street, Cambridge CB2 3DZ, UK

The past decade has witnessed significant advances in our understanding of human evolution; discoveries during that period have provided extensive new evidence of fossil hominids, whilst developments in dating techniques and the geological sciences have yielded a wealth of information permitting the reconstruction of the environment, ecology and behaviour of past hominid communities. The impact of these developments has not been limited to providing additional evidence to chart the patterns of human evolution; they have opened up new avenues of investigation and altered the conceptual framework within which the fossil evidence is analysed and evaluated. Some of these theoretical and investigative changes are discussed by Wood (1981). Fossil evidence of postcranial anatomy and approaches for investigating the evolution of truncal erectness and bipedalism are similarly dealt with by Aiello & Day (1982). This paper therefore focusses primarily upon craniodental material assigned to *Homo*, and contextual evidence pertinent to its evaluation.

AIMS AND DEFINITIONS

Constructing an adequate definition of the genus *Homo* is one of the thornier problems of palaeoanthropology. The limitations of static Linnean nomina, particularly their inadequacy for characterising evolutionary processes involving spatial variation and temporal change, are now generally recognised and the once prevalent excessively typological approach to fossil taxa has been largely abandoned. Granted the arbitrary nature of any taxonomic division, most recent discussions have centred upon the most appropriate (i.e. useful) point at which to effect separation. The traditional approach has been to use *Homo* and other hominid taxa in a grade sense, and the associated phylogenies have been termed 'evolutionary' (Simpson, 1975) or, less elegantly, 'stratophenetic' (Gingerich, 1978).

Disaffection with this approach and, in particular, its inevitable corollary that 'an australopithecine mother must have given birth to a *Homo* child' (Campbell, 1978), has led some workers to advocate a cladistic approach (see Wood, 1981). It is not appropriate to discuss this in detail here: suffice it to note that the claimed objectivity of cladistic systematics generally involves circular reasoning (Gingerich, 1978), and is equally arbitrary in its taxonomic distinctions. If grade classifications necessarily involve the taxonomic separation of temporally sequent populations, clade ones inevitably lead to the splitting of single species at their nodal points. Cladistic analysis depends critically upon the identification of multiple character states and their polarity (i.e. from primitive to derived). This is difficult enough when the group under investigation includes an array of clearly closely related extant species (e.g.

cercopithecoids); it is much more so when the group is represented only by a single extant species and the fossil record is fragmentary and incomplete, as with Hominidae.

For these and other reasons I, like Walker (1976), 'prefer to classify things on the basis of what they look like rather than on what they might evolve into if, by any chance, we happen to have our lineages correctly documented'. I therefore use *Homo* and other taxa in a grade sense in the remainder of this paper.

Various criteria other than morphological have been offered as a basis for defining *Homo*. Several workers have advocated a cultural (e.g. association of fossils with undoubted artefacts) or chronological boundary, or a combination of chronological and morphological criteria. For example, Campbell (1973) advocates defining *Homo* as those non-robust australopithecine populations $\leqslant 1.3$–1.5 My old, whilst Boaz & Howell (1977) consider the genus to have an antiquity of 2.3 My, a view shared by Tobias (1978). This figure is apparently based upon the reported potassium–argon (K–Ar) date of 1.9 ± 0.4 My from Modjokerto (Java), itself subject to uncertainties (see below). Campbell's boundary is based upon the appearance of culture-related traits which indicate 'a new hominid adaptive plateau' in response to environments characterised by marked seasonality. This definition is not directly demonstrable from the fossil material *per se*, but depends upon the recognition and evaluation of particular traits – an inferential and subjective process and, as such, likely to vary between workers.

Combinations of morphological, cultural and temporal criteria, whilst superficially attractive, therefore raise more problems than they solve. For example, what is the optimal compound of different kinds of data, and should a specimen which morphologically approximates to *Homo* be excluded if its age exceeds the posited lower limit of the genus, or if it lacks cultural association?

For all the admitted inadequacies, therefore, the most satisfactory basis for defining *Homo* remains solely morphological. Various such definitions are available in the literature, and I do not intend to consider them in detail here. Two well known examples are Le Gros Clark (1964) and Leakey, Tobias & Napier (1964). Walker (1976) outlines the main cranial contrasts between *Australopithecus* and *Homo* and their morphological concomitants, whilst the most complete recent characterisation known to me is that of Howell (1978). In summary, compared with *Australopithecus*, early specimens referred to *Homo* show features phenetically closer to later human populations in the size and proportions of the dentition, the size and shape of the dental arcade, the depth and thickness of the mandibular corpus and height of the ramus, the structure of the middle face (moderate/strongly developed supra-orbital torus; anteriorly projecting nasal bones; nasal floor sharply delineated from the alveolar plane of the maxilla; zygomatic process with an inferior margin below, or posterior to, the inferior margin of the orbit), and an expanded, strongly constructed neurocranium.

It is worth noting that fossil specimens are individually assigned to taxa, whereas it is the populations from which they are derived which are of primary concern in phyletic studies. Early hominid populations whose mean parameters would justify their inclusion within *Homo* are likely to have included individuals whose characteristics could fall at or beyond the limits of the genus. It may eventually prove possible, given appropriate morphological, chronological and spatial data, to aggregate specimens into samples from which realistic estimates of population parameters may be derived. Unfortunately, we are as yet far from that stage, and current studies of the initial evolution of *Homo* are perforce based upon isolated or almost isolated specimens when compared with the later stages of evolution within the genus.

EARLY HOMO

The documented evidence for the evolution of the genus *Homo* falls predominantly – perhaps entirely – within the Quaternary era (Pleistocene and Holocene). The earliest specimens assigned to the genus (whether formally or informally) are from east Africa, particularly the sites at Olduvai Gorge (Tanzania) and Koobi Fora (Kenya), supplemented by more limited material from Omo (Ethiopia) and the Sterkfontein Valley (South Africa). The material, which is often associated with remains of robust australopithecines, is highly variable and, as yet, incompletely described. Further attribution has been made in some cases, usually to the still unfortunately poorly known species *H. habilis* (Leakey *et al.*, 1964), of which the Olduvai type and paratypes have not been fully described. The recovery of specimens from Omo and extensive remains from Koobi Fora has led to comparisons with, and some necessary reassessment of, the Olduvai material although all current evaluations are provisional. The most useful recent reviews are Wood (1978) and Howell (1978). A brief summary of the more complete specimens attributed to early *Homo* follows.

Olduvai

The classic *H. habilis* material is characterised by relatively capacious ($\geqslant 600\,\text{cm}^3$) but lightly constructed crania (OH 7, 13, 24) from Bed I and Lower II (1.8–?1.5 My) associated with teeth and masticatory remains of small-to-moderate size (Fig. 6.1), a fragmentary but more rugged cranium (OH 16) with well defined supraorbital torus, postorbital narrowing and a nuchal ridge is known from the top of Bed I or Lower Bed II (Fig. 6.1) whilst there is an undoubted *H. erectus* cranium (OH 9) from Upper Bed II (?1.2 My) (see Fig. 6.2).

Omo

From the upper levels (member G dated at 1.84 My) is a fragmented cranium and cheek teeth (L 894–1). This appears to have possessed a relatively flat face with parabolic dental arcade, weak supraorbital torus, expanded parietal and occipital areas and relatively large endocranial volume when compared with *A. africanus*. It has consequently been considered an early member of the genus *Homo* (Boaz & Howell, 1977).

Koobi Fora

The large number of specimens from East Turkana exhibit a range of morphological variation unsurpassed elsewhere. The remains are intercalated between volcanic tuffs which assist in dating; the major division is between the Lower and Upper Members of the Koobi Fora formation, the boundary of which is the KBS tuff or its lateral correlates; those from the Upper Member are again ordered by their stratigraphic relationship to subsequent tuffs (Walker & Leakey, 1978; Leakey & Leakey, 1978).

Remains from the Lower Member include a calvarial fragment (ER 3732), a fragmented juvenile cranium and teeth (ER 1590) and a relatively complete cranium (ER 1470) (Fig. 6.2). This includes most of the vault, part of the base and much of the face including the maxilla. The cranial capacity is large ($775\,\text{cm}^3$) with lateral and vertical expansion of the frontal, and moderately developed supraorbital and nuchal

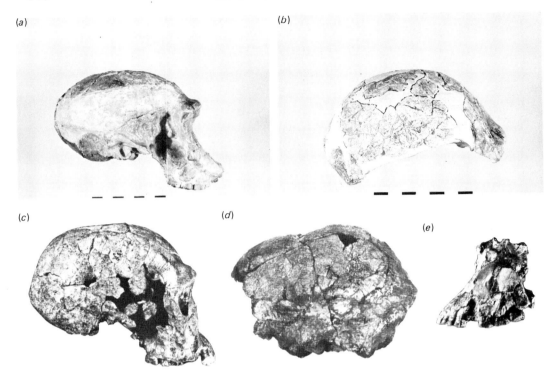

Fig. 6.1. Early *Homo*: (*a*) Olduvai, Tanzania. Bed I: OH 24. (*b*) Olduvai, Tanzania. Bed II. OH 16. (*c*) Koobi Fora, Kenya. KNM-ER 1813. (*d–e*) Koobi Fora, Kenya. KNM–ER 1805.

tori. ER 1590 is less complete and lightly constructed (although this may be a function of its immaturity); cranial capacity was probably greater than that of ER 1470.

Specimens from the Upper Member (Fig. 6.1) include the relatively rugged ER 1805, consisting of a calvarium, a mid/lower facial fragment and palate and damaged mandibular corpus. The stoutly constructed cranium is platycephalic, with slight mid-line thickening and a low but distinct sagittal crest as well as a prominent nuchal crest delimiting a broad flat planum. ER 1813 is a virtually complete specimen lacking only the zygomatic arch and a small part of the cranial base. By comparison with the other Turkana specimens the neurocranium is small, lightly constructed and remarkably like that of *A. africanus*, although rather larger (500 cm³). The mid/lower face, however, is relatively orthognathic, contrasting markedly with the morphology of many *africanus* specimens, whilst the palate is parabolic and the teeth small.

ER 3733 (Fig. 6.3) is a complete, virtually perfect cranium of rugged construction and an estimated cranial capacity of 900 cm³. It has been assigned to *H. erectus* (Walker & Leakey, 1978). Other, less complete, crania (e.g. ER 3883) suggest the presence of further *erectus* specimens at Turkana, whilst maxillary and mandibular remains provide additional evidence of the genus *Homo* (Wood, 1978).

The chronology of the Turkana material has been a vexatious issue since its discovery. Hominid remains from the Upper Member are relatively securely dated at 1.3–1.6 My but there has been much uncertainty over the date of the KBS tuff which delimits the Lower Member and which effectively calibrates the specimens therein. The tuff was initially dated by the ^{40}Ar/^{39}Ar technique at 2.61 ± 0.26 My, a figure

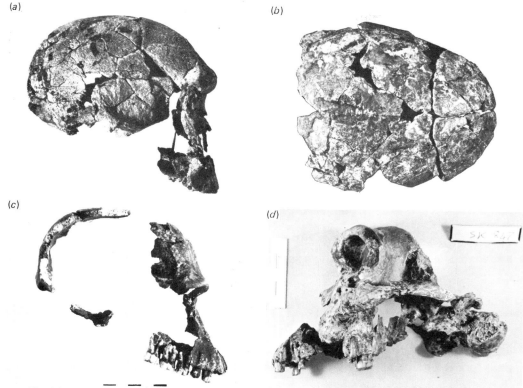

Fig. 6.2. Early *Homo*: (*a*) Koobi Fora, Kenya. KNM-ER 1470. (*b*) Koobi Fora, Kenya. KNM-ER 1590. (*c*) Sterkfontein, South Africa. STW 53. Swartkrans, S. Africa. SK 847.

subsequently refined to 2.42 ± 0.01 My. The conventional K–Ar method yields 1.6–1.82 My. A discrepancy of such magnitude would have far-reaching implications when assessing alternative hominid phylogenies. Palaeomagnetic evidence is consistent with either figure; some fission track age estimates agree with the older date, others with the younger. Detailed faunal correlations, based upon extensive sampling at Omo, Koobi Fora and Olduvai, together with geochemical analysis of tuffs at Omo and Turkana suggest that a date of *c.* 1.8 My is most likely for the KBS tuff, thereby supporting the conventional K–Ar range estimate. More data are needed before the issue is finally resolved, but the balance of current evidence strongly supports the later age estimate for the KBS tuff: recent reviews are in Bishop (1978) and Drake *et al.* (1980).

Most recently, further fieldwork (Brown & Cerling, 1982; Cerling & Brown, 1982) suggests that some marker tuff correlates have been misidentified, and that the geological sequence for the Turkana region needs extensive revision. However, it is unlikely to alter the age estimates for the majority of hominid fossils from the later parts of the sequence. This recent work provides further support for the equivalence of some of the later Omo deposits with those at Turkana, thereby confirming the younger age of the KBS tuff.

South Africa

Of broadly comparable age and morphology are specimens from Swartkrans and Sterkfontein (Tobias, 1978) (Fig. 6.4). Cranio-facial material (SK 847) demonstrates

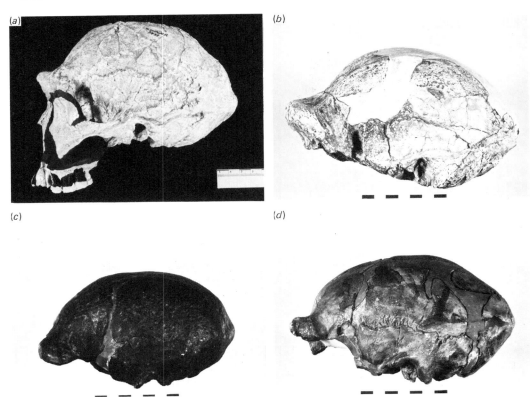

Fig. 6.3. *Homo erectus*: (*a*) Koobi Fora, Kenya. KNM-ER 3733. (*b*) Olduvai, Tanzania. Bed II: OH 9. (*c*) Sangiran, Indonesia. Sangiran I. (*d*) Choukoutien (Pekin), China. Pekin L2.

the existence at Swartkrans of a second hominid, contemporary with the robust australopithecines and not dissimilar from some of the East African gracile specimens. It possesses a pronounced supraorbital torus distinct from the frontal squama, anteriorly projecting nasal bones, a sharply delineated nasal aperture and has a relatively small dentition.

More recently, Tobias & Hughes (see Tobias, 1978) have recovered a partial cranium, including much of the maxilla, face and vault from the artefact-bearing member 5 at Sterkfontein. The specimen is small and lightly built, although the endocranial volume appears relatively large and there is little postorbital constriction of the frontal. The nasal bones project only slightly, but the inferior margin of the nasal aperture and the maxilla are like SK 847. The cheek teeth are heavily worn, displaying the heliocoidal occlusal plane considered characteristic of *Homo* (Tobias, 1980), whilst the premolars are three-rooted – a phenomenon almost unknown in *A. africanus* but occurring in some other specimens of early *Homo*.

Current evidence therefore indicates the widespread presence in southern and eastern Africa of relatively lightly constructed hominids showing cerebral expansion over *Australopithecus* populations, and whose cranio-facial and dental characteristics justify their incorporation within *Homo*. On the other hand, the morphological parameters of the populations from which they derive are poorly known, and it is not clear whether more than one lineage is being sampled. For example, interpretation of the Turkana material ranges from the parsimonious view that all specimens – robust australopithecines apart – can be assigned to one lineage and that the variability reflects a compound of limited sampling, sexual dimorphism and temporal change, to schemes which infer the existence of multiple taxa.

Walker & Leakey (1978) suggest that three clusters are represented in the Upper Member at Koobi Fora – robusts (e.g. ER 406), graciles (ER 1813) and *erectus* (ER 3733). In the Lower Member, three clusters are again discernible – robusts, graciles and early *Homo* (ER 1470). Wood (1978) argues for grouping ER 1470, 1590 and 3732, largely on similarities in neurocranial proportions and capacity; ER 1813 is considered separate from this cluster since it differs substantially in endocranial capacity (from ER 1470) and dental proportions (from ER 1590) and instead is grouped with ER 1805, whilst ER 3733 is distinctive and represents a third morphotype. Yet other groupings are possible: e.g. Howell (1978) associates ER 1470, 1590, 3732 and 1813 as one group (*habilis*) and ER 1805 and 3733 as another (*erectus*).

With the recovery of ER 1470 and 1590 from below the KBS tuff initially dated as 2.6 My, the fossil evidence suggested the early derivation of a large-brained *Homo* lineage *c.* 3.0 My, perhaps subsequently evolving into *erectus*. Such a pattern rendered unlikely the incorporation within that lineage of the smaller, more lightly built and apparently much later cranial material of the Olduvai *habilis* specimens, and suggested to many a polyphyletic radiation of early hominids in the later Pliocene/basal Pleistocene.

The increasing body of evidence supporting a later (1.6–1.8 My) date for the KBS tuff considerably modifies this picture. It does not, of course, definitely exclude a multiplicity of lineages, but it renders more probable alternative, phyletically more economical schemes, whilst also indicating the broad contemporaneity of the Olduvai and Turkana material, thereby increasing the probability that they represent comparable evolutionary phenomena. Similarly, Sterkfontein member 5 and Swartkrans are considered on faunal grounds to be of equivalent age (1.5–2.0 My) and the specimens probably sample a population in the Sterkfontein (Blaauwbank) valley comparable to that represented by some of the East African material. At both major East African sites undoubted *erectus* crania (OH 9, ER 3733) are present in the upper levels, whilst other specimens, although not obviously included within *erectus* as currently defined, show similarities with that taxon. OH 16 and ER 1805 fall into this category, as possibly does ER 1470 at least in terms of its cranial capacity and some of its vault dimensions. This may indicate that we are sampling a *Homo* lineage prior to the stabilisation of an *erectus* morphology, and which shows a correspondingly wide range of cranial variation, perhaps reflecting a burst of rapid evolutionary change ('tachytely'). However, the extremely gracile specimens from Turkana and Olduvai (OH 13, OH 24/ER 1813) do not readily fit into such a scheme and show few, if any, characteristics which indicate that they represent proto-*erectus* populations. To accommodate them within the same lineage as, for example, ER 1470 requires a remarkable range of variation, and it is probably necessary to posit that the few fossil specimens available effectively sample the upper and lower limits of the population range in many cranial characters – in itself an improbable situation.

The present evidence therefore does not overwhelmingly favour any one scheme; it is certainly possible, for example, to adduce arguments for the allocation of ER 1813 and OH 24 to *Australopithecus*. One difficulty is that different workers use taxa such as *Australopithecus* and *Homo* as clades and grades (Wood, 1981), which inevitably influences the composition of these and the resulting phylogenies. Another major problem is that whilst it is relatively straightforward to distinguish between 'robust' and 'non-robust' categories, the absence in the latter group of features characterising the former does not, of course, guarantee biological homogeneity. The limited nature of the fossil specimens and their isolated occurrence renders grouping difficult, and yet the reconstruction of phylogeny depends critically upon the initial assignment of specimens to various morphological clusters.

The investigation of allometric variation in extant primates (Wood, 1981) in conjunction with morphometric analysis of the fossil specimens offers the most promising approach to this problem, since it should assist in refining the probabilities for allocating specimens. At this time the possibility remains open that there were two or more contemporaneous non-robust hominid lineages, and that the genus *Homo* (in the sense of a grade) may be polyphyletic, at least in its earlier stages.

HOMO ERECTUS

After the diversity of the early material it is something of a relief to consider the relatively well defined chronospecies *H. erectus*. The last two decades have added significantly to our knowledge of this taxon, extending over the greater part of the Pleistocene and much of the Old World. The classic Javanese material from Trinil, Sangiran (Fig. 6.3) and Modjokerto has been supplemented by the recovery of further specimens from the Sangiran dome area of Central Java whilst new finds have been made at Choukoutien and Lantian, China. In Europe, *erectus* remains are known from Heidelberg and Bilzingsleben (Germany); whilst in Africa, specimens from Rabat, Ternifine, Sidi Abderrahman, Olduvai, Koobi Fora and Swartkrans document the presence of *erectus* across the greater part of that continent. The taxon was clearly geographically diverse and, on the basis of chronometric estimates, temporally long-lived.

The more recently recovered Javanese material has, like the early finds, been uncovered as a result of the activities of local villagers acting as collectors, a situation not conducive to controlled excavation. There is consequently a dearth of the stratigraphic and contextual information which is available for the African fossils. All specimens consist of cranial fragments and teeth; postcranial elements are totally lacking, probably due to non-recognition. Stratigraphically the fossils are from the Pucangan (Poetjang or Djetis Beds) or the Kabuh Formation (Boundary and Trinil Beds). Although the area of recovery is volcanic and therefore accessible to K–Ar dating, absolute dates are few: the site of Modjokerto yields a date of 1.9 ± 0.4 My from the horizon considered to be that from which the *erectus* infant cranium was recovered in 1936, whilst the Middle and Upper Trinil beds are dated at 0.83 My and 0.5–0.7 My respectively. Two useful reviews are those by Pilbeam (1975) and Sartono (1975). Faunal assemblages suggest a basal-to-late Lower Pleistocene placement for the *erectus* material and a tropical, predominantly forested or wooded, environment.

The morphologically comparable *erectus* cranium from Lantian (Shensi province, China) is from a Lower Pleistocene horizon, the fauna of which is similar to the Javanese Djetis faunas therefore possibly > 1 My, although recent Chinese estimates suggest dates of 0.75–0.8 My (Howells, 1980). If correct, this date has implications for the age of the Javanese fossils.

Although fewer in number, the available *erectus* remains from Africa are generally better preserved, and have usually been recovered under more controlled conditions of excavation. This is particularly so of the East African specimens, one of which (ER

3733) is the most complete *erectus* cranium known. Others (OH 9, OH 12, ER 3883) although more fragmentary, are undistorted. The Koobi Fora specimens are probably 1.3–1.5 My old, Olduvai H 9 about 1.1 My old; allowing for dating errors they are thus of broadly comparable age to the early Javanese material, whilst *erectus* material from Olduvai Bed IV (OH 12, OH 22, OH 28: 0.7–?1.0 My) would be of Lower Trinil age.

Fragmentary (and undiagnostic) cranial remains associated with Acheulian artefacts at el Ubeidiya, Israel, were originally thought to be *H. habilis*, but were later widely accepted as *H. erectus*. A recent faunal analysis (Repenning & Fejfor, 1982) suggests that the site may be much older than previously thought, thus re-opening the possibility that the material is *habilis*, or that there are *erectus* remains outside Africa antedating the earliest specimens from that continent. However, caution is needed: faunal correlations are notoriously subject to uncertainties, and the minimal age estimates urged by Repenning & Fejfor are compatible with the Ubeidiya material being approximately the same age as the early African *erectus* crania.

In South Africa, some of the material from Swartkrans originally assigned to 'Telanthropus' has subsequently been included within *erectus*. It includes a mandible (SK 15), two lower premolars and a proximal radius fragment derived from a pocket of secondary breccia (Member 2 of Butzer) which on faunal evidence is about 5 My old. Perhaps of broadly comparable age are the earliest 'Atlanthropus' remains from North Africa; these appear to be the parietal, mandibular and dental remains from Ternifine, Algeria. Other, younger *erectus* material is known from quarries at Sidi Abderrahman, Morocco, whilst the crania and maxillary remains from Salé and Rabat are probably not much more than 0.2 My old.

A similar chronological span is perhaps covered by the sparse early hominid material from Europe. Apart from the Mauer (Heidelberg) mandible, only cranial fragments (frontal, occipital) from Bilzingsleben, and possibly the Vertesszollos occipital (see below), suggest the presence of *erectus* in Europe. All are relatively late (post Matuyama), with Bilzingsleben as recent as 0.2 My, but there is archaeological evidence pointing to earlier hominid occupation of Europe, at least during warmer periods. The cave of Vallonet (France), and the sites of El Aculadero (Spain) and Besse-sur-Issole (France) all attest to hominid presence in at least southern Europe during the later Lower/early Middle Pleistocene (Bordes & Thibault, 1977).

The most extensive sample of *erectus* material is still that from Choukoutien (Pekin) largely recovered before the last war, but supplemented by more recent discoveries (Fig. 6.3). Dating is uncertain; amino acid racemisation indicates 0.3 My and at least two estimates based on wide-ranging faunal correlations suggest a comparable age. However, these were derived from the imposition of a four-fold European glacial framework upon the site's geology; the identification of multiple climatic oscillations renders such a scheme improbable, quite apart from the uncertainty inherent in long-range faunal correlations. The Choukoutien (CKT) fauna has undoubted similarities with the later Trinil (? Boundary Beds) fauna, which would suggest a date of 0.5–0.6/My. A palaeomagnetic reversal (?Brunhes/Matuyama) has apparently been identified low in the CKT section, below the hominid deposits (J. K. Woo, personal communication) and would support such a date.

The preceding summary demonstrates the spatial and temporal diversity of *erectus*, the taxon covering a minimum of 1.0 My. Not surprisingly, the material is also morphologically highly variable, being characterised cranially by little more than its relatively constant neurocranial shape – platycephalic vault, often with mid-sagittal reinforcement, thick cranial bones, prominent supra-orbital torus and extensive nuchal area.

The earliest specimens appear to be those from East Africa and Indonesia. The Javanese crania share certain characteristics: the cranial vault is low, with a pronounced supra-orbital torus, narrow retreating frontal and marked parietal flattening. The occipital is sharply angulated with an extensive, flat, nuchal area delineated by a prominent nuchal torus which is continuous laterally with the supra-mastoid crest. Maximum cranial width is low down at the level of the meati; the cranial bones are generally thick, but there is additional reinforcement of the frontal and parietals in the median sagittal plane, producing a keel or ridge, often accentuated by parasagittal depressions. Cranial capacity ranges between 775 cm³ to just over 1000 cm³. Almost all specimens consist of calvaria or fragments thereof, but 'Pithecanthropus VIII' (Sartono, 1975) from the Kabuh formation at Sangiran includes the face and palate, although these are much distorted and compressed by fossilisation. This specimen has a relatively large cranial capacity (about 1030 cm³) and shows resemblances to the later Ngandong (Solo) sample (Fig. 6.4) – similarities which have led Sartono (1975) to propose a relatively complex phylogeny for the Indonesian hominids, including the presence of large- and small-brained *erectus* populations in the Middle Pleistocene. Since the similarities between 'Pithecanthropus VII' (P. VIII) and the Solo material merely reflect the retention of primitive ('plesiomorphous') *erectus* features in the latter population, and bearing in mind the great variation of cranial capacity in hominoids, it seems more reasonable to regard P. VIII as a member of a population with the same endocranial parameters as those sampled by the other *erectus* specimens rather than representative of a new subspecies.

The recovery of undoubted *erectus* from sub-Saharan Africa along with other early members of the genus *Homo* has stimulated comparisons between these and the Javanese specimens, and re-examination of the morphological diversity of that material. An early, pioneering, comparison of Olduvai and Sangiran specimens was that of Tobias & von Koenigswald (1964) who considered that OH 7 (the type of *habilis*) was dentally similar to the 'Meganthropus' material, and OH 13 like 'Pithecanthropus IV' and the Sangiran B mandible. Subsequently von Koenigswald has argued that these latter specimens, together with others, represent a more primitive hominid, *Homo modjokertensis*. These and other comparisons have led to suggestions that *habilis*, or other morphologically primitive non-*erectus* hominids, are represented in the Sangiran fossil record; the tendency of Indonesian workers (e.g. Sartono, 1975) to utilise multiple taxa to categorise the specimens has also fostered an impression of phyletic diversity among the Javanese material.

However, the existence of *habilis* or other early *Homo* species (other than *erectus*) outside Africa has yet to be convincingly demonstrated. Whilst there are undoubted similarities in dental and gnathic features between certain specimens from East Africa and Indonesia, such characteristics are not necessarily specific, since early hominids show considerable overlap in dental dimensions. This is well illustrated by the 'Meganthropus' material: considered by Tobias & von Koenigswald to be morphologically equivalent to Olduvai Bed I *habilis*, it has also been cited by Robinson (1953) as evidence of *A. robustus* in southeast Asia. There are, in fact, significant differences between the Asian and African fossils: in particular, there is no evidence from Java of hominids with the lightly constructed neurocrania characteristic of the classic *habilis* material (e.g. OH 7, OH 13, OH 24), and no African specimens, except those formally assigned to *erectus* (and possibly the as yet unassigned ER 1805/OH 16), approach the Javanese crania in platycephaly, cranial thickness, torus development and nuchal expansion. Material from both areas exhibits considerable morphological diversity, especially in cranial capacity and dental dimensions, but this needs to be evaluated on a regional basis before comparisons can be drawn between the two geographically separated sets of crania. Until that time, the most economical interpretation is that the Javanese specimens represent a single species, the differences reflecting individual variability and change over time.

The lack of definite evidence for hominid precursors of *erectus* in southeast Asia and elsewhere points increasingly towards sub-Saharan Africa as the focus for the initial evolution and establishment of this morphotype, claims for Ubeidiya (Repenning & Fejfor, 1982) notwithstanding. The underlying selection pressures are obscure, but morphometric analysis currently in progress suggests that derivation of an *erectus* cranial morphology from that exhibited by early East African *Homo* does not require any rapid or dramatic evolutionary mechanism; neither does the fossil record require the sudden entry of *erectus* into that area, having evolved elsewhere, as has been suggested on the basis of the archaeological evidence.

The available chronology suggests virtual contemporaneity of the earliest African, southeast Asian and Chinese *erectus*, indicating a relatively rapid radiation and dispersal over much of the tropical Old World. This is almost certainly spurious: the errors inherent in dating at this time range allow at least 0.2–0.3 My between numerically identical dates, which ethnographic parallels indicate is a more than sufficient interval for the observed distribution from African source. Moreover, virtually all of the very small number of early dates from other regions are disputed, with younger alternative estimates having been suggested for a variety of reasons. If these are correct, the time available for dispersal from Africa becomes even greater. The distinctive features of the Javanese specimens may then reasonably be considered to be a consequence of strongly directional selective forces interacting with a restricted gene pool (founder effect) at the limits of hominid distribution in the Lower Pleistocene.

The environmental factors associated with this radiation are unknown, but it presumably implies some increase in population numbers; the greater body size and robusticity of *erectus* compared with earlier *Homo* were probably important factors in facilitating the expansion since they would result in greater strength (thereby making accessible new food resources?) and improved thermoregulation in cooler environments. The adaptive significance of this is attested by the penetration of *erectus* communities into higher latitudes during the later Lower/early Middle Pleistocene.

Later *erectus* crania differ from the early specimens in numerous respects. I have attempted elsewhere (Bilsborough, 1976) to summarise these differences and to argue that they are of considerable importance in assessing the pattern of evolution within the taxon. Early *erectus* populations have a cranium dominated by a powerful masticatory apparatus with large palate, stout mandibular corpus and ramus, strongly constructed zygomatic arch and broad, open articular fossae. The relatively small neurocranium is low, flattened and medially buttressed, whilst the nuchal musculature was extensive and powerful to balance the heavy anterior cranial segment. The anterior teeth were strongly implanted and, in some individuals at least, the canines projecting, whilst posterior dental proportions were primitive ($M_1 < M_2 < M_3$).

Later *erectus* crania show much reduced facial and masticatory regions – no larger than those of early *sapiens* specimens – articular fossae of modern size and proportions, reduced non-projecting anterior teeth, and molar dimensions which fall within the range of modern populations. Cranial capacity, which is considerably greater than in the earlier specimens (950–1225+ cm³) similarly falls within the modern range. Indeed, later *erectus* samples phenetically resemble *sapiens* more closely than they do early *erectus*, and the distinction between the two morphotypes is generally accepted to be arbitrary, and dictated by convenience rather than fundamental phyletic considerations.

HOMO SAPIENS

Until recently the earliest specimens assigned to *sapiens* were from late Middle Pleistocene deposits in higher latitudes. The best known of these – the Steinheim (Fig. 6.4) and Swanscombe crania – both derive from a warm interval, usually considered the Holstein interglacial, and are generally dated at 0.2–0.25 My. However, the identification of multiple climatic oscillations casts doubt on the integrity of the 'Holsteinian', and the dates may require revision. This is further suggested by more recent discoveries: Petralona, Greece (cranium); Vertesszollos, Hungary (occipital); and Arago, France (cranio-facial fragment and mandible).

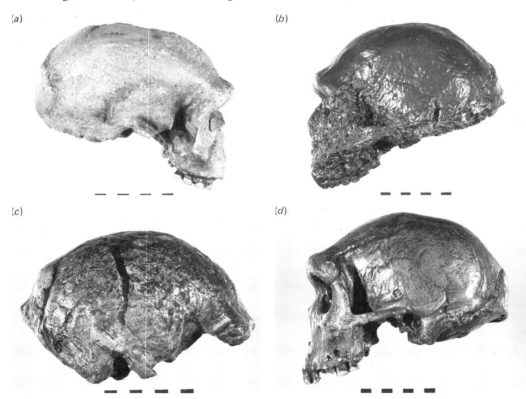

Fig. 6.4. Early *Homo sapiens*: (*a*) Steinheim, Germany. (*b*) Petralona, Greece. (*c*) Ngandong (Solo), Indonesia. Solo 9. (*d*) Broken Hill (Kabwe), Zambia.

The Petralona specimen (Stringer, Howell & Melentis, 1979) in particular provides important evidence of the cranial morphology of European early *sapiens* populations (Fig. 6.4). Originally considered to be of Upper Pleistocene age and labelled 'Neanderthal', its age is now known to be ≥0.3 My, whilst cleaning has revealed the non-Neanderthal features of this, the most complete cranium known from the earlier Middle Pleistocene. The bones of the vault are extremely thick but pneumatised, with voluminous sinuses; cranial capacity is about 1200 cm³. The supra-orbital torus is massive, the nuchal area extensive and bordered by a distinct torus, whilst the lower face is flat and broad with stout zygomatic arches which shelve into the alveolar border of the maxilla in a manner reminiscent of some Neanderthals.

The remains recovered from living floors at Arago are dated at 0.2–0.3 My and are associated with a Tayacian flake industry and a fauna which indicates a dry, cold steppe environment, perhaps at the beginning of a glacial phase. They reveal a similarly robust facial morphology with prominent brow ridge, prognathous inflated maxilla and stout mandible (Fig. 6.5).

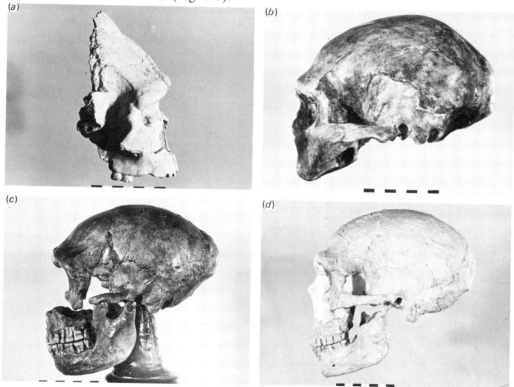

Fig. 6.5. *Homo sapiens*: (*a*) Arago (Tautavel), France. Arago 21. (*b*) Mt Circeo, Italy. (*c*) La Quina, France. (*d*) Amud, Israel. Amud 1.

The Vertesszollos occipital is older (> 0.4 My) but also derives from occupation horizons indicating a cool, open environment. It resembles *H. erectus* in the possession of a marked nuchal ridge and has been included by some within that taxon. However the bone's dimensions exceed those of *erectus* specimens, and the cranial capacity has been estimated at about 1400 cm³.

These *sapiens* remains possess many features in common with later *erectus* specimens, particularly in facial, dental and jaw proportions and general robusticity, but the neurocranial bones are generally bigger, lighter and more spherical than in typical *erectus*, reflecting endocranial volumes which fall at or beyond the upper limit of *erectus* crania. Mid-sagittal keeling and an occipital torus, where present, are generally less marked than in *erectus*, and maximum cranial width is well above the auditory meati, as masticatory forces diminish and the external as well as internal contour of the vault increasingly reflects brain proportions. Several fragmentary specimens dating from later phases of the 'Riss Saale' glacial complex and Eem interglacial indicate the continuation of this rugged cranio-facial morphology within European *sapiens* populations until $\leqslant 0.1$ My.

The enlarged sample now available strongly indicates the appearance of a *sapiens* morphology considerably earlier (at least 0.1–0.2 My) than was thought only a few years ago. However, later Middle Pleistocene European populations were clearly variable cranially, and the Bilzingsleben cranium suggests the co-existence of later *erectus* and early *sapiens* morphotypes, underlining the artificiality of the taxonomic distinction. The early age of this material may possibly indicate a European origin for the initial *sapiens* morphology. If so it would perhaps provide the best hominid example of the punctuated equilibrium model of evolutionary change, where a morphological variant initially restricted to the geographical limit of the species becomes established over the entire range. However, important new material from Africa pointing to the early appearance of *sapiens* on that continent, throws considerable doubt on this interpretation, suggesting that a 'phyletic gradualism' model may be more appropriate, with gradual change in the human gene pool over wide areas of the Old World.

Analysis of later Pleistocene human evolution in Africa has long suffered from the lack of a reliable chronology. The morphologically archaic subspecies *H. sapiens rhodesiensis*, characterised by massive face, pronounced supra-orbital torus, moderate-to-large cranial capacity and a long, relatively low vault with retreating frontal and angulated occipital with prominent nuchal torus has long been known from Kabwe (Broken Hill) Zambia (Fig. 6.4), Eyasi in Tanzania, and Saldanha (Hopefield) South Africa. Stratigraphic controls are lacking for all these specimens and dating, which has generally relied upon faunal and/or cultural association, traditionally suggested a late age (40 000–50 000 B.P.) for the material; the inevitable conclusion was that an advanced *erectus*/archaic *sapiens* morphology obtained in sub-Saharan Africa long after disappearing elsewhere.

Improved dating techniques, and the recovery of further specimens now render this view improbable. Revised age estimates suggest that Kabwe and Saldanha are over 0.1 My, Saldanha perhaps substantially so (Rightmire, 1979). Furthermore, the important find of a partial cranium having affinities with Kabwe and Petralona in mid-Pleistocene deposits at Bodo D'Ar, Ethiopia provides further evidence of the early occurrence of an archaic *sapiens* morphology (Conroy *et al.*, 1978); also possibly referable to this morphotype is the N'dutu cranium considered by its describers to be advanced *erectus*. Dating of this specimen is by correlation of deposits with those at nearby Olduvai Gorge, and indicates an age of 0.2–0.4 My. These specimens therefore suggest the occurrence of transitional *erectus*/*sapiens* populations in sub-Saharan Africa at least as early as those currently known elsewhere, and await confirmation by further discoveries.

Hominid fossils from the later Pleistocene (< 0.1 My) differ from those of previous periods in several ways. Specimens are separated by relatively short time intervals and morphological contrasts are less extensive than among earlier fossils, so that individual and polytypic differences contribute more to the observed variation than previously. One is, in effect, focussing upon the fine detail of human evolution, and a different order of interpretation is required from the broad phylogenies of the earlier Pleistocene. Observed changes are likely to reflect a compound of population variation and replacement, gene flow as well as phyletic change, so that unifactorial interpretations are likely to be inadequate: a local 'punctuated equilibrium' model may well accord with 'phyletic gradualism' at the continental or supra-continental level.

Most studies of human evolution in the later Pleistocene have focussed on the European and Middle Eastern material since this is the most extensive and best documented. However, studies of the interrelationships of early last glacial circum-Mediterranean communities have been hampered by, as much as anything else, the lack of precision in defining the term 'Neanderthal'. The paper by Brose & Wolpoff (1971) advocating a universal Neanderthal phase in human evolution illustrates the problem: those by Howells (1974) and Santa Luca (1978) attempt to illuminate the problem by providing more precise definitions. Mann & Trinkaus (1974) provide a useful check list of Neanderthal fossils *sensu lato*; the most recent review is that of Trinkaus & Howells (1979).

Most investigators have focussed on the distinctive cranial morphology of the Neanderthals – especially the projecting face with its voluminous orbits and nose, inflated maxillary/zygomatic region and anteriorly situated dental arcade, the long, flat neurocranium with occipital 'bunning' and relatively unflexed basicranium (Fig. 6.5), and several authors (Bilsborough, 1973; Stringer, 1974; Howells, 1975) have used multivariate techniques to investigate this. Such approaches are valuable in providing measures of total morphological pattern and as aids to analysing the interplay of otherwise isolated characters, but it cannot be claimed that they have unambiguously resolved problems of interpretation, nor fulfilled all the methodological claims earlier made for them by some workers. Not surprisingly the relationships expressed by multivariate statistics differ according to the technique used and the assumptions upon which it is based: some treat isolated specimens as unique, others assign them to pre-determined groups; some express total variation, others partition this into size and shape components. However, the use of these methods does appear to have fostered a greater awareness among workers of both the pattern of variation in Neanderthal fossils and the questions of interpretation posed by the application of such techniques.

The report by Santa Luca (1978) provides a complementary approach by grouping Neanderthal fossils by discontinuous morphological traits of the auditory/mastoid region and the torus/supra-iniac area of the occipital. The results accord with biometrical investigations in showing clustering of European/Middle Eastern specimens and their separation from African and Asian material. The thrust of these (and other) studies has been towards adequately characterising the cranial morphology and providing a refined definition of Neanderthal; the recovery of relatively complete early *H. sapiens* specimens (see above) has facilitated this, and stimulated attempts to distinguish between those features of Neanderthals which are confined to the group, and those which are shared with preceding or contemporary *sapiens* populations (see e.g., Stringer, 1974, 1978).

Much controversy has been generated by attempts to reconstruct the language capability of Neanderthal (Lieberman, Crelin & Klatt, 1972) which suggested that it was only about 10% as extensive as that of modern man, with an inability to produce vowels A,I,O,U and consonants G and K. This conclusion has been considered by some to parallel, and perhaps underlie, the archaeological observation that the Mousterian industries associated with Neanderthals are relatively limited in their range of expression compared with the great diversity of tool forms and the expansion of bone working and art seen in the Upper Palaeolithic assemblages associated with anatomically modern humans.

The vocal reconstruction is a three-fold process involving (a) reconstruction of the Neanderthal vocal tract from surviving basicranial evidence, (b) comparison of the reconstruction with modern human and pongid tracts, (c) computer simulation of language capability based upon the vocal tract comparisons. The approach has been severely criticised at each level of analysis on the basis of the fragmentary nature of the basicranium in Neanderthal fossils and the relevance of the evidence for vocal tract reconstruction (Siegal & Carlisle 1974; Burr, 1976), the evolutionary assumptions made, and the vocalisation model generated (Wind, 1978). My own view is that the limited anatomical evidence available does not permit detailed reconstruction of language capacity, a more fruitful approach to which is likely to be via consideration of the relevant archaeological evidence. The relatively constant production techniques associated with a diversity of tool forms within the Mousterian complex, the evidence for elaborate social organisation and ritualistic behaviour, for effective systematic hunting and the range of environments exploited by Mousterian communities are all powerfully suggestive, not of an impoverished linguistic capacity in Neanderthals, but of a communication level similar to our own.

Relatively little attention has recently been paid to the Neanderthal postcranium – perhaps a natural consequence of Strauss and Cave's demonstration of the errors in Boule's reconstruction of Neanderthal posture through failing to take account of pathological deformation. A notable exception here is Trinkaus (1981) whose studies have illuminated aspects of Neanderthal shoulder and hindlimb anatomy, but there is still need for a comprehensive re-evaluation of the Neanderthal trunk and limb material.

There have been important recent advances in our knowledge of circum-Mediterranean Neanderthal communities. The descriptions of the Amud (Israel) specimen (Fig. 6.5) and the Shanider (Iraq) material (Stewart, 1977; Stringer & Trinkaus, 1981) have added significantly to our knowledge of Neanderthal morphology in that area, whilst renewed excavations at Mount Carmel and Djebel Qafseh (Vandermersch, 1972) suggest that communities of Neanderthal and morphologically more modern individuals were separated by only very short time intervals, if not actually contemporaneous. The Amud and Shanidar specimens, whilst displaying a basically classic morphology, share a number of differences from the European material and somewhat more modern traits (less voluminous orbits and nasal aperture, rather higher, more rounded cranial vault, more linear build). Broadly Mousterian industries extend westwards along the North African littoral, and fragmentary Neanderthal remains are known from Hau Fteah (Libya) and Jebel Ir(g)houd (Morocco) (Howell, 1978). Two crania are known from this site, both with long cranial vaults and some occipital bunning, but also possessing vertically orientated frontals; the more complete specimen has a facial region of relatively modern morphology: they do, in fact, rather resemble the Skhul (Fig. 6.6) and Djebel Qafseh specimens, and are excluded by some workers from Neanderthal sensu stricto, who argue that their similarities to the group merely reflect the retention of archaic sapiens characteristics (Fig. 6.6).

There have been few finds of Neanderthals in European Russia and Asia, although archaeological evidence indicates the presence of humans over much of the present USSR, including high latitudes of Siberia, during the last glaciation (McBurney, 1976). It appears that the intensely cold, but dry, climate of the last glacial promoted the spread of steppe/tundra conditions with an associated rich arctic fauna (mammoth,

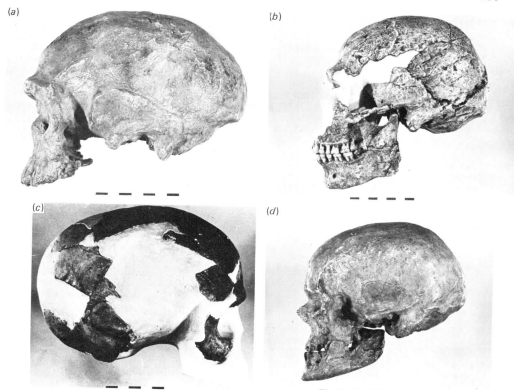

Fig. 6.6. *Homo sapiens*: (*a*) Djebel Ir(g)houd, Morocco. Djebel Ir(g)houd 1. (*b*) Mt Carmel, Israel. Skhul 5. (*c*) Border Cave, South Africa. Border Cave 1. (*d*) Cromagnon, France. Cromagnon 1.

woolly rhino) which facilitated human occupation of northerly regions with a continental climate. The colonisation of such environments would expose human groups to new and intensely directional selection pressures which may have strongly influenced human morphology.

Several authors have noted similarities between western classic Neanderthals and those of eastern Europe, and even between western European Neanderthals and recent Asiatic populations. The total spectrum of anatomical variation and its geographical distribution suggest a broadly Neanderthal morphology in the circum-Mediterranean, Middle East and European/Asiatic Russia regions, within which the distinctive features of the European classic Neanderthals perhaps represent a geographically and ecologically more defined grouping. This may have its focus in middle/high latitudes of eastern Europe and the USSR, with its presence along the Atlantic seaboard due to westward movement of human groups consequent upon faunal migration as a response to climatic change: as the arctic fauna moved west/south-westwards during the last glaciation, so may the classic Neanderthals.

Support for this view is provided by the fact that European Neanderthals date from the early part of the last glaciation, not the succeeding warmer interstadial. However, further morphological studies and the recovery of well dated specimens from geographically intermediate regions will be necessary to validate this suggestion. Despite intensive searches little human fossil material is known from western Europe during mid-Wurm, i.e. the interval between the early Wurm Neanderthals and the morphologically modern specimens of later Wurm (Cromagnon, Combe Capelle etc.) (Fig. 6.6). Archaeological evidence indicates continuity of occupation, although the small number of sites known may indicate a drop in population numbers and/or shift during the climatic amelioration towards habitation of more open sites rather than rock shelters.

The recent recovery of apparent Neanderthal skeletal remains from a Châtelperon-nian horizon at St Césaire (ApSimon, 1980) falls within this interval, and is important in indicating the persistence of a Neanderthal morphology down to 30 000–35 000 B.P. and its association with an 'Upper Palaeolithic' blade industry. This discovery, and other fragmentary finds in central and eastern Europe have stimulated debate about the pattern of replacement of Neanderthal morphology by an anatomically modern one (e.g. ApSimon, 1980, 1981; Wolpoff, 1980, 1981; Stringer, Kruszynski & Jacobi, 1981). Despite the finds of recent years, available specimens are still too few, too fragmentary, and insecurely dated to provide enough data to allow a choice between the alternative schemata, but there does at least seem to be greater awareness of the kinds of question to be asked, and the kinds of evidence required to answer them. Much of the voluminous literature on the 'Neanderthal problem' seems to have been generated largely by the failure of earlier workers to recognise that the broad evolutionary concepts applicable to the major phases of hominid evolution are simply inappropriate applied to geographically restricted populations localised within brief time intervals.

Although skeletal evidence has steadily accumulated over the last half-century, the investigation of the evolution of *H.s. sapiens* in sub-Saharan Africa has long been hampered by lack of a reliable chronological framework. This period of stasis has been ended by several important recent developments. New age determinations indicate substantially greater antiquity for industrial variants associated with anatomi-cally modern remains (Rightmire, 1975; Howell, 1978) whilst direct dates are available for a few of the more recently excavated specimens. As a consequence there is now evidence pointing to dates of 60 000–100 000 B.P. for several specimens which are predominantly or entirely modern in their morphology. These include crania from the Kibish formation, Omo (100 000–130 000 B.P.), Border Cave (Fig. 6.6) Florisbad (44 000–110 000 B.P.) and Klasies River mouth (70 000–80 000 B.P.), South Africa.

The two Omo calvaria (Day, 1972) are from apparently contemporary deposits, but differ from one another morphologically and metrically. Both have large cranial capacities (over 1400 cm³), with one specimen having relatively thick cranial bones, a long low vault with retreating frontal and a prominent torus in the median portion of the occipital. The other specimen is thinner, with a high vault, no occipital torus, a more vertical frontal and no mid-sagittal keeling. Initially considered in view of their comparable age to be drawn from one population, subsequent analysis suggests that they may represent different groups.

The well known Florisbad cranium may possibly be comparable to the Omo material. Other specimens from southern Africa of broadly equivalent age are the rugged crania from Border Cave (?90 000–100 000 B.P.) and the slightly built, fragmen-tary but more reliably dated remains from Klasies River mouth (⩾ 70 000 B.P.: Rightmire, 1979). These last specimens are of anatomically modern individuals and have far-reaching evolutionary implications for they antedate by a considerable margin comparable finds elsewhere. If the dating is confirmed by subsequent discovery it indicates the evolution of a flat-faced, globular neurocranium *sapiens* morphology in sub-Saharan Africa earlier than elsewhere. The changes revealed by the more extensive fossil record in western Europe, the Middle East and Asia would then mirror the parochial effects of rapid morphological transition compounded from change *in situ*, gene flow and population movement.

A comparable, although chronologically later, pattern is revealed by the sparse remains from the Far East. There are relatively few later Pleistocene human remains currently known from China although the renewed palaeontological activity of recent years may soon prove fruitful. In Indonesia the long-known but poorly dated Ngandong crania point to the existence within the Upper Pleistocene of a rugged cranial morphology with endocranial values within the *sapiens* range but proportions reminiscent of *erectus* specimens from that region. The earliest claimed *H.s. sapiens* is the cranium from Niah cave (Borneo) dated to 40 000 B.P. However, only sufficient charcoal was present in the deposit for a single ^{14}C assay, which reduces the reliability of the dating.

The most significant recent developments in this region have been within the field of Australian prehistory. The discoveries of the last decade have more than doubled the known period of human occupation of the continent to *c.* 30 000 B.P., with most sites concentrated in southeast Australia, especially New South Wales. Morphologically modern skeletal remains are known from sites at Lake Mungo (25 000–30 000 B.P.) whilst there is increasing archaelogical evidence from this time range. The similarity of these skeletons to those of modern aborigines is all the more remarkable when contrasted with the much later (9000–13 000 B.P.) Kow Swamp specimens. These are much more rugged, large-faced crania with curiously flattened, retreating frontals, enormous jaw dimensions, and prominent nuchal ridging. Numerous specimens are known from the large site, pointing to the persistence of a rugged cranial morphology at a late (Holocene) date in Australia and consequently extreme anatomical variation (Thorne, 1976).

Several interpretations have been proposed to account for this phenomenon (Thorne, 1976). The recent recovery of a similar cranium from Cossack, western Australia (Freedman & Lofgren, 1979) provides striking evidence that the Kow Swamp morphotype is not confined to southeast Australia, but as yet there is too little skeletal evidence from the interior of the continent to enable us to reconstruct population relationships across Australia, or to assess the degree of late Pleistocene contact with the islands of southeast Asia.

The presence by 30 000 B.P. of anatomically modern communities in western Europe and southeast Australia – opposite points on the periphery of human distribution in the Upper Pleistocene – indicates that whatever the complexities of detail revealed by the local fossil record, a *H.s. sapiens* morphology was well established over large areas of the Old World by that time, and may be expected to have a correspondingly greater antiquity in regions closer to the centre of the species range.

Such geographically distant finds thus provide further, indirect, support for the suggestive early dates from sub-Saharan Africa (see above). Whatever the detailed pattern, recent discoveries indicate a significantly longer duration for anatomically modern *H. sapiens* than was recognised only a few years ago.

THE PATTERN OF HUMAN EVOLUTION

In recent years there has been considerable debate about the nature of evolutionary change, and the patterns revealed by the fossil record. In particular, the notion of punctuated equilibria (Eldredge & Gould, 1972) has been presented as an alternative to the orthodoxy of 'phyletic gradualism'. A useful discussion of the two models is in Vrba (1980); Wood (1981) provides a briefer statement. The differences between the two models have, on occasion, been overstated, and in their most extreme forms neither is likely to attract many adherents. However, there does appear to be a real difference between the two in the significance accorded to anagenetic evolution (change within a lineage without speciation).

Phyletic gradualists recognise such a phenomenon and, indeed, may accord it a major role, whereas the punctuated equilibria model denies its existence, apparent examples being attributed instead to random, short term fluctuations about a stable mean, or to speciation events observed by a deficient fossil record. On this interpretation the only significant evolutionary change is that associated with allopatric speciation events.

In a stimulating and provocative review Gould & Eldredge (1977) claimed that hominid evolution provided a particularly clear demonstration of punctuated equilibria. Cronin et al. (1981) attempt to refute this view by arguing that the hominid fossil record is more consistent with a phyletic gradualism model.

Despite claims to the contrary, hominids are unlikely to serve as test cases for determining the general veracity of evolutionary models; the fossil record is too meagre and the material too contentious. Both the analyses referred to above are forced to rely upon very small samples – in some cases individual specimens – often insecurely dated. It is axiomatic that evolutionary change is a property of populations, not individuals, and severely limited knowledge of the parameters of those populations will clearly bias the pattern of evolutionary change recognised from the fossil record, as may chronological inaccuracies. For some crucial sets of specimens, even minor errors in dating may result in the direction of evolutionary change being misidentified! Other groups, with more complete fossil records than Hominidae, will have to be used to determine the validity of these contrasting models of phyletic change.

Despite these caveats, sufficient fossil material is available to discern the broad pattern of evolutionary change in hominids, although not with total resolution. My own interpretation, which should be evident from much of the above, is that the earlier stages were polyphyletic, with indications of speciation events. The spectacular discoveries of the last decade or so have revealed the complexity of morphological variation among Pliocene and basal Pleistocene Hominidae, and promoted greater awareness of this polyphyly. The pattern revealed is consistent with the punctuated equilibria model, but does not conclusively demonstrate its applicability to hominids, since phyletic gradualism also accords a prominent role to change through speciation events.

By contrast, the accumulating fossil evidence of the last 1.5 My indicates a broadly anagenetic i.e. phyletic gradualistic model, with no conclusive evidence of punctuated equilibria. As noted above, local fossil records may accord with such a pattern at a parochial level, suggesting demic or subspecific replacement, whilst still being consistent with indications of gradualism at the species level.

With further improvements of dating techniques, and the recovery of specimens continuing apace, the next decade should see many of the present ambiguities of the fossil record resolved, and the emergence of a much clearer and more detailed reconstruction of the pattern of evolution within the genus *Homo*.

Some of the interpretations offered above are based upon work supported by Cambridge University, King's College, Cambridge, and the Boise Fund, Oxford.

REFERENCES

Aiello, L. & Day, M. H. (1982). The evolution of locomotion in the early Hominidae. In *Progress in Anatomy*, vol. 2, ed. R. J. Harrison & V. Navaratnam, pp. 81–98. Cambridge University Press.

ApSimon, A. (1980). The last neanderthal in France? *Nature (London)*, **287**, 271–2.

ApSimon, A. (1981). Matters arising. *Nature (London)*, **289**, 823–4.

Bilsborough, A. (1973). A multivariate study of evolutionary change in the hominid cranial vault and some evolution rates. *Journal of Human Evolution*, **2**, 387–403.

Bilsborough, A. (1976). Patterns of evolution in Middle Pleistocene hominids. *Journal of Human Evolution*, **5**, 423–39.

Bishop, W. W. (ed.). (1978). *Background to Early Man in Africa*. Edinburgh: Scottish Academic Press.

Boaz, N. & Howell, F. C. (1977). A gracile hominid cranium from upper member G of the Shungura Formation, Ethiopia. *American Journal of Physical Anthropology*, **46**, 92–108.

Bordes, F. & Thibault, C. (1977). Thoughts on the initial adaptation of hominids to European glacial climates. *Quaternary Research*, **8**, 115–27.

Brose, D. S. & Wolpoff, M. H. (1971) Early upper Paleolithic man and late middle Paleolithic tools. *American Anthropologist*, **73**, 1156–94.

Brown, F. H. & Cerling, J. E. (1982). Stratigraphical significance of the Tulu Bor Tuff of the Koobi Fora Formation. *Nature (London)*, **299**, 212–15.

Burr, D. B. (1976). Neanderthal vocal tract reconstruction. A critical appraisal. *Journal of Human Evolution*, **5**, 285–90.

Campbell, B. G. (1973). A new taxonomy of fossil man. *Yearbook of Physical Anthropology*, **17**, 194–201.

Campbell, B. G. (1978). Some problems in hominid classification and nomenclature. In *Early Hominids of Africa*, ed. C. Jolly, pp. 567–81. London: Duckworth.

Cerling, T. E. & Brown, F. H. (1982). Tuffaceous marker horizons in the Koobi Fora region of the Lower Omo valley. *Nature (London)*, **299**, 216–20.

Clark, W. E. Le Gros (1964). *The Fossil Evidence for Human Evolution*. Chicago University Press.

Conroy, G.; Jolly, C.; Cramer, D. & Kalb, J. (1978). Newly discovered fossil hominid skull from the Afar depression, Ethiopia. *Nature (London)*, **276**, 67–70.

Cronin, J. E., Boaz, N. T., Stringer, C. B. & Rak, Y. (1981). Tempo and mode in hominid evolution. *Nature (London)*, **292**, 113–22.

Day, M. H. (1972). The Omo human skeletal remains. In *The Origin of Homo sapiens*, ed. F. Bordes, pp. 31–6. Paris: UNESCO.

Drake, R. E., Curtis, G. H., Cerling, T. E., Cerling, B. W. & Hampel, J. (1980). KBS tuff dating and geochronology of tuffaceous sediments in the Koobi Fora and Shungura Formations, East Africa. *Nature (London)*, **283**, 368–72.

Eldredge, N. & Gould, S. J. (1972). Punctuated equilibria: an alternative to phyletic gradualism. In *Models in Paleobiology*, ed. T. J. M. Schopf, pp. 82–115. San Francisco: Freeman.

Freedman, L. & Lofgren, M. (1979). Human skeletal remains from Cossack, western Australia. *Journal of Human Evolution*, **8**, 283–99.

Gingerich, P. (1978). Phylogeny reconstruction and the phylogenetic position of *Tarsius*. In *Recent Advances in Primatology*, vol. 3, *Evolution*, ed. D. J. Chivers & K. A. Joysey, pp. 249–56. London: Academic Press.

Gould, S. J. & Eldredge, N. (1977). Punctuated equilibria: the tempo and mode of evolution reconsidered. *Palaeobiology*, **3**, 115–51.

Howell, F. C. (1978). Hominidae. In *Evolution of African Mammals*, ed. V. J. Maglio & H. B. S. Cooke, pp. 154–248. Boston: Harvard University Press.

Howells, W. W. (1974). Neanderthals: names, hypotheses and scientific method. *American Anthropologist*, **76**, 24–38.

Howells, W. W. (1975). Neanderthal man: facts and figures. In *Paleoanthroplogy. Morphology and Paleoecology*, ed. R. H. Tuttle, pp. 389–408. The Hague & Paris: Mouton.

Howells, W. W. (1980). *Homo erectus* – who, why, where: a survey. *Yearbook of Physical Anthropology*, **23**, 1–23.

Leakey, L. S. B., Tobias, P. V. & Napier, J. R. (1964). A new species of the genus *Homo* from Olduvai Gorge. *Nature (London)*, **202**, 7–9.

Leakey, M. G. & Leakey, R. E. (eds.). (1978) *Koobi Fora Research Project 1. The Fossil Hominids and an Introduction to their Context. 1968–1974*. Oxford University Press.

Lieberman, P., Crelin, E. J. & Klatt, D. H. (1972). Phonetic ability and related anatomy of the newborn and adult human, Neanderthal man and the chimpanzee. *American Anthropologist*, **74**, 287–307.

McBurney, C. B. M. (1976). *Early Man in the Soviet Union: The Implications of some Recent Discoveries*. London: British Academy.

Mann, A. & Trinkaus, E. (1974). Neanderthal and Neanderthal-like fossils from the Upper Pleistocene. *Yearbook of Physical Anthropology*, **17**, 169–93.

Pilbeam, D. R. (1975). Middle Pleistocene hominids. In *After the Australopithecines*, ed. K. Butzer & G. Isaac, pp. 809–56. The Hague & Paris: Mouton.

Repenning, C. A. & Fejfor, O. (1982). Evidence for earlier date of Ubeidiya, Israel, hominid site, *Nature (London)*, **299**, 344–7.

Rightmire, G. P. (1975). Problems in the study of late Pleistocene Man in Africa. *American Anthropologist*, **77**, 28–52.

Rightmire, G. P. (1979). Implications of Border Cave skeletal remains for later Pleistocene human evolution (and comments following). *Current Anthropology*, **20**, 23–35.

Robinson, J. T. (1953). *Meganthropus*, Australopithecines and Hominids, *American Journal of Physical Anthropology*, **11**, 1–38.

Santa Luca, A. P. (1978). A re-examination of presumed Neanderthal fossils. *Journal of Human Evolution*, **7**, 619–36.

Sartono, S. (1975). Implications arising from Pithecanthropus VIII. In *Paleoanthropology. Morphology and Paleoecology*, ed. R. H. Tuttle, pp. 327–60. The Hague & Paris: Mouton.

Siegal, M. I. & Carlisle, R. C. (1974). Some problems in the interpretation of Neanderthal speech capabilities: a reply to Leiberman. *American Anthropologist*, **76**, 319–23.

Simpson, G. G. (1975). Recent advances in methods of phylogenetic inference. In *Phylogeny of Primates*, ed. W. P. Luckett & F. S. Szalay, pp. 3–20. New York & London: Plenum.

Stewart, T. D. (1977). The Neanderthal skeletal remains from Shanidar Cave, Iraq: a summary of findings to date. *Proceedings of the American Philosophical Society*, **121**, 121–65.

Stringer, C. B. (1974). Population relationships of later Pleistocene hominids: a multivariate study of available crania. *Journal of Archaeological Science*, **1**, 317–42.

Stringer, C. B. (1978). Some problems in Middle and Upper Pleistocene hominid relationships. In *Recent Advances in Primatology*, vol. 3, *Evolution*, ed. D. J. Chivers & K. A. Joysey, pp. 395–418. London: Academic Press.

Stringer, C. B., Howell, F. C. & Melentis, J. K. (1979). The significance of the fossil hominid skull from Petralona, Greece. *Journal of Archaeological Science*, **6**, 235–53.

Stringer, C. B., Kruszynski, R. C. & Jacobi, R. M. (1981). Matters arising. *Nature (London)*, **289**, 823–4.

Stringer, C. B. & Trinkaus, E. (1981). The Shanidar Neanderthal crania. In *Aspects of Human Evolution*, ed. C. B. Stringer, pp. 129–65. London: Taylor & Francis.

Thorne, A., (1976). Morphological contrasts in Pleistocene Australians. In *The Origin of the Australians*, ed. R. L. Kirk & A. G. Thorne, pp. 95–112. Canberra: Australian Institute for Aboriginal Studies.

Tobias, P. V. (1978). The earliest Transvaal members of the genus *Homo* with another look at some problems of hominid taxonomy & systematics. *Zeitschrift für Morphologie und Anthropologie*, **69**, 225–65.

Tobias, P. V. (1980). The natural history of the heliocoidal occlusal plane and its evolution in early *Homo*. *American Journal of Physical Anthropology*, **53**, 173–88.

Tobias, P. V. & von Koenigswald, G. H. R. (1964). A comparison between the Olduvai hominines and those of Java, and some implications for hominid phylogeny. *Nature (London)*, **204**, 515–18.

Trinkaus, E. (1981). Neanderthal limb proportions and cold adaptation. In *Aspects of Human Evolution*, ed. C. B. Stringer, pp. 187–224. London: Taylor & Francis.

Trinkaus, E. & Howells, W. W. (1979). The Neanderthals. *Scientific American*, **241**, 94–105.

Vandermersch, B. (1972). Récentes découvertes de squellettes humains à Qafzeh (Israel): essai d'interprétation. In *The Origin of Homo sapiens*, ed. F. Bordes, pp. 49–54. Paris: UNESCO.

Vrba, E. (1980). Evolution species and fossils: how does life evolve? *South African Journal of Science*, **76**, 61–84.

Walker, A. (1976). Remains attributable to *Australopithecus* in the East Rudolf succession. In *Earliest Man and Environments in the Lake Rudolf Basin: Stratigraphy, Paleoecology and Evolution*, ed. Y. Coppens, F. C. Howell, G. Isaac & R. E. F. Leakey, pp. 484–9. Chicago University Press.

Walker, A. & Leakey, R. E. F. (1978). The hominids of East Turkana. *Scientific American*, **239**, 44–56.

Wind, J. (1978). Fossil evidence for primate vocalisations? In *Recent Advances in Primatology*, vol. 3, *Evolution*, ed. D. J. Chivers & K. A. Joysey, pp. 87–92. London: Academic Press.

Wolpoff, M. H. (1980). *Paleoanthropology*. New York: Knopf.

Wolpoff, M. H. (1981). Matters arising. *Nature (London)*, **289**, 823.

Wood, B. A. (1978). Classification and phylogeny of East African hominids. In *Recent Advances in Primatology*, vol. 3, *Evolution* ed. D. J. Chivers & D. A. Joysey, pp. 351–72. London: Academic Press.

Wood, B. A. (1981). Human origins: fossil evidence and current problems of analysis and interpretation. In *Progress in Anatomy*, vol. 1, ed. R. J. Harrison & R L. Holmes, pp. 229–45. Cambridge University Press.

7 The primary afferent nociceptive neuron

A. D. HOYES

Department of Anatomy, St Mary's Hospital Medical School, London W2 1PG, UK

INTRODUCTION

Pain, or nociception as it is now increasingly styled, is possibly the most fundamental and important of all peripheral sensations. It plays a crucial role in protection against injury and represents the primary mechanism for the signalling to the central nervous system of tissue damage. The role of pain in protection is perhaps most clearly exemplified by the condition of syringomyelia, in which the development of progressive cavitation and gliosis in the region of the central canal of the spinal cord interrupts the projection pathways for both pain and temperature sensation. Although the patient retains touch sensation in the affected areas, because of loss of nociceptive input to the higher regions of the central nervous system, repeated trauma is suffered from, for example, burning by cigarette ends. The primacy of pain as a signalling device for tissue damage (whether arising from trauma, inflammation due to chemical or bacterial or other infective agents or to invasion of the tissues by neoplasia) is indicated by the fact that a high proportion of the patients consulting their physicians complain of some kind of pain.

Despite its importance in peripheral sensation, until recently our understanding of the mechanisms by which pain impulses are generated at the periphery and are projected to higher levels of the central nervous system was limited. The classic studies of Keele & Armstrong (1964) on the human blister base, the development and application of single fibre and intracellular recording techniques and the enunciation of the gate control theory of Melzack & Wall (1965) have been followed by a dramatic and almost explosive increase in research on pain generation and projection mechanisms. As in any other situation of this kind, a comprehensive synthesis of this information has yet to be accomplished, but it is now reasonable to assume that, within a few years, it will be possible to provide a much more thorough and essentially holistic account of the mechanisms involved in pain sensation.

THE PRIMARY AFFERENT NEURON

The primary afferent neuron is the first of a series of three neurons which, in classical terms, are involved in the projection of sensory information from the periphery to the cerebral cortex. Except for those associated with some of the special sense organs, the cell bodies of the primary neurons are located in the dorsal root ganglia of the spinal nerves or the ganglia of the cranial nerves and are pseudo-unipolar in type. The peripheral branch of the single process which arises from the neuron conducts impulses from the periphery and, in terms of the usual classification

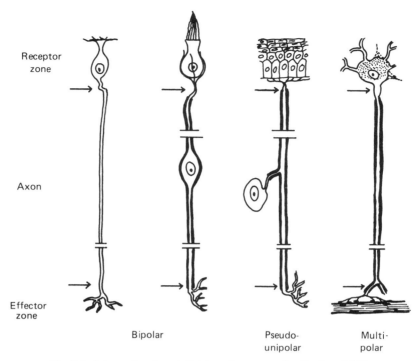

Fig. 7.1. Scheme for the subdivision of neurons after Bodian (1962).

of neuronal processes, should be regarded as a dendrite. The central branch of the perikaryal process runs through the dorsal roots or the roots of the cranial nerves into the central nervous system, where it establishes synaptic contact with the secondary afferent neuron.

Although the peripheral process of the primary afferent neuron should be classified as a dendrite, it has the structural characteristics of an axon and is often myelinated. It is, indeed, normally regarded as an axon. In an attempt to overcome this and other problems in the classification of neuronal processes, Bodian (1962) proposed that the neuron should be divided into three zones. A modified form of this scheme is illustrated in Fig. 7.1. Its principal advantage is that, because it avoids the use of the neuronal perikaryon as a focus for impulse transmission in the processes, it allows all processes with the structural features of axons to be classified as such. Its principal disadvantage is that it makes no allowance for the presynaptic or prejunctional input at the ends of axons which has been demonstrated in many parts of the nervous system. It is, nevertheless, a useful way of looking at neurons and it is surprising that it has not been more widely accepted.

The perikarya of the secondary afferent neurons are located in the dorsal horn of the spinal cord or in the nuclei of the cranial nerves in the brain stem. According to classical concepts, the axons of the secondary neurons which transmit pain and thermal sensations project from the spinal cord through the spinothalamic or anterolateral pathway (Fig. 7.2) and from the brain stem through the ventral secondary ascending tract of the Vth nerve to the posterior part of the ventral nucleus of the thalamus, where they establish synaptic contact with the tertiary afferent neurons. The axons of the tertiary afferent neurons project through the internal

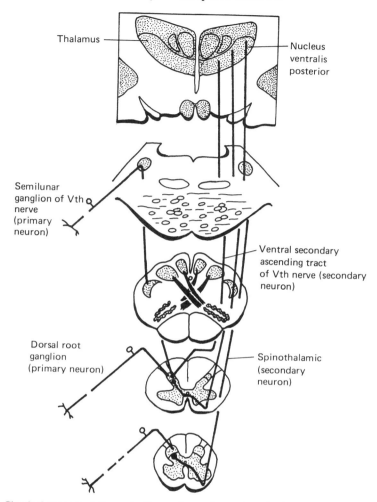

Fig. 7.2. Classical concept of the projection pathways for nociceptive impulses from the periphery to the thalamus.

capsule to the primary sensory area in the post-central gyrus of the cerebral hemisphere.

It is now clear that the classical concept of the pain projection pathway is, at the very least, a gross oversimplification. There is, for example, a substantial body of evidence that the primary afferent neurons transmit not only directly to the secondary afferent neurons, but also to internuncial neurons. The modulation, by these internuncial neurons, of input into the secondary afferent neurons is a fundamental aspect of the gate control theory. There is also evidence that many of the axons transmitting pain impulses in the anterolateral pathway terminate either in the brain stem reticular formation or the phylogenetically older intralaminar nuclei of the thalamus. These projections provide a mechanism for input of nociceptive information into the limbic system. This system is involved in emotional responses, and it is reasonable to suppose that it contributes to the affective responses which represent one of the major problems in experimental assessment of pain in man. Whether in fact pain impulses are projected from the ventral nucleus of the thalamus to the post-central gyrus has also been seriously questioned, and there is now physiological evidence that the thalamocortical projection passes through the posterior nucleus of the thalamus to a second sensory area located within the lateral fissure (see Mountcastle, 1980).

THEORIES OF PERIPHERAL SENSATION

Together with touch, warmth and cold, pain represents one of the major modalities of sensation. As pointed out by Sinclair (1981), in the hands of some observers, each of the modalities can be shown to merge imperceptibly into one another. There is, however, general acceptance that each of the modalities represents a specific type of peripheral sensation. Almost all research work on sensory processing from the periphery is based upon the existence of the modalities as separate entities. Such considerations are also central to the two major extant theories of peripheral sensation. One of these theories, the pattern theory, derives from the earlier intensive theory and assumes that perception of sensations referable to particular modalities is determined by the pattern of projection of impulses from particular parts of the periphery on the central nervous system. The second theory, the specificity theory, dictates that each modality of sensation is associated with a separate population of primary afferent neurons which are at least preferentially sensitive to stimuli associated with that modality.

The history and development of the theories of sensation has been fully reviewed by both Bonica (1980) and Sinclair (1981). Both the pattern and specificity theories still have their adherents, but it is probably true to say that, at the present time, the specificity theory has more credence.

TYPES OF PAIN

Primary afferent nociceptive neurons are widely distributed in the skin as well as in deeper structures such as muscle and the viscera. In the skin, noxious stimuli evoke two kinds of response. Of these, one reaches consciousness much more rapidly than the other and is typically described as being 'pricking' in quality. The second is conducted through the projection pathways at a much slower rate and is usually recorded as being 'burning' in quality.

Analysis of the responses elicited in cutaneous afferent axons by mechanical as well as other forms of stimuli has established the existence of fundamental differences in the types of neuron responsible for fast, pricking and slow, burning pain. These studies have been extensively reviewed, in particular by Perl (1971, 1980) and Iggo (1980). The neurons responsible for both types of pain are excited by mechanical stimuli which are much more intense than those responsible for excitation of the various types of cutaneous ending which are now classified as low threshold mechanoreceptors and which, in general, can be regarded as being responsible for the sensation of touch. Because responses are normally elicited in these neurons only by mechanical stimuli of sufficient intensity to produce tissue damage, it is widely considered that such damage is a prerequisite for excitation of the neurons.

It has been shown that pricking or pinching the skin elicits responses in axons which are lightly myelinated, and which conduct at speeds of between 10 and > 40 m s^{-1} (Burgess & Perl, 1967). This range brackets the Aδ peak of the compound action potential, but does not correspond directly to it. For this reason, the common designation of this type of nociceptive afferent as Aδ in type is not strictly accurate, and it is possible that the neurons should be classified simply as lightly myelinated. Because of their particular stimulus parameters, these neurons are classified as high threshold mechanoreceptors. The punctate location in the skin, the rapid adaptation and the high speed of conduction in the axons of these neurons are all in overall agreement with the concept that they are responsible for the fast, pricking type of pain.

Examination of the responses of cutaneous unmyelinated (C) axons to stimulation has shown that, in addition to axons sensitive to mechanical stimuli of low intensity and to thermal stimuli, the cutaneous plexuses contain substantial numbers of unmyelinated axons which respond to mechanical stimuli of the kind of intensity required to produce tissue damage (Bessou & Perl, 1969). Because these neurons also respond to noxious thermal and to a variety of chemical stimuli, they are classified as polymodal nociceptors. In humans, examination of the responses from axons in cutaneous nerves (Torebjörk, 1974) has provided strong support for the concept that the polymodal nociceptors are responsible for slow, burning pain. As in experimental animals, these neurons are slowly adapting and are sensitive to both noxious thermal and chemical stimuli.

The precise location of the receptors for the two types of pain which can be elicited from the skin has not been fully and conclusively established. Waterston's (1933) studies suggested that the epidermis itself is insensitive to noxious stimuli, and that pain is elicited only by stimulation of dermal nerves. The whole question of the presence of intraepidermal axons separate from those associated with the Merkel cell has been widely and extensively debated. The difficulty in demonstrating the intraepidermal axons (which have been clearly demonstrated with the light micro-scope in silver stained preparations) in material prepared for electron microscopy may, however, be attributed to technical factors, and especially to the much lower density of the axons in the epidermis than in the dermal plexuses. Kruger, Perl & Sedivec (1981) have, however, recently identified intraepidermal axons by electron microscopy in punctate areas of skin from which physiological responses of the type observed in high threshold mechanoreceptors had previously been demonstrated. These axons were found to possess a myelin sheath prior to entering the epidermis.

Pain arising in deep structures, and in particular from the viscera, is less well localised than cutaneous pain and tends to radiate (Procacci, Zoppi & Maresca, 1979). In skeletal muscle and joints, the available evidence indicates that nociceptive stimuli are conducted, as in skin, by unmyelinated and myelinated axons (see Yaksh & Hammond, 1982). The location of the receptors in muscles, joints and viscera, and their patterns of response to stimulation have been less extensively studied than have nociceptive axons in the skin. One of the problems in investigating the distribution of nociceptive axons in visceral structures is that they are intimately associated with autonomic efferent axons which, as in the case of the polymodal nociceptor, are also unmyelinated.

STRUCTURE OF RECEPTORS

The search for a structurally distinct type of axon mediating nociceptive responses has been influenced to a considerable extent by the existence of the pattern and specificity theories of sensation. The pattern theory requires the existence in the periphery of only one type of receptor subserving all modalities of sensation.

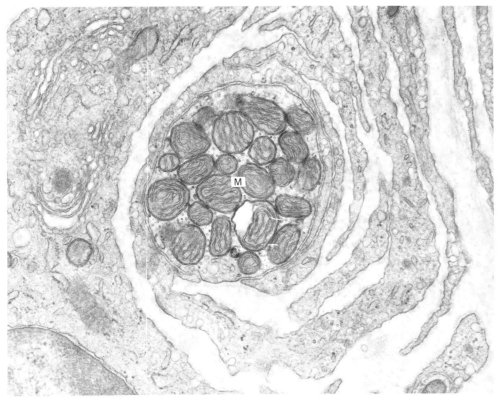

Fig. 7.3. Mitochondria-containing mechanosensitive nerve ending (M) in guinea-pig foot skin. The ending is surrounded by a loose capsule of connective tissue cells. × 28 000.

Ultrastructural examination of structures known to be sensitive only to mechanical stimuli, such as muscle spindles and encapsulated endings (e.g. the Pacinian corpuscle), has shown that the afferent axons possess terminals which contain numerous, usually rather closely packed, mitochondria and few, if any, vesicles. Similar endings have been identified in a variety of other situations and in both less well encapsulated and free nerve endings (Fig. 7.3). In skin, the terminals are particularly numerous in the nerves associated with hair follicles. In the viscera, they tend to occur in clusters, suggesting that they are formed at the ends of multiple terminal branches of a single axon (Fig. 7.4). Except in structures such as the carotid sinus, where they display considerable variation in fine structure (Knoche, Addicks & Schmitt, 1974), the endings are not easy to identify by electron microscopy in visceral structures. Their infrequent occurrence in thin sections (in relation to the terminals of autonomic efferent post-ganglionic axons) may, however, not be a true reflection of their overall density in such plexuses. This is because, in contrast to the terminals of autonomic efferent axons – which occur at intervals along the last part of the axons – the terminals of these axons probably occur only at the ends of their branches.

The specificity theory requires that the receptors of axons mediating different modalities of sensation exhibit different sensitivities to different forms of stimuli. Because it is in all probability related more to the nature of the receptors on axonal membranes than to any other factor, modality specificity in primary afferent neurons

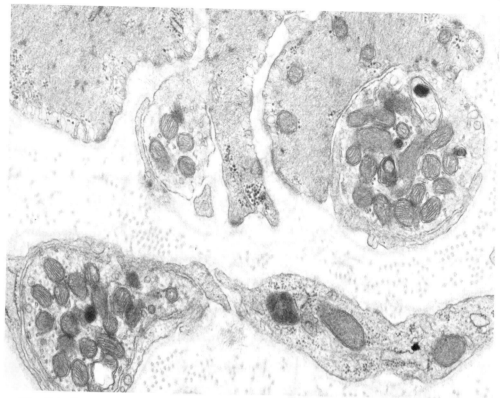

Fig. 7.4. Group of mitochondria-containing nerve endings in the trachealis muscle of the guinea-pig. × 35 000.

need not be associated with any substantial degree of diversity in the structure of the axon terminals. Modality specificity may also be related to a number of other factors. These include the location and cell and tissue relationships of the axonal terminals. One example of this is the termination of axons in the epidermis in relation to Merkel cells. In this situation, it is possible that the Merkel cell is the primary stimulus transducer, the response in the axon being elicited by secondary mechanisms and associated with the release and interaction at receptors on the axons of transmitters stored in the Merkel cell granules. Another example is the termination of nociceptive axons within the epidermis or in the dermis. Such considerations have already been discussed with regard to the axons responsible for fast, pricking pain which, according to the evidence presented by Kruger *et al.* (1981), terminate in the epidermis. The persistence of a Schwann cell investment around these axons, until after they enter the epidermis, clearly isolates them from the effects of chemicals released into the dermis as a result of a noxious stimulus and restricts their firing to situations in which, aside from direct trauma, they are excited by substances released from the epidermal cells themselves. Axons which terminate in the dermis may be subject not only to the effects of direct mechanical stimuli, but also to all of the different pain-producing chemicals. These include those which are released from mast cells and other structures, including blood vessels and autonomic efferent axons.

Modality specificity in primary afferent neurons may be determined by factors such as the nature of the receptors on the axonal membranes and the location of the

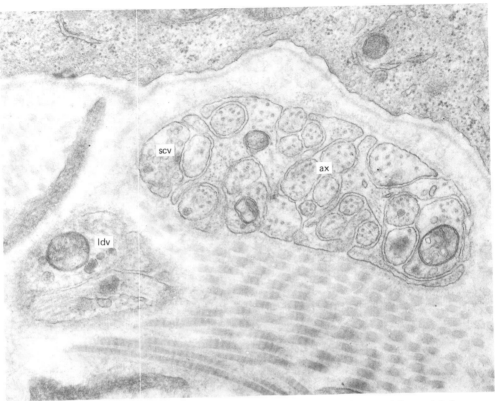

Fig. 7.5. Subepithelial nerves of the rat ureter showing a terminal profile containing mainly large dense-cored vesicles (ldv) and a terminal profile containing mainly small clear vesicles (scv). The remaining axon profiles (ax) contain mainly microtubules and represent sections through pre- or inter-terminal regions of the axons. × 34 500.

terminals. It could, therefore, reasonably be argued that nociception is also mediated by axons with terminals containing mainly mitochondria, similar to those found in encapsulated mechanoreceptors (such as Pacinian corpuscles), and as free nerve endings in structures such as the carotid sinus and around hair follicles. Recent work on the nerve plexuses of the urinary tract, and other visceral structures such as the trachea, has suggested that this is not the case, and that nociception is mediated by a population of axons with an ultrastructurally distinct type of vesicle-containing terminal. Examination of the subepithelial plexus of the rat ureter showed that the nerves contain large numbers of unmyelinated axons with terminals which (instead of containing numerous, usually closely packed small vesicles and only occasional large dense-cored vesicles present in the terminals of autonomic efferent axons) contain mainly large dense-cored vesicles (Hoyes, Bourne & Martin, 1975; Figs. 7.5, 7.6). The terminals of these axons also contain some small clear vesicles, but these are typically few in number and are usually widely dispersed in the axoplasm (Figs. 7.5, 7.6). In addition, the terminals frequently contain at least small amounts of glycogen. Another feature is that, after effective perfusion fixation, the terminals show little evidence of the enlargement or varicosity that is characteristic of the terminals of autonomic efferent axons.

Although they were not recognised in our earlier studies (Hoyes *et al.*, 1975), more

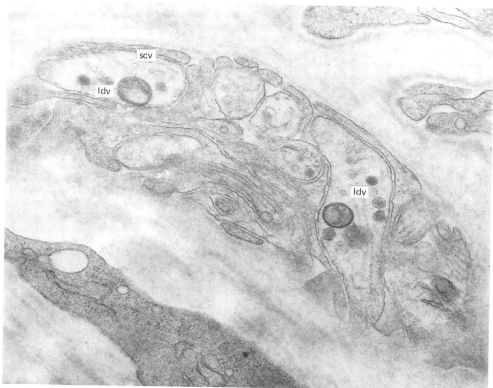

Fig. 7.6. Subepithelial nerve of the rat ureter showing terminal profiles containing mainly large dense-cored vesicles (ldv). One of the profiles also contains scattered small clear vesicles (scv). × 35 000.

recent work has shown that, in addition to axons with terminals containing mainly large dense-cored vesicles, the subepithelial nerves of the rat ureter contain small numbers of axons with terminals in which there are the numerous closely packed small vesicles found in the terminals of autonomic efferent axons. The proportion of such axons in the nerves has been assessed from counts of the frequency of their terminals in random ultrathin sections, and is probably less than 3%. Rather larger numbers of axons with terminals of this type are present in the muscular plexuses, but other studies (Hoyes, Bourne & Martin, 1976) have shown that, even in these plexuses, most of the axons are of the type comprising the principal constituent of the subepithelial plexus. A similar contribution of axons with terminals containing mainly large dense-cored vesicles has been demonstrated in as yet unpublished studies on the subepithelial and muscular plexuses of the guinea-pig ureter.

The presence in peripheral axon terminals of accumulations of vesicles has frequently been regarded as evidence that the axons are efferent. The distribution of axons with terminals containing mainly large dense-cored vesicles in the ureteric plexuses, and in particular their presence in large numbers in the subepithelial nerves, nevertheless suggested that they are in fact afferent. Direct evidence of the afferent identity of these axons has been obtained from quantitative electron microscopical studies on the structurally similar axons in the tracheal nerve plexuses. In the guinea-pig (Hoyes & Barber, 1978), the axons are concentrated in the plexus in

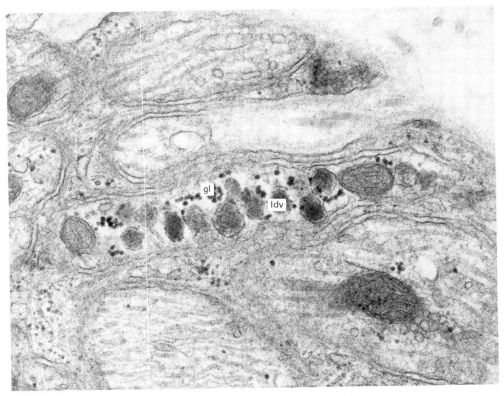

Fig. 7.7. Axon terminal containing mainly large dense-cored vesicles (ldv) and scattered glycogen granules (gl) in a submucous nerve of the guinea-pig trachea. × 57 000.

the submucosa (Fig. 7.7), where they are closely associated with adrenergic axons. In the rat and the cat, the axons frequently enter and terminate within the epithelium (Hoyes & Barber, 1981a; Das, Jeffery & Widdicombe, 1978). In both animals, the origin of the axons directly from the vagus nerve has been established by degeneration studies. In these studies (Hoyes & Barber, 1981a; Das, Jeffery & Widdicombe, 1979) it was shown that, after unilateral section of the vagus nerve below the nodose ganglion, there is extensive degeneration of the axons in the epithelium of the ipsilateral side of the trachea. Quantitative analysis showed that, rather than being derived from other nerves, the small number of normal axons which remained in the epithelium of the ipsilateral side of the trachea after section of the vagus are probably derived from the contralateral vagus nerve. To exclude the possibility that the axons are derived from neurons with perikarya located in the brainstem or from neurons with perikarya in ganglia such as the superior cervical ganglion, from which they enter the vagus through branches arising from the nodose ganglion, the effect on the number of axons in the tracheal epithelium of section of the vagus nerve above the nodose ganglion and of section of the branches which arise from the ganglion was compared with that of section of the vagus below the nodose ganglion. The absence of any reduction in the number of intraepithelial axons after section of these nerves not only excludes both of these possibilities, but also, since axonal degeneration within the short survival times used in the experiments occurs only after isolation of the axons from the neuronal perikarya, also constitutes *prima facie* evidence of the location of the axons in the nodose ganglion (Hoyes, Barber & Jagessar, 1982a). Because there is no evidence of the presence of efferent neuronal perikarya in the nodose ganglion, these observations also provide direct evidence that the axons in the epithelium of the trachea are afferent in nature.

The involvement in nociception of the axons with terminals containing mainly large dense-cored vesicles (identified in the ureteric plexuses) is supported by several lines of evidence. One of these relates to their pattern of distribution in other structures which, at least in humans, are known to contain large numbers of pain afferents (e.g. the cornea). Ultrastructural examination of the corneal nerve plexuses in the rat (Hoyes & Barber, 1976a) and in other mammals (Hoyes & Barber, 1977) has shown that, in the avascular part of the cornea, a high proportion of the axons possess terminals similar to those found in the nerves of the ureter. These studies also showed that, as in the ureter, the terminals are spaced at intervals along the last part of the axons.

In the skin, the presence of axons with terminals containing mainly large dense-cored vesicles of the type found in the ureteric plexuses is less well established. Cauna (1973) found that, in hairy skin, the unmyelinated nerve fibres branch repeatedly as they approach the epidermis to form a complex defined as a penicillate nerve ending. In glabrous skin, Cauna (1980) found that the nerve endings are somewhat simpler and have a much smaller spatial distribution than the penecillate endings. In both situations, the axons were accompanied by Schwann cell processes but, as in the ureter, there were frequently areas in which the Schwann cell investment of the axons was incomplete. Although, except where the axons entered the epidermis, there was no evidence of total loss of the Schwann cell investment, the existence of parts of the axons separated from the surrounding connective tissue only by the basal lamina of the Schwann cell provides a series of loci in which the axons can be directly stimulated by chemicals released into this tissue. In both hairy and glabrous skin, the axons contained a variety of vesicles, but rarely showed any clear evidence of terminals containing the accumulations of large dense-cored vesicles seen in the ureteric nerves. Our own observations on rat and guinea-pig skin have also shown that axon terminals containing accumulations of such vesicles are much less easy to identify in cutaneous nerves than in the nerves of the cornea or in visceral nerve plexuses in structures such as the ureter.

The apparent absence of numerous vesicle-containing terminal areas in the unmyelinated axons of cutaneous nerves may be due to a variety of factors. As in other situations, these may be partly technical. One of the most interesting aspects of analysis of the structure of the axons identified in the ureteric plexuses is that they are highly susceptible to the effects of imperfect fixation. In inadequately perfused material or material subjected to immersion fixation, the axons are often dilated and show either a clumping or dispersal of the large dense-cored vesicles. Dilatation is most evident after cold fixation with fixatives containing paraformaldehyde. In this context, it is of interest that Weddell & Zander (1951) found that the corneal nerve fibres show no evidence of focal enlargement during short-term incubation *in vitro*, but rapidly develop such enlargements when fixed in formalin. These observations are consistent with our own findings on the axons in the ureter. We have also shown that, in material fixed in osmium tetroxide and in fixatives which do not contain glutaraldehyde, the density of the cores of the large vesicles is substantially reduced and is sometimes lost (Hoyes & Barber, 1976b). Such considerations may account, in part, for the failure of Cauna (1973, 1980) to identify more than very small numbers of large dense-cored vesicles in cutaneous nerve endings.

An alternative possibility is that, in contrast to those in other tissues such as the cornea and ureter, the terminals of unmyelinated nociceptive axons in the skin are much less numerous and are restricted either to the ends of the axons or to a much shorter segment of the last part of the axons. Under such circumstances, the terminals would be much less frequently observed in ultrathin sections, especially since the nerves in the skin are more widely dispersed and generally less numerous than in structures such as the ureter. A further possibility is that, irrespective of the presence of smaller numbers of terminals on the axons, the vesicle content of these regions is substantially lower than in visceral axons.

The evidence currently available is not sufficient to provide an adequate assessment of the extent to which these factors are responsible for the infrequent occurrence of terminal areas in the unmyelinated axons in cutaneous nerve plexuses, and it is clear that much further work will be required on this aspect of the innervation of the skin before any definite conclusions can be reached on the relationships between such axons and those found in the viscera. Such evidence as is available from the work of Cauna (1973, 1980) and from our own unpublished work on laboratory mammals is, however, consistent with the existence of at least a degree of similarity in the structure of the axons to those identified in the corneal and other nerve plexuses.

Although the evidence on the identity of the unmyelinated axons in the skin with those classified in our studies on the cornea and both the trachea and ureter is not conclusive, the work of Macintosh (1975) and Kruger et al. (1981) indicates that the axons which terminate in the epidermis do possess terminals which contain substantial numbers of large dense-cored vesicles. Although the studies undertaken by Kruger et al. (1981) indicate that the intraepidermal axons are responsible for fast, pricking pain rather than the slow, burning type of pain (generally considered to be mediated by unmyelinated axons), a close structural similarity in the terminals of the two types of nociceptive afferent neuron is not surprising, especially if it is assumed that the response parameters of the neurons are determined by the location of the terminal areas of the axons.

The distribution and location of axons with terminals of the type found in the ureteric plexuses, in muscles and joints, and in viscera other than the trachea, have not been determined. In the trachea, there are substantial differences in their distribution in the guinea-pig from those in the rat and the cat. Whereas in the latter species the axons frequently terminate in the epithelium, in the guinea-pig intra-epithelial axons are rarely (if ever) observed; most of the axons with terminals containing mainly large dense-cored vesicles are found in the plexus of nerves which, in this species, is located in the loose connective tissue of the submucosa (Hoyes & Barber, 1978; Fig. 7.7). This difference in the location of the axons in relation to the epithelium is also reflected in the ureter where, in the guinea-pig, both intraepithelial axons are less numerous and the subepithelial plexus is less well developed than in the rat.

The reasons for these differences are not clear. One possibility is that they are determined by differences in the nature and timing of the development of the plexuses. In the ureter, the muscular and mucosal plexuses are formed by extension into the wall of branches of the large nerves in the adventitia. In the rat, this process takes place mainly in the immediate post-natal period; the development of axons with terminals containing mainly large dense-cored vesicles also precedes that of axons with the small-vesicle-containing terminals – which are regarded as those of auto-nomic efferent axons (A. D. Hoyes & P. Barber, unpublished observations). The

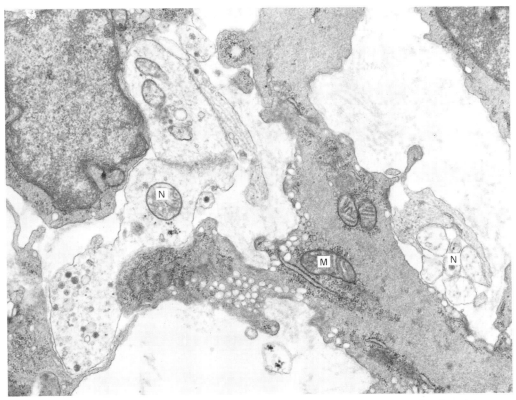

Fig. 7.8. Small nerves (N) in the muscle coat of a 2-day-old rat showing close approximation of the axons to a developing muscle cell (M). × 21 000.

migration of the nerves through the muscle coat is also accompanied by the development of a close structural relationship between the axons and the muscle cells (Fig. 7.8). The functional significance of this relationship (which persists for only a short period of time) is unknown, but is suggestive of some form of trophic interaction between the axons and the muscle cells. The pattern of development of the ureteric plexuses in the guinea-pig and in other species has not been analysed in detail, but it seems reasonable to postulate that the degree of development – both of the subepithelial plexus and of intraepithelial axons – is determined by the number and extent of migration of the branches of the adventitial nerves into the wall and the temporal relationship of their migration to the development of the muscle coat.

Although the precise location of nociceptive afferent axons in most deeper structures is largely unknown, there is some evidence that they are associated primarily with small blood vessels. A primarily perivascular location of free nerve endings in skeletal muscle in the cat was reported by Stacey (1969). In the ureteric arterioles, there is also evidence of a substantial contribution of axons with terminals containing mainly large dense-cored vesicles to the perivascular plexuses (Hoyes & Barber, 1981c). The extent of the contribution of these axons to the innervation of cutaneous arterioles has still to be determined, but their presence in the perivascular plexuses would be expected from the extensive arteriolar dilatation which is responsible for the flare observed in the triple response. A relationship between axons of this type and small blood vessels has also been observed in the human parietal peritoneum

(A. D. Hoyes & R. Bourne, unpublished observations). In humans, the parietal peritoneum has a substantial blood supply and there is a well developed capillary plexus beneath the mesothelium. In the rat, the parietal peritoneum does not seem to possess either a direct blood supply or an innervation.

The evidence, derived from studies on the cornea and on other structures containing large numbers of nociceptive afferents, on the role in nociception of the axons with terminals containing mainly large dense-cored vesicles is largely circumstantial. More direct evidence on the identity of these axons and their function in nociception has been obtained from studies with capsaicin. Capsaicin is the pungent substance present in capsicum, and was once used in the form of a tincture as a counter-irritant. In the human blister base, capsaicin induces an initial sharp pain response which is followed by a period of insensitivity to further stimuli (Dash & Deshpande, 1976).

When capsaicin is injected into rats, there is also a prolonged loss of sensitivity to noxious stimuli, and this is accompanied by loss of the flare associated with the triple response (Jancsó, Jancsó-Gábor & Scolcsányi, 1967). Although loss of sensitivity to noxious stimuli after injection of capsaicin has been attributed to desensitisation of the pain afferents, there is evidence that it may be due to degeneration of the axons. In neonatal animals, capsaicin induces degeneration in the small neurons in dorsal root ganglia (Jancsó, Kiraly & Jancsó-Gábor, 1977) and a permanent reduction in the number of unmyelinated axons in peripheral nerves (Scadding, 1980). In the rat, it has been shown that, even in the adult, there is degeneration of the axons with terminals containing mainly large dense-cored vesicles (Hoyes & Barber, 1981b).

There is, on the other hand, no evidence of a similar degree of degeneration of the axons in the cornea (Scolcsanyi, Jancso-Gabor & Joo, 1975). In the trachea, the degeneration of the axons is also incomplete (Hoyes et al., 1982a). It has been suggested that this is due to diffusion of capsaicin into the epithelium in insufficient amounts to evoke total degeneration of the axons. The central part of the cornea is avascular, and it is possible that the reported absence of degeneration of the corneal nerves after treatment with capsaicin is also due to inadequate penetration of capsaicin into the dense connective tissue which comprises the corneal stroma.

Because the subepithelial plexus of the rat ureter contains very few axons other than those possessing terminals containing mainly large dense-cored vesicles, it is particularly suitable for quantitative electron microscopic analysis of the effects of noxious stimuli on the axons. Examination of the subepithelial nerves in specimens of ureter exposed to capsaicin during incubation in oxygenated Krebs–Ringer bicarbonate buffer revealed major changes in both the diameter and vesicle content of the axons (Hoyes & Barber, 1979; Fig. 7.9). In these studies, the specimens were exposed to capsaicin at a concentration of 2×10^{-4} g ml^{-1} for 5 minutes. More recent work has shown that the changes develop within 2 minutes of exposure to capsaicin at concentrations as low as 2×10^{-6} g ml^{-1}. This concentration corresponds closely to that shown to evoke pain responses when capsaicin is instilled into the conjunctival sac (Heubner, 1925). Similar changes in the fine structure of the axons have been observed after exposure to acetylcholine for 2 minutes at a concentration of 10^{-4} g ml^{-1} (P. Barber, unpublished observations). This concentration also corresponds closely to the threshold concentration of acetylcholine required to elicit pain responses in the human blister base (Keele & Armstrong, 1964).

After exposure to both capsaicin and acetylcholine, there was a significant increase in the diameter of the axons and an increase in the number per 100 axon profiles of

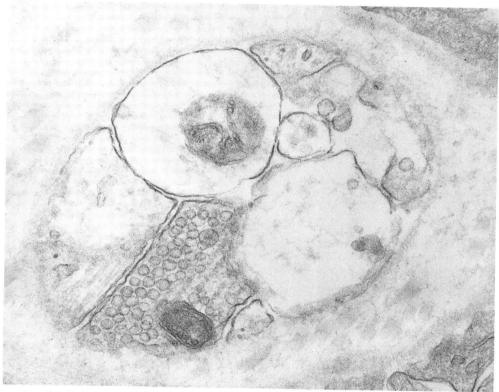

Fig. 7.9. Subepithelial nerve of the rat ureter showing dilated, 'empty' axons in a specimen incubated *in vitro* in capsaicin. The axon terminal containing small clear vesicles (scv) is structurally normal. × 68 500.

large dense-cored vesicles. In specimens treated with capsaicin, there was also a significant decrease in the number per 100 axon profiles of small clear vesicles. The use in these studies of counts of vesicles per 100 axon profiles is subject to error arising from the presence in the sections of some obliquely sectioned axons, but provides a direct indication of the changes in the vesicle content of the axons. Application of more sophisticated stereological procedures, based on estimates of volume density of the vesicles, would in themselves require a correction for section thickness and – unless also corrected for the changes in axon volume – the figures obtained could not be used to provide a direct indication of the effect of stimulation on the overall numbers of vesicles in the axons.

Although the changes in the fine structure of the axons in the subepithelial nerves of the ureter observed after exposure *in vitro* to both capsaicin and acetylcholine occur at concentrations which correspond to the threshold concentrations required to induce pain responses in human cutaneous axons, they persist for a number of minutes and clearly cannot be related directly to the membrane depolarisation which is responsible for initiation of the action potential in the axons. They may, however, be associated with the after-discharges which have been recorded in the axons of cutaneous polymodal nociceptors after peripheral stimulation (Perl, 1980) and with a prolonged and at least partial depolarisation of the membrane of the axon terminals. A possible explanation for the increase in axonal diameter is that the membrane depolarisation is accompanied by a substantial increase in the permeability of the membrane and by influx of water into the axons under the influence of the osmotic gradient created by the presence of a higher concentration of protein in the axoplasm than in the surrounding medium. In this context, it is of interest that studies *in vitro* currently being undertaken on the ureteric plexuses of the guinea-pig with capsaicin have provided evidence that the increase in diameter occurs both in the terminal-bearing and in the preterminal regions of the axons. This is in sharp contrast to the degeneration of the axons induced by treatment *in vivo* with capsaicin, which is confined to the terminal-bearing regions of the axons (Hoyes & Barber, 1981*b*).

The reduction in small vesicles in the axons observed after exposure *in vitro* to capsaicin can be most readily explained by exocytosis of the vesicles at the axonal membrane. The increase in large dense-cored vesicles is less easy to explain. It is possible, however, that it is due to the formation of new vesicles by endocytosis at the axonal membrane. If this is the case, the process of formation of the vesicles may contribute to the removal of receptors from the surface and to the prolonged insensitivity of the axons to further stimulation which is observed after treatment even with low doses of capsaicin. The increase in large dense-cored vesicles which follows treatment with acetylcholine may also be related to the development of a similar, but much less long-lasting period of insensitivity to further stimulation (see Keele & Armstrong, 1964).

Until recently, the nature of the contents of the vesicles in the axons classified as nociceptive afferents was unknown. There is now evidence from electron immuno-cytochemical studies that they contain the undecapeptide, substance P. This was first isolated by von Euler & Gaddum (1931) and is one of an extensive group of peptides which have been identified in peripheral neurons, especially in the gastrointestinal tract. In the ureter of the guinea-pig, substance-P-like immunoreactivity has been demonstrated in the lumina of large dense-cored vesicles in axon terminals similar to those identified in the subepithelial nerves of the rat ureter (Sikri *et al.*, 1981). Clear-cut evidence of the presence of immunoreactivity in the scattered small clear vesicles (which are also present in the axon terminals) has not been obtained, but the occurrence of a major reduction in the amount of substance-P-like immunoreactivity in the ureteric plexuses after treatment *in vitro* with capsaicin may be related to the loss of these vesicles which is seen after treatment with capsaicin in material processed for conventional electron microscopical examination. Substance-P-like immunoreac-tivity has also been demonstrated in the corneal nerves (Miller *et al.*, 1981), as well as in the nerves in the skin, where, in common with those in the ureter, it is depleted by treatment with capsaicin (Gamse, Holzer & Lembeck, 1980).

Although there is now a substantial body of evidence to support the view that the axons with terminals containing mainly large dense-cored vesicles identified in the ureter and other structures are those of primary afferent neurons involved in nociception, it has been postulated that axons with such terminals subserve other functions. Burnstock (1972) suggested that the axons are those of efferent neurons responsible for the non-cholinergic, non-adrenergic responses which can be elicited by nerve stimulation in a variety of structures, but in particular in the gastrointestinal tract. Because many of these responses are mimicked by ATP, Burnstock (1972) proposed that the neurons employ ATP as a transmitter. ATP is a purine, and he therefore classified the neurons as purinergic neurons.

One aspect of experimental studies involving field stimulation and other forms of peripheral nerve stimulation that has so far received relatively little attention is that, in addition to causing orthodromic activation of the axons of efferent neurons, such stimulation excites afferent axons in the nerves; the resulting antidromic activation of the terminals of these axons may be accompanied by release from the terminals of substances such as substance P or ATP. Release of one or more substances of this kind on antidromic activation of primary afferent nociceptive neurons is a prerequisite for involvement of the neurons in producing the arteriolar vasodilatation responsible for the flare observed in the triple response. The dilatation of the axons in the subepithelial nerves of the ureter which is seen after exposure to capsaicin can be attributed to fundamental changes in the physiology of the axonal membranes, and could well be accompanied by release from the axons of ATP.

The role of substance P in producing the vascular responses which occur during the triple response are less clear-cut. While intravenous infusion of substance P has been shown to produce extensive peripheral vasodilatation (Burcher *et al.*, 1976), intra-arterial injection has been reported to produce little change in peripheral vascular resistance, but to have marked effects on pressor responses to nerve stimulation (Hedqvist & von Euler, 1976). There is, on the other hand, evidence that substance P is extremely potent in producing plasma extravasation from capillary plexuses (Lembeck, Gamse & Juan, 1976). There is evidence from studies on the skin (Hagermark, Hökfelt & Pernow, 1978) and on chromaffin cells (Livett *et al.*, 1979) that the vascular effects of substance P may be due partly to release of histamine and partly to prejunctional action on adrenergic axons in the arteriolar perivascular plexuses.

It has also recently been suggested (Håkanson *et al.*, 1981) that neurons containing regulatory peptides other than substance P also possess axon terminals containing mainly large dense-cored vesicles. These peptides include vasoactive intestinal polypeptide (VIP), enkephalin and bombesin, all of which are present in axons in the intramural plexuses of the gut (Schultzberg *et al.*, 1980). Axon terminal profiles containing mainly large dense-cored vesicles can also often be seen in thin sections of the nerves in these plexuses. There is, moreover, evidence from our studies with capsaicin of only very small amounts of axonal degeneration in these plexuses (Hoyes & Barber, 1981*b*). The validity of the hypothesis that all forms of peptidergic neuron possess axon terminals containing mainly large dense-cored vesicles is, however, questionable. It has been observed on a number of occasions that, in the gut plexuses, there is frequently focal accumulation of both large dense-cored and small vesicles in the axon terminals; quantitative evidence of the existence of such accumulation and of concentration of the large dense-cored vesicles at the ends of the axon terminals has recently been obtained from studies on the myenteric plexuses of the mouse and hamster stomach (Hoyes *et al.*, 1982*b*). Since ultrathin sections may pass through areas of the terminals containing accumulations of either type of vesicle, it is clearly extremely difficult in such situations to distinguish different types of terminal on the basis of their vesicle content. Although there is clear evidence of the presence of regulatory peptides within the lumen only of large dense-cored vesicles, VIP has recently been demonstrated in axon terminals which also contain substantial numbers of small vesicles (Johansson & Lundberg, 1981). Because it is now widely accepted that only small vesicles in peripheral axon terminals are involved in transmitter release, the location of peptides such as VIP in terminals of this type is also in agreement with the role in neurotransmission which has frequently been postulated for them.

STIMULUS PARAMETERS OF RECEPTORS

The peripheral axons of primary afferent nociceptive neurons can be excited by a wide variety of physical and chemical stimuli. Physical methods of stimulation, such as heat, have been widely used in experimental studies on pain in man. Although there is some evidence that direct mechanical stimulation results in depolarisation of nociceptive axons (see Yaksh & Hammond, 1982), in most of these studies the stimuli were applied at mid-axon levels rather than to the terminal regions of the axons. They also fail to produce the series of action potentials which the studies of Collins, Nulsen & Shealy (1966) indicate are necessary to elicit a pain response in human peripheral nerves. These observations suggest that the pain responses which result from direct mechanical stimuli, if not from other forms of physical stimulation (e.g. heat), are due to excitation of the axons by chemicals released into the tissues as a consequence of the damage induced by the stimuli.

Most of the evidence on the nature of chemicals which stimulate primary afferent nociceptive neurons has been obtained from studies on human cutaneous nerves. In these studies, the chemicals are either injected into the skin or are applied to the base of a blister raised by cantharidin, a technique which was developed and applied extensively by Keele & Armstrong (1964). Of the chemicals which stimulate nociceptive axons, some (such as capsaicin) are exogenous. Others may be released either from damaged cells, from the blood or from other structures (e.g. efferent nerve fibres). Cellular damage may release into the tissues a wide variety of chemicals which directly stimulate the axons. Although the nature of these substances is largely unknown, they include substantial quantities of potassium. There is clear evidence from a variety of studies that potassium excites nociceptive afferent neurons (see Keele & Armstrong, 1964). The threshold concentrations for stimulation are, however, fairly high, and there is doubt as to whether (other than in exceptional circumstances) tissue concentrations of the ion would be raised sufficiently to excite the axons directly.

Other chemicals which are often considered to be involved in excitation of nociceptive axons following release by tissue damage include acetylcholine, 5-hydroxytryptamine, histamine and bradykinin. In both the skin and the subepithelial nerves of the ureter, fairly low concentrations of acetylcholine produce responses in nociceptive axons. There is also evidence from studies on the cornea that depletion of acetylcholine is followed by a reduction in the sensitivity of the cornea to surface stimulation (Fitzgerald & Cooper, 1971). In addition to its presence in autonomic post-ganglionic efferent axons, acetylcholine is present in high concentration in the corneal epithelium. Therefore, its release following tissue damage could well be a major factor in the stimulation of axons subserving pricking pain of the type mediated by lightly myelinated axons, as well as producing the burning pain associated with the unmyelinated polymodal nociceptor. 5-Hydroxytryptamine is as potent a stimulator of cutaneous nociceptive axons as acetylcholine (Keele & Armstrong, 1964), and may well be released by damage into the tissues from structures such as platelets (in which it is present in high concentrations) in sufficient amounts to induce responses in pain afferents.

The effect of histamine on cutaneous nociceptive axons has been extensively studied by Rosenthal (1977), who has reported that it elicits pain responses at concentrations as low as 10^{-18} g ml^{-1}. These concentrations are substantially lower than those of acetylcholine and 5-hydroxytryptamine which are required to stimulate the axons –

which are of the order of 10^{-5} g ml^{-1} (Keele & Armstrong, 1964). Other authors, notably Emmelin & Feldberg, (1947), have been unable to demonstrate that histamine excites pain afferents directly. However Emmelin & Felberg (1947) found that pain is produced on injection of acetylcholine and histamine together, in concentrations similar to those present in nettle hair fluid. In the ureter, the axons of the subepithelial nerves also show no evidence of the changes observed after treatment with capsaicin or acetylcholine following treatment with histamine, even at concentrations as low as 10^{-3} g ml^{-1} (Barber & Hoyes, 1982). However, when treatment with histamine is combined with treatment with subthreshold concentrations of acetylcholine, dilatation of the axons and changes in their content of large dense-cored vesicles are observed at histamine concentrations as low as 10^{-21} g ml^{-1} (P. Barber, unpublished observations).

The evidence that nociceptive axons are stimulated by combinations of histamine and acetylcholine suggests that at least some of the chemicals normally considered to stimulate nociceptive axons directly merely sensitise them to other stimuli. The evidence obtained from the studies on the ureteric nerves suggests that, under normal conditions, histamine is a sensitiser rather than a stimulator of such axons. It also suggests that, at subthreshold concentrations, acetylcholine acts as a sensitiser of the axons. Similar mechanisms probably operate with prostaglandin, which has been shown to potentiate the action of bradykinin on nociceptive axons (Ferreira, 1972). There is in addition, evidence from the work of authors such as Matthews (1976) that noradrenaline sensitises nociceptive axons to other forms of stimulation. In this context, it is pertinent that, both in the submucous plexus of the guinea-pig trachea and the human parietal peritoneum (Hoyes & Barber, 1978; A. D. Hoyes & R. Bourne, unpublished observations), the axons defined on the basis of their terminal vesicle content as those of nociceptive axons are closely associated with adrenergic axons. Similar considerations apply to the arteriolar perivascular plexuses of the ureter, in which the axons are also present in substantial numbers, and in which adrenergic axons represent the principal component of the nerves (Hoyes & Barber, 1981c).

THE PERIPHERAL AXON

The terminals of the unmyelinated axons classified as those of nociceptive neurons have been shown (from studies on the ureter and other structures where such axons are common) to be spaced at intervals along the last part of the axon. Although, in this respect, the axons resemble those of autonomic efferent postganglionic neurons, the terminals are probably more widely spaced, and the inter-terminal regions are approximately twice the length of the terminals (Hoyes & Barber, 1977). In perfusion-fixed material, the mean diameter of the axons in the subepithelial plexus of the rat ureter, in which it is probable that the majority of the axons have already entered their terminal-bearing segments, is less than 300 nm. The diameter of the inter-terminal segments is, however, often as low as 100 nm. The diameter of the preterminal segments of these axons has not yet been determined, but this figure is well below the range of diameters of unmyelinated axons in other tissues (Ochoa, 1976). The reduction in the diameter of the axons in their terminal-bearing regions which is suggested by these figures may be due either to tapering of the axons or to limited amounts of branching, similar to that reported by Cauna (1973, 1980) in unmyelinated axons in the skin.

Except for the difference in diameter, the structure of the inter-terminal regions of the axons is similar to that of the preterminal parts of the axons. Both contain fairly evenly spaced microtubules, occasional sacs of smooth endoplasmic reticulum and mitochondria, but very few vesicles. Because all types of myelinated and unmyelinated axon possess the same ultrastructural features, identification of different types of peripheral axon by electron microscopy is necessarily based upon the demonstration of the particular features of their terminals and can be undertaken effectively only in plexuses in which a substantial proportion of the axons have already entered their terminal-bearing regions.

THE NEURONAL PERIKARYON

The cell bodies of the primary afferent nociceptive neurons are located in the dorsal root or cranial nerve ganglia. They are pseudo-unipolar in type, and both the peripheral axon and the central axon are connected to the neuronal perikaryon by a single, often highly coiled, stem process. Classic descriptions of the cells in the dorsal root ganglia suggest that they are divisible on the basis of their size, cytoplasmic density and fine structure into two separate populations (see Lieberman, 1976). The large neurons, classified as A neurons, have a light cytoplasm and the small B neurons have a cytoplasm which is much more dense. Ultrastructural studies have revealed a number of differences in the organisation of the endoplasmic reticulum and the neurofilaments in the two types of neuron, but the possibility that these are related to the use of suboptimal fixation and preservation procedures cannot be discounted.

Pineda, Maxwell & Kruger (1967) were unable to demonstrate clear-cut differences in the cytoplasmic organisation of large and small cells in the trigeminal ganglion following perfusion fixation with a glutaraldehyde–paraformaldehyde mixture. Because it represents the best and most effective method of achieving the concentrations of fixative required to effect fixation in the immediate vicinity of the cells in the shortest possible time, perfusion fixation can be regarded as providing the optimum conditions for preservation of neurons as well as other tissue cells. Our own studies, which have been undertaken on dorsal root and pelvic ganglia, indicate that the temperature at which the fixative is perfused may also be critical to establishment of optimum fixation and that at $4\,^{\circ}C$ and room temperature cellular structure may be dramatically different from that in material fixed by perfusion at $37\,^{\circ}C$.

Irrespective of the absence of distinct and reproducible differences in the ultrastructure of neurons of different sizes, there are a number of lines of evidence which support the view that the B neurons include those involved in nociception. An association between perikaryal size and axon diameter has been demonstrated by quantitative analysis in both adult and developing ganglia (see Lieberman, 1976). Histochemical studies have also shown that there are major differences in the enzyme content of the B neurons as compared with A neurons, and in particular of cholinesterase and phosphatases (Lieberman, 1976). Of particular interest in this context is the presence in the B neurons of fluoride-resistant acid phosphatase, an enzyme which is probably specifically associated with primary afferent nociceptive neurons (Kynihar, 1971). Further support for the view that the B neurons include those involved in nociception is provided by studies with capsaicin. Subcutaneous injection of capsaicin has been reported to produce mitochondrial and other changes in these neurons in adult rats (Scolcsányi et al., 1975) and to induce total degeneration in the neurons in the neonatal rat (Jancsó et al., 1977).

There is also evidence from immunofluorescence studies of the preferential location of substance P in B neurons (Hökfelt *et al.*, 1975). Although substance P may be used as a transmitter in primary nociceptive neurons, it is a peptide and must be synthesised at perikaryal levels and transmitted down the axon to its site of release. The presence of the peptide in the perikaryon is therefore not unexpected. However, Chan-Palay & Palay (1977) found that, in sensory neurons, substance P is located in structures resembling lysosomes. Such a location of the peptide is consistent with its involvement in neurotransmission only if it is assumed that excess production at perikaryal levels is followed by elimination of the transmitter by incorporation into lysosomes prior to its transport down the axon.

If, on the other hand, it is assumed that the admittedly enigmatic mechanisms which operate to control and coordinate neuronal function and metabolism are so adjusted to provide a balance between synthesis and utilisation (both of structural proteins and either proteins or peptides which are released at the axon terminals during impulse transmission) the existence of high concentrations of peptide transmitters in the perikaryon similar to those present in the axon terminals, where they are probably stored in accumulations of vesicles, is highly debatable. The possibility cannot be excluded that the presence of peptides such as substance P in perikaryal lysosomes represents part of a process of elimination of the peptides which, after attachment to receptors on the axons, are then transported by retrograde flow to the perikaryon in a manner similar to that demonstrated for horseradish peroxidase (see Mesulam, 1982). Under such circumstances, it cannot be assumed that the presence of the peptides in the perikaryon is related to their synthesis in the neuron.

THE CENTRAL AXON

There is evidence, in particular in the case of neurons with unmyelinated axons, that the central axon of pseudo-unipolar neurons is of smaller diameter than the peripheral axon (Ha, 1970). There is also some evidence that dorsal roots proximal to the ganglion contain more axons than those distal to the ganglion (see Lieberman, 1976). As in the periphery, these differences may be related to branching of the axons. The extent to which they are related to differences in the rate and pattern of transport of substances along the axons as compared with the peripheral axons is unknown. Accumulation of transmitters, and especially of peptide transmitters, at the central synapses of the axons implies, however, that there is some mechanism for preferential transport along the central axons.

The fine fibres in the dorsal roots enter the spinal cord through their lateral divisions. Within the cord, the central axons of the primary nociceptive neurons branch in the tract of Lissauer and distribute to the dorsal horn over approximately three segments. Although it has been suggested that the tract of Lissauer consists largely of the axons of intersegmental neurons, recent studies in the monkey have shown that 80% of the axons in the tract are those of primary afferent neurons (Coggeshall *et al.*, 1981). The site of termination of the primary afferent nociceptive neurons within the dorsal horn has been extensively studied and reviewed, notably by Kerr (1975), Perl (1980), Wall (1980) and Yaksh & Hammond (1982). Although there is no universal agreement on the exact site of termination of the axons in the dorsal horn, it is generally agreed that the unmyelinated axons of polymodal nociceptors terminate in lamina I and in at least the outer part of lamina II. Kerr (1975) postulated that the nociceptive axons synapse on the dendrites of the neurons in lamina I, and that inhibitory input into these neurons is mediated by synapses on the perikarya of the neurons. Similar patterns of termination of excitatory and inhibitory synapses have been reported on α-motor neurons (Conradi, 1976).

The site of termination in the dorsal horn of the lightly myelinated axons of the high threshold mechanoreceptors is less clearly established that that of unmyelinated axons. There is fairly good evidence for termination of these axons in lamina II and some evidence for their termination in laminae I, III and V (Wall, 1980). One of the main problems with such patterns of termination is that it has been shown that, in addition to those in lamina I, some of the neurons in lamina V respond specifically to stimulation of both polymodal nociceptors and high threshold mechanoreceptors. Transmission to lamina V neurons from the axons of high threshold mechanoreceptors may be achieved directly through synapses on dendrites of the neurons which extend into the outer laminae of the dorsal horn, but it seems probable that transmission to these neurons of information from polymodal nociceptors is mediated through internuncial neurons (see Wall, 1980).

There is a substantial body of evidence that transmission from primary afferent nociceptive neurons to neurons in the dorsal horn is mediated by the undecapeptide, substance P. This evidence, which has recently been reviewed by Nicoll, Schenker & Leeman (1980), is based upon an impressive array of physiological and pharmacological as well as immunocytochemical studies. The immunocytochemical studies undertaken by authors such as Barber *et al.* (1979) indicate that substance-P-like immunoreactivity is concentrated in the outer laminae of the dorsal horn and is located in synapses containing both small vesicles and large dense-cored vesicles. As in the periphery, immunoreactivity to substance P is located within the lumina of the large dense-cored vesicles. It is also found in substantial quantities on the membranes of the small vesicles. Although Barber *et al.* (1979) discussed the possible involvement of the large dense-cored vesicles in transmission at the synapses, it is doubtful whether these vesicles play such a role in most synapses. The location of immunoreactivity on the membranes of the small vesicles rather than within the lumen of the vesicles may also be related to diffusion of the peptide from within the lumen during fixation and processing. In this context, it is necessary to bear in mind that substance P is a small peptide and its precise localisation by fixation cannot be assumed. The presence of substance P in the small vesicles would also be in better agreement with current concepts of involvement of these vesicles in synaptic transmission than the postulate of Barber *et al.* (1979) that transmission is mediated by release of transmitter from the large dense-cored vesicles.

I am indebted to Dr Diana Kershaw for assistance with the illustrations and to Mrs Pauline Barber, with whom much of the work on the endings of nociceptive afferent neurons documented in this account was undertaken.

REFERENCES

Barber, P. & Hoyes, A. D. (1982). The *in vitro* effects of histamine dihydrochloride on the subepithelial nerves of the rat ureter. *Journal of Anatomy*, **134**, 625.
Barber, R. P., Vaughn, J. E., Slemmon, J. R., Salvaterra, P. M., Roberts, E. & Leeman, S. E. (1979). The origin, distribution and synaptic relationships of substance P axons in rat spinal cord. *Journal of Comparative Neurology*, **184**, 331–52.
Bessou, P. & Perl, E. R. (1969). Response of cutaneous sensory units with unmyelinated fibres to noxious stimuli. *Journal of Neurophysiology*, **32**, 1025–43.
Bodian, D. (1962). The generalised vertebrate neuron. *Science*, **137**, 323–6.

Bonica, J. J. (1980). Introduction. In *Pain*, ed. J. J. Bonica, *Research Publications of the Association for Research in Nervous and Mental Disease*, vol. 58, pp. 1–18. New York: Raven Press.

Burcher, E., Atterhög, J.-H., Pernow, B. & Rosell, S. (1976). Cardiovascular effects of substance P: effects on the heart and regional blood flow in the dog. In *Substance P*, ed. U. S. von Euler & B. Pernow, pp. 261–8. New York: Raven Press.

Burgess, P. R. & Perl, E. R. (1967). Myelinated afferent fibres responding specifically to noxious stimulation of the skin. *Journal of Physiology*, **190**, 541–62.

Burnstock, G. (1972). Purinergic nerves. *Pharmacological Reviews*, **24**, 509–81.

Cauna, N. (1973). The free penicillate endings of the human hairy skin. *Journal of Anatomy*, **115**, 277–88.

Cauna, N. (1980). Fine morphological characteristics and microtopography of the free nerve endings of the human digital skin. *Anatomical Record*, **198**, 643–56.

Chan-Palay, V. & Palay, S. L. (1977). Ultrastructural identification of substance P cells and their processes in rat sensory ganglia and their terminals in the spinal cord by immunocytochemistry. *Proceedings of the National Academy of Sciences, USA*, **74**, 4050–4.

Coggeshall, R. E., Chung, K., Chung, J. M. & Langford, L. A. (1981). Primary afferent axons in the tract of Lissauer. *Journal of Comparative Neurology*, **196**, 431–42.

Collins, W. F., Nulsen, F. E. & Shealy, C. N. (1966). Electrophysiological studies of peripheral and central pathways conducting pain. In *Pain*, ed. R. S. Knighton & P. R. Dunke, pp. 33–45. Boston; Little, Brown & Co.

Conradi, S. (1976). Functional anatomy of the anterior horn motor neuron. In *The Peripheral Nerve*, ed. D. N. Landon, pp. 279–329. London: Chapman & Hall.

Das, R. M., Jeffery, P. K. & Widdicombe, J. G. (1978). The epithelial innervation of the lower respiratory tract on the cat. *Journal of Anatomy*, **126**, 123–31.

Das, R. M., Jeffery, P. K. & Widdicombe, J. G. (1979). Experimental degeneration of intra-epithelial nerve fibres in cat airways. *Journal of Anatomy*, **128**, 259–67.

Dash, M. S. & Deshpande, S. S. (1976). Human skin nociceptors and their chemical responses. In *Advances in Pain Research and Therapy*, ed. J. J. Bonica & D. Albe-Fessard, pp. 47–51. New York: Raven Press.

Emmelin, N. & Feldberg, W. (1947). The mechanisms of the sting of common nettle (*Urtica urens*). *Journal of Physiology*, **106**, 440–55.

Ferreira, S. H. (1972). Prostaglandins, aspirin-like drugs and analgesia. *Nature New Biology*, **240**, 200–3.

Fitzgerald, G. G. & Cooper, J. R. (1971). Acetylcholine as a possible sensory mediator in rabbit corneal epithelium. *Biochemical Pharmacology*, **20**, 2741–8.

Gamse, R., Holzer, P. & Lembeck, F. (1980). Decrease of substance P in primary afferent neurones and impairment of neurogenic plasma extravasation by capsaicin. *British Journal of Pharmacology*, **68**, 207–13.

Ha, H. (1970). Axonal bifurcation in the dorsal root ganglion of the cat: a light and electron microscopic study. *Journal of Comparative Neurology*, **140**, 227–40.

Hagermark, O., Hökfelt, T. & Pernow, B. (1978). Flare and itch induced by substance P in human skin. *Journal of Investigative Dermatology*, **71**, 233–5.

Håkanson, R., Leander, S., Sundler, F. & Uddman, R. (1981). P-type nerves: purinergic or peptidergic? In *Cellular Basis of Chemical Messengers in the Digestive System*, ed. M. I. Grossman, M. A. B. Brazier & J. Lechago, pp. 169–200. New York: Academic Press.

Hedqvist, P. & von Euler, U. S. (1976). Effects of substance P on some autonomic neuroeffector junctions. In *Substance P*, ed. U. S. von Euler & B. Pernow, pp. 89–96. New York: Raven Press.

Heubner, W. (1925). Zur Pharmakologie der Reizstoffe. *Archiv für experimentelle Pathologie und Pharmakologie*, **107**, 129–54.

Hökfelt, T., Kellerth, J. O., Nilsson, G. & Pernow, B. (1975). Experimental immunohistochemical studies on the localisation and distribution of substance P in cat primary sensory neurons. *Brain Research*, **100**, 235–52.

Hoyes, A. D. & Barber, P. (1976a). Ultrastructure of the corneal nerves in the rat. *Cell and Tissue Research*, **172**, 133–44.

Hoyes, A. D. & Barber, P. (1976b). Parameters of fixation of the putative pain afferents in the ureter: preservations of the dense cores of the large vesicles in the axonal terminals. *Journal of Anatomy*, **122**, 113–20.

Hoyes, A. D. & Barber, P. (1977). Ultrastructure of corneal receptors. In *Pain in the Trigeminal Region*, ed. B. J. Anderson & B. Matthews, pp. 1–12. Amsterdam: Elsevier/North-Holland Biomedical Press.

Hoyes, A. D. & Barber, P. (1978). Fine structure and composition of the submucous nerve plexus of the guinea-pig trachea. *Cell and Tissue Research*, **190**, 301–16.

Hoyes, A. D. & Barber, P. (1979). *In vitro* effect of capsaicin on the subepithelial nerves of the rat ureter. *Journal of Anatomy*, **128**, 438–9.

Hoyes, A. D. & Barber, P. (1981a). Morphology and response to vagus nerve section of the intra-epithelial axons of the rat trachea. A quantitative ultrastructural study. *Journal of Anatomy*, **132**, 331–9.

Hoyes, A. D. & Barber, P. (1981b). Degeneration of axons in the ureteric and duodenal nerve plexuses of the adult rat following *in vivo* treatment with capsaicin. *Neuroscience Letters*, **25**, 19–24.

Hoyes, A. D. & Barber, P. (1981c). Quantitative ultrastructural studies on arteriolar innervation in the rat ureter. *Microvascular Research*, 165–74.

Hoyes, A. D., Barber, P. & Jagessar, H. (1981). Effect of capsaicin on the intraepithelial axons of the rat trachea. *Neuroscience Letters*, **26**, 329–34.

Hoyes, A. D., Barber, P. & Jagessar, H. (1982a). Location in the nodose ganglion of the perikarya of neurons whose axons distribute in the epithelium of the rat trachea. *Journal of Anatomy*, **134**, 265–71.

Hoyes, A. D., Bourne, R. & Martin, B. G. H. (1975). Ultrastructure of the submucous nerves of the rat ureter. *Journal of Anatomy*, **119**, 123–32.

Hoyes, A. D., Bourne, R. & Martin, B. G. H. (1976). Ureteric vascular and muscle coat innervation in the rat. *Investigative Urology*, **14**, 38–43.

Hoyes, A. D., Grant, K., Barber, P. & Jagessar, H. (1982b). Distribution and diameter of large dense-cored vesicles in axon terminals in the myenteric ganglia of the mouse and hamster stomach. *Neuroscience Letters*, **30**, 19–24.

Iggo, A. (1980). Electrophysiology of cutaneous sensory receptors. In *The Skin of Vertebrates*. ed. R. I. C. Spearmen & P. A. Riley, *Linnaean Society Symposium Series* No. 9. pp. 255–70. London: Academic Press.

Jancsó, G., Kiraly, E. & Jancsó-Gábor, A. (1977). Pharmacologically induced selective degeneration of chemosensitive primary sensory neurones. *Nature (London)*, **270**, 741–3.

Jancsó, N., Jancsó-Gábor, A. & Scolcsányi, J. (1967). Direct evidence for neurogenic inflammation and its prevention by denervation and by pretreatment with capsaicin. *British Journal of Pharmacology and Chemotherapy*, **31**, 138–51.

Johansson, O. & Lundberg, J. M. (1981). Ultrastructural localisation of VIP-like immunoreactivity in large dense-core vesicles of 'cholinergic-type' nerve terminals in cat exocrine glands. *Neuroscience*, **6**, 847–62.

Keele, C. A. & Armstrong, D. (1964). *Substances Producing Pain and Itch*. London: Edward Arnold.

Kerr, F. W. L. (1975). Neuroanatomical substrates of nociception in the spinal cord. *Pain*, **1**, 325–56.

Knoche, H., Addicks, K. & Schmitt, G. (1974). A contribution regarding our knowledge of pressoreceptor fields and the sinus nerve based on electron microscopic findings. In *Symposium: Mechanoreception*, ed. J. Schwartzkopf, pp. 57–74. Opladen: Westdeutscher Verlag.

Kruger, L., Perl, E. R. & Sedivec, M. J. (1981). Fine structure of myelinated mechanical nociceptor endings in hairy cat skin. *Journal of Comparative Neurology*, **198**, 137–54.

Kynihar, E. (1971). Fluoride-resistant acid phosphatase system of nociceptive dorsal root afferents. *Experientia*, **27**, 1205–7.

Lembeck, F., Gamse, R. & Juan, H. (1976). Substance P and sensory nerve endings. In *Substance P*, ed. U. S. von Euler & B. Pernow, pp. 169–82. New York: Raven Press.

Lieberman, A. R. (1976). Sensory ganglia. In *The Peripheral Nerve*, ed. D. N. Landon, pp. 188–278. London: Chapman & Hall.

Livett, B. G., Kozuzek, V., Mizobe, F. & Dean, D. M. (1979). Substance P inhibits nicotinic activation of chromaffin cells. *Nature (London)*, **278**, 256–7.

Macintosh, S. R. (1975). Observations on the structure and innervation of the rat snout. *Journal of Anatomy*, **119**, 537–46.

Matthews, B. (1976). Effects of sympathetic stimulation on the response of intradental nerves to chemical stimulation of dentin. In *Advances in Pain Research and Therapy*, ed. J. J. Bonica & D. Albe-Fessard, pp. 195–203. New York: Raven Press.

Melzack, R. & Wall, P. D. (1965). Pain mechanisms: a new theory. *Science*, **150**, 971–80.

Mesulam, M.-M. (1982). Principles of horseradish peroxidase neurochemistry and their applications for tracing neural pathways – axonal transport, enzyme histochemistry and light microscopical analysis. In *Tracing Neural Connections with Horseradish Peroxidase*, ed. M.-M. Mesulam, pp. 1–151. Chichester: John Wiley & Sons.

Miller, A., Costa, M., Furness, J. B. & Chubb, I. W. (1981). Substance P immunoreactive sensory nerves supply the rat iris and cornea. *Neuroscience Letters*, **23**, 243–9.

Mountcastle, V. B. (1980). Pain and temperature sensibilities. In *Medical Physiology*, 14th edn, vol. 1, ed. V. B. Mountcastle, pp. 391–427. St Louis: C. V. Mosby Co.

Nicoll, R. A., Schenker, C. & Leeman, S. E. (1980). Substance P as a transmitter candidate. *Annual Review of Neuroscience*, **3**, 227–68.

Ochoa, J. (1976). The unmyelinated nerve fibre. In *The Peripheral Nerve*, ed. D. N. Landon, pp. 106–58. London: Chapman & Hall.

Perl, E. R. (1971). Is pain a specific sensation? *Journal of Psychiatric Research*, **8**, 273–87.

Perl, E. R. (1980). Afferent basis of nociception and pain: evidence from the characteristics of sensory receptors and their projections to the spinal dorsal horn. In *Pain*, ed. J. J. Bonica, *Research Publications of the Association for Research in Nervous and Mental Disease*, vol. 58. pp. 19–61.

Pineda, A., Maxwell, D. S. & Kruger, L. (1967). The fine structure of neurons and satellite cells in the trigeminal ganglion of the cat and monkey. *American Journal of Anatomy*, **121**, 461–88.

Procacci, P., Zoppi, M. & Maresca, M. (1979). Experimental pain in man. *Pain*, **6**, 123–40.

Rosenthal, S. R. (1977). Histamine as the chemical mediator for cutaneous pain. *Journal of Investigative Dermatology*, **69**, 98–105.

Scadding, J. W. (1980). The permanent anatomical effects of neonatal capsaicin on somatosensory nerves. *Journal of Anatomy*, **131**, 473–482.

Schultzberg, M., Hökfelt, T., Nilsson, G., Terenius, L., Rehfeld, J. F., Brown, M., Elde, R., Goldstein, M. & Said, S. (1980). Distribution of peptide- and catecholamine-containing neurons in the gastro-intestinal tract of the guinea-pig: immunohistochemical studies with antisera to substance P, vasoactive intestinal polypeptide, enkephalins, somatostatin, gastrin/cholecystokinin, neurotensin and dopamine β-hydroxylase. *Neuroscience*, **5**, 689–744.

Scolcsányi, J., Jancsó-Gábor, A. & Joo, F. (1975). Functional and fine structural characteristics of the sensory neuron blocking effect of capsaicin. *Naunyn-Scmiedeberg's Archiv für experimentelle Pathologie und Pharmakologie*, **287**, 157–69.

Sikri, K. L., Hoyes, A. D., Barber, P. & Jagessar, H. (1981). Substance P-like immunoreactivity in the intramural nerve plexuses of the guinea-pig ureter: a light and electron microscopical study. *Journal of Anatomy*, **133**, 425–42.

Sinclair, D. (1981). *Mechanisms of Cutaneous Sensation*. Oxford University Press.

Stacey, M. J. (1969). Free nerve endings in skeletal muscle of the cat. *Journal of Anatomy*, **105**, 231–54.

Torebjörk, H. E. (1974). Afferent C units responding to mechanical thermal and chemical stimuli in human non-glabrous skin. *Acta Physiologica Scandinavica*, **92**, 374–90.

von Euler, U. S. & Gaddum J. H. (1931). An unidentified depressor substance in certain tissue extracts. *Journal of Physiology*, **72**, 74–87.

Wall, P. D. (1980). The role of substantia gelatinosa as a gate control. In *Pain*, ed. J. J. Bonica, *Research Publications of the Association for Research in Nervous and Mental Disease*, vol. 58, pp. 205–32. New York: Raven Press.

Waterston, D. (1933). Observations on sensation. The sensory functions of the skin for touch and pain. *Journal of Physiology*, **77**, 251–7.

Weddell, G. & Zander, E. (1951). The fragility of non-myelinated nerve terminals. *Journal of Anatomy*, **85**, 242–50.

Yaksh, T. L. & Hammond, D. L. (1982). Peripheral and central substrates involved in the rostrad transmission of nociceptive information. *Pain*, **13**, 1–86.

8   The neonatal development of autonomic innervation of the rat iris

D. C. DAVIES
Department of Anatomy, St Mary's Hospital Medical School, London W2 1PG, UK

INTRODUCTION

The iris, which constitutes the most anterior part of the vascular tunic of the eye, is situated in a more or less frontal plane in the albino rat. It appears as a thin annular diaphragm situated in front of the lens and ciliary body, separating the anterior and posterior chambers of the eye. It inserts into the scleral spur via its attachment to the middle of the anterior surface of the ciliary body, and the pupillary margin rests on and is supported by the anterior surface of the lens. The pupil is an almost circular aperture in the centre of the iris, located slightly to the nasal side and possibly slightly inferiorly.

The size of the pupil, and thus the amount of light passing through the eye to the retina, is reflexly regulated by the two muscular components of the iris, the sphincter and dilator pupillae. The sphincter pupillae forms a ring around the pupillary border near the posterior surface of the iris. It consists predominantly of circularly arranged, intertwining, smooth muscle fibres separated by vascularised connective tissue. Contraction of these sphincter fibres results in constriction of the pupil (miosis). The dilator pupillae comprises a thin sheet of smooth muscle fibres which lies between the stroma of the iris and the pigmented epithelium. The dilator fibres are arranged mainly radially, taking their origin in the ciliary body and extending centrally to near the pupillary margin where the dilator and sphincter pupillae fuse. Contraction of these dilator fibres results in dilatation of the pupil (mydriasis).

The sphincter pupillae and dilator pupillae are atypical for muscle, in that they arise from the neural ectoderm rather than from the mesoderm. In the albino rat, the iris first appears on the 18th day of gestation, as a double-layered structure budded off from the anterior rim of the optic cup (see Lai, 1972*a*, *b*). Myofilaments can first be observed in differentiating cells of the anterior epithelium of the iris, near to the pupil in the region of the developing sphincter pupillae, on the 19th day of gestation. Myofilaments do not appear in the cells of the anterior epithelium at the site of the dilator pupillae until a day later (20th day of gestation). The differentiation of these muscle cells continues postnatally so that by the 12th day *post partum* the sphincter muscle is fully developed, resembling that of the adult. However, the dilator muscle does not achieve this stage of maturity until 18–20 days *post partum*.

THE CLASSICAL VIEW OF THE AUTONOMIC INNERVATION OF THE IRIS

The iris musculature receives its motor innervation from the autonomic nervous system. Traditionally the sphincter pupillae was considered to be controlled solely by fibres from the IIIrd cranial nerve, originating in the paired Edinger–Westphal nuclei (Crouch, 1936) which constitute part of the oculomotor nucleus. These parasympathetic IIIrd nerve fibres synapse in the ciliary ganglion and the post-ganglionic fibres follow the short ciliary nerves to the iris. The dilator pupillae was thought to be innervated purely by sympathetic fibres via the superior cervical ganglion (Loewenfeld, 1958; Niesel, 1961). This pathway comprises three divisions: (a) the central neuron in the brain stem and cervical spinal cord; (b) the pre-ganglionic cholinergic sympathetic neuron which originates in the thoracic spinal cord and ascends in the neck via the stellate ganglion to the superior cervical ganglion; (c) the post-ganglionic adrenergic neuron in the superior cervical ganglion whose axon penetrates the base of the skull and enters the orbit and finally the iris via the long ciliary nerves. The sphincter and dilator pupillae were considered to be simply antagonistic in their activity, the sphincter being the more powerful since topical application of histamine (which stimulates both dilator and sphincter muscle fibres) results in marked miosis (Appenzeller, 1970).

ANATOMICAL STUDIES OF THE INNERVATION OF THE IRIS

Joseph (1921) and Poos (1927) suggested that the classical view of a simple antagonistic double innervation of the iris musculature was not accurate, and that the sphincter pupillae receives a dual nerve supply (i.e. excitatory from parasympathetic fibres of the IIIrd cranial nerve and inhibitory from cervical sympathetic fibres). The true nature of the innervation of the iris musculature was, however, not elucidated for a number of years.

The development of the formaldehyde-induced fluorescence method for catecholamines (Falck et al., 1962) facilitated the visualisation of the adrenergic terminal innervation of the iris musculature, which is readily discernible in section and in whole-mount 'stretch' preparations (Falck, 1962; Malmfors, 1965). The adrenergic innervation of the dilator muscle, which in the rat is only one cell thick (Nilsson, 1964), has been shown (Malmfors, 1965) to comprise a network of varicose fibres distributed uniformly over the anterior surface of the muscle but not penetrating between the individual muscle cells. The varicosities, which measured about 1 μm in diameter, were more strongly fluorescent than the intervening segments.

Malmfors (1965) also observed that the adrenergic innervation of the iris musculature continued to the pupillary margin over the sphincter pupillae where the fluorescent fibres penetrated between the muscle cells. Malmfors (1965) established, by means of denervation experiments, that all or practically all of the adrenergic fibres in the eye of the rat (and a number of other animals investigated) originate from ipsilateral cervical ganglion cells and that very few such cells are localised peripherally to the superior cervical ganglion. This indicated that the adrenergic innervation of the sphincter (as well as that of the dilator pupillae) is sympathetic, originating in the superior cervical ganglion. Moreover, Malmfors & Sachs (1965) have demonstrated by fluorescence histochemistry that the same sympathetic adrenergic neuron can innervate both muscles of the iris. Thus, by inference, the effect on the dilator must be excitatory and that on the sphincter probably inhibitory. The adrenergic innervation of the rat sphincter pupillae has been confirmed both by fluorescence histochemical (Ehinger, 1966) and ultrastructural studies (Hökfelt, 1966; Tranzer & Thoenen, 1967). However, it must be noted that Ivens et al. (1973) claimed that the rat sphincter pupillae does not receive any adrenergic innervation.

Acetylcholinesterase-containing presumptive cholinergic parasympathetic fibres have been observed in the dilator pupillae of the rat (Ehinger & Falck, 1966) as well as in the sphincter pupillae. These fibres were observed to run both in close association with and separate from the predominant adrenergic fibres of the dilator pupillae. The ultrastructural studies of Hökfelt (1966, 1967) revealed cholinergic as well as adrenergic terminals in the dilator pupillae of the albino rat. Thus, most authors now agree that in the albino rat, and in most other mammals studied, both the sphincter and dilator pupillae receive a mixed adrenergic sympathetic and cholinergic parasympathetic innervation.

ELECTROPHYSIOLOGICAL AND PHARMACOLOGICAL STUDIES OF THE IRIS INNERVATION

A concept of active adrenergic relaxation of the sphincter pupillae was proposed by Hess, Koella & Szabo (1950) and Rüegg & Hess (1953) who observed that isolated sphincter muscle not only contracts as a result of the application of acetylcholine but also relaxes in response to noradrenaline. Schaeppi & Koella (1964a) provided support for this idea with their demonstration of the induction of almost pure relaxation of atropinised cat sphincter pupillae by high frequency electrical stimulation. Such stimulation was found to be ineffective in inducing sphincter muscle relaxation after chronic sympathetic denervation. Thus, these observations indicate that relaxation of the sphincter pupillae can be induced by excitation of sympathetic nerve terminals. The findings of Burn & Rand (1958) and those of Schaeppi & Koella (1964a) that tyramine (a noradrenaline releasing agent) causes a marked relaxation of normal sphincter muscle, but is ineffective when applied to sympathetically denervated muscle, are compatible with this view.

After investigating the effects of dichloroisoproterenol (a β-adrenergic receptor blocker) and phentolamine (an α-receptor blocker) Schaeppi & Koella (1964a) proposed that β-adrenergic receptors mediate active relaxation of the sphincter pupillae and that, *in vitro* at least, they are activated predominantly by high frequency electrical stimulation. In addition to the principal excitatory cholinergic innervation of the cat sphincter pupillae, these authors also reported the presence of a minor α-adrenergic receptor mediated contractile component, mainly activated by low frequency electrical stimulation.

Schaeppi & Koella (1964b) also examined the innervation of the feline dilator pupillae and confirmed that it is largely supplied by excitatory noradrenergic fibres. However, on the basis of pharmacological experiments using phentolamine and dichloroisoproterenol, they concluded that this noradrenergic innervation is two-fold in its effect. They reported that electrical stimulation could activate both α-adrenergic receptors, causing contraction of dilator fibres, and β-adrenergic receptors, causing relaxation. However, high frequency stimulation promoted α-receptor mediated fibre contraction whereas low frequency stimulation favoured β-receptor mediated relaxation. The presence of both α- and β-adrenergic receptors in feline dilator pupillae has been confirmed by Alphen, Robinette & Macri (1964) and Ehinger, Falck & Persson (1968).

A cholinergic relaxing mechanism has also been proposed for the dilator pupillae. Schaeppi & Koella (1964b) found that the application of high frequency electrical stimulation to chronically sympathetically denervated dilator strips caused relaxation, or transient contraction followed by relaxation, of dilator muscle fibres. These responses were enhanced by neostigmine and reduced by atropine. These authors considered that the transient contraction of the sympathetically denervated dilator strips was due to contamination of the preparation with aberrant sphincter pupillae muscle fibres, but that the relaxation was due to a cholinergic mechanism acting on true dilator muscle fibres. Ehinger *et al.* (1968) also demonstrated that dilator pupillae relaxation can be elicited by electrical stimulation or the administration of acetylcholine after sympathectomy and that this response can be abolished by atropine or parasympathetic denervation.

Therefore, in agreement with the classical view, the principal excitatory innervation of the spincter pupillae is cholinergic and that of the dilator pupillae adrenergic. However, the innervation of the mammalian iris musculature now appears to be more complex than this, with pupillary diameter being controlled by at least six interlinked components. It seems likely that the sphincter pupillae contracts by means of a primary cholinergic and a secondary α-adrenergic system, and relaxes by means of a β-adrenergic system. An α-adrenergic system is predominant in contraction of the dilator pupillae while a β-adrenergic and a cholinergic system mediate its relaxation. Pupil diameter must therefore reflect a dynamic balance between these systems.

THE NEONATAL DEVELOPMENT OF THE RAT IRIS INNERVATION

Specific catecholamine fluorescence is visible for the first time in the developing sympathetic chains of the albino rat towards the end of the second week of gestation (Champlain *et al.*, 1970; Owman, Sjöberg & Swedin, 1971). At this stage of development Champlain *et al.* (1970) described two loosely arranged rows of fluorescent cells situated one on each side of the spinal cord, with two further groups of more intensely fluorescent cells in the thoracic and lumbar regions. The fluorescence intensity in these regions increased rapidly during the beginning of the third week of gestation so that the paravertebral sympathetic ganglia, including the superior cervical ganglion which supplies the sympathetic innervation of the iris, became visible by the middle of the third week of gestation.

At birth, however, the principal neurons in the superior cervical ganglion, which contains its full neuronal complement at this stage (Davies, 1978), exhibit only a weak fluorescence (Eränkö, 1972a; Davies, 1979). This fluorescence, which was uniformly distributed throughout the neuronal cytoplasm, increases in intensity until about the 12th day *post partum* (Davies, 1977). Thereafter a second granular mode of amine storage, localised mainly at the perikaryonal periphery, becomes evident. This granular fluorescence causes a further increase in the overall fluorescence intensity exhibited by the principal neurons in the superior cervical ganglion up to the end of the third week *post partum*. Radiochemical assays were conducted (Davis, 1977) to determine the levels of noradrenaline (after Coyle & Henry, 1973; Cuello, Hiley & Iversen, 1973) and tyrosine hydroxylase activity (after Hendry & Iversen, 1971) in the superior cervical ganglion. Tyrosine hydroxylase is the rate-limiting enzyme in noradrenaline biosynthesis (Levitt *et al.*, 1965) and, in the superior cervical ganglion, it is localised in adrenergic neurons (Black, Hendry & Iversen, 1971a). The results concur with the estimations of fluorescence intensity, indicating that mature transmitter levels are attained by the end of the third week of life, when ultrastructural studies first reveal definitive sympathetic neurons (Davies, 1977).

Fluorescent nerve fibres (from neurons in the superior cervical ganglion) have been reported to be visible for the first time in the iris of the albino rat on the 21st

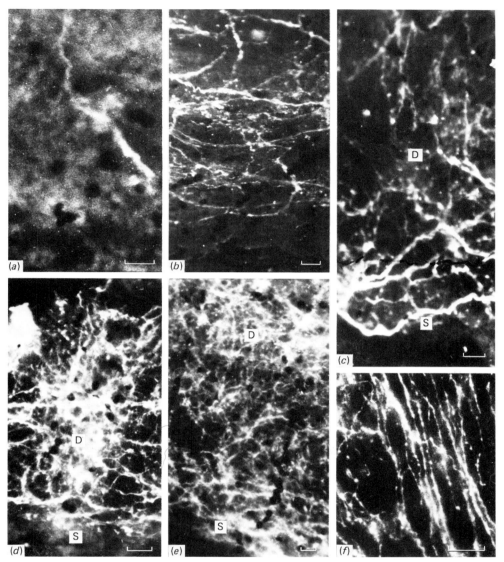

Fig. 8.1. Fluorescence micrographs showing the development of catecholamine-containing nerve fibres in the neonatal rat iris. D, dilator pupillae; S, sphincter pupillae. (*a*) 18 day foetus; the preparation includes both the developing ciliary body and iris. (*b*) 19 day foetus; ciliary body and iris. (*c*) Newborn iris. (*d*) 4 day iris. (*e*) 7 day iris. (*f*) 21 day dilator pupillae showing fluorescent varicosities. All scale bars represent 20 μm. (Photomicrograph kindly supplied by K. Tervo, T. Tervo and A. Palkama.)

(Lai, 1976) and 18th (Tervo, Tervo & Palkama, 1978) day of gestation (Fig. 8.1*a*). The earlier visualisation of fluorescent fibres by Tervo *et al.* (1978) could have been due to their use of the more sensitive glyoxilic acid method for the demonstration of catecholamines compared with the formaldehyde vapour method since, at the ultrastructural level, Lai (1976) did observe some axons containing dense-cored vesicles at 20 days of gestation, or it could have resulted from differences in the strains of rats used. On the 19th day of gestation Tervo *et al.* (1978) reported a large increase in both the number and fluorescence intensity of nerve fibres in the iris (Fig. 8.1*b*).

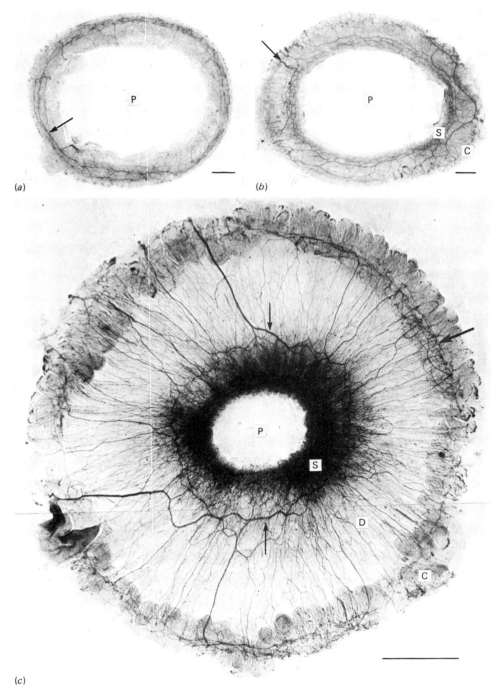

Fig. 8.2. The development of acetylcholinesterase-containing nerve fibres in the neonatal rat iris, demonstrated by the thiocholine technique. P, pupil; S, sphincter pupillae; D, dilator pupillae; C, ciliary body. (*a*) Newborn whole-mounted iris. A complete circle of acetylcholinesterase-containing nerves (arrow) is present around the pupil and gives off fine branches towards it. (*b*) 3 day iris. A loose circular network of acetylcholinesterase-containing nerves is apparent in the region of the sphincter pupillae and this is joined by numerous acetylcholinesterase-containing

At birth (Fig. 8.1*c*) the fluorescent fibre density had increased further, especially at the dilator–sphincter interface. On the fourth day *post partum*, the dilator innervation was further elaborated (Fig. 8.1*d*) and terminal varicosities could be observed for the first time. On the fifth day of life Lai (1976) observed some fluorescent nerve fibres to be superimposed on the anterior surface of the dilator pupillae. On the seventh day, the dilator innervation had increased further and was accompanied by a well-developed network of fluorescent fibres in the sphincter pupillae (Fig. 8.1*e*). This adrenergic sphincter innervation increased so that, by the ninth day *post partum*, some fluorescent fibres were seen to have penetrated the sphincter muscle itself (Lai, 1976). Although Lai (1976) observed that by 14 days *post partum* the fluorescent nerves in the iris had a similar pattern to that in the adult, Tervo *et al.* (1978) found that fluorescent nerve density continued to increase up to approximately three weeks of age (Fig. 8.1*f*). Eventually, by 30 days, Lai (1976) states that 'fluorescent nerves were plentifully distributed among sphincter muscle cells and superimposed on the anterior surface of the dilator muscle cells'.

The presence of acetylcholinesterase in a nerve fibre in the iris musculature is not conclusive proof that it is a true parasympathetic cholinergic nerve, since sympathetic (Eränkö, 1972*b*) and sensory (Kalina & Wolman, 1970) nerves may also contain acetylcholinesterase. Indeed, a number of trigeminal sensory nerve fibres which contain acetylcholinesterase have been demonstrated in the iris (Huhtala *et al.* 1976). It must also be borne in mind that acetylcholinesterase may have some as yet unknown developmental role in the nervous system (Silver, 1971), since its activity is greater in some regions of the immature central nervous system than in their adult counterparts (Krnjević & Silver, 1966). Nevertheless, since parasympathetic cholinergic fibres are by far the predominant source of acetylcholinesterase activity in the iris musculature, it remains a useful marker for cholinergic neurotransmission in this case at least, as long as its limitations are understood.

Little is known about the neonatal development of the post-ganglionic parasympathetic neurons in the ciliary ganglion but the development of their processes and acetylcholinesterase activity in the iris has been studied. Using light microscopy, Lai (1976) first observed acetylcholinesterase-positive nerve fibres of varying diameter in the 21 day foetal rat iris, situated about half way between the ciliary body and the pupillary margin. In the newborn rat iris, the number of acetylcholinesterase-containing nerve fibres and their reaction intensity increased and they were arranged to form a circle surrounding the pupil and giving off finer branches towards it (Fig. 8.2*a*). A loose network of acetylcholinesterase-positive nerve fibres was present in the sphincter pupillae by the third day *post partum* (Fig. 8.2*b*) and, by the fifth day, acetylcholinesterase-positive nerve fibres were also evident in the dilator pupillae. By the eighth day of life, a dense network of acetylcholinesterase-containing nerve fibres was apparent in the sphincter pupillae and by day 14, the number of acetylcholinesterase-containing fibres had increased substantially to give a pattern similar to that found in the adult (Fig. 8.2*c*). In a similar study, Tervo *et al.* (1978) reported that acetylcholinesterase-containing nerve fibres first became visible in the

nerve bundles (arrow) originating from the region of the ciliary body. (*c*) 14 day iris. A network of acetylcholinesterase-containing fibres has developed in the dilator pupillae. Large acetylcholinesterase-stained nerve bundles arise from the ciliary region and join the circular plexus in the area of the sphincter pupillae (small arrows). A plexus of acetylcholinesterase-containing nerves is also present between the ciliary body and the root of the iris (bold arrow) All scale bars represent 200 µm. (Photomicrograph kindly supplied by Y.-L. Lai.)

rat iris on the 19th day of gestation. The number of such fibres increased rapidly over the next two days so that, at birth, a well defined sphincter pupillae with a dense innervation could be distinguished from the much more sparsely innervated dilator pupillae. The number of acetylcholinesterase-containing nerve fibres and the intensity of the reaction increased, especially in the sphincter pupillae, until the adult pattern of innervation was achieved between two and three weeks *post partum* (Tervo *et al.*, 1978).

Lai (1976) also investigated the development of acetylcholinesterase-containing nerve fibres in the rat iris at the ultrastructural level. These studies showed that small acetylcholinesterase-containing nerve bundles first penetrated between the sphincter muscle cells on the ninth day *post partum*. At 11 days *post partum*, acetylcholinesterase-containing nerves were first observed to become superimposed on the anterior surface of the muscle cells of the dilator pupillae. Although the density of the acetylcholinesterase-containing nerve network in the dilator pupillae continued to increase with age, up to the 17th day *post partum* most of these fibres were still situated in the iris stroma. It was not until 30 days that the number of acetylcholinesterase-containing fibres superimposed directly on the dilator muscle became comparable with the number in the adult. Thus, although at the light microscope level the adult pattern of innervation appeared to be achieved between the 14th and 21st days of life (Lai, 1976; Tervo *et al.*, 1978), ultrastructural studies revealed that this does not in fact occur until 30 days *post partum* (Lai, 1976).

THE POSTNATAL DIFFERENTIATION OF ADRENOCEPTIVE AND CHOLINOCEPTIVE RESPONSIVENESS IN THE RAT IRIS

Although the iris musculature has a complex innervation, it is a useful model for studying the innervation of effector tissue since its thinness and its ease of visualisation and removal facilitate pharmacological, physiological and histological investigation. The effects of transmitter substances and other pharmacological agents can easily be studied after topical application, with the advantage that the contralateral eye can often be used as a control. Alterations in pupil diameter can serve as an index of the effect of such agents on the iris musculature.

In the previous section, the neonatal development of the autonomic innervation of the rat iris musculature was discussed. A second factor which governs the functional differentiation of an effector tissue is the development of its ability to respond to the stimulation provided by its innervation, i.e. the rate of maturation of its receptor systems. With this in view, Davies & Navaratnam (1979) investigated the postnatal differentiation of the α- and β-adrenergic and cholinergic receptor systems in the rat iris as reflected by their mediation of changes in pupil diameter.

Before pupil diameter could be used as an index of the development of receptor responsiveness, it was necessary to determine basal values of pupil diameter for each stage of development since pupil size increases considerably as a result of normal growth processes during the first month of life. These baseline data were obtained by inactivating the iris musculature pharmacologically and measuring the resultant 'paralysed' pupil diameter at each stage of development by superimposing a graduated (0.1 mm division) strip of cellulose acetate over the eye in a manner similar to that of Langham & Diggs (1972). All measurements were made in the horizontal meridian, since the pupil, which is circular at birth, tends to become slightly elliptical with age and hence its diameter varies slightly with the axis of measurement. It is necessary to use such a baseline of 'paralysed' pupil diameter since in the normal untreated pupil, the stress of the experimental situation (handling, light, anaesthesia etc.) induces a variable degree of miosis. Thus the iris musculature in a series of anaesthetised rat pups was inactivated by successive topical application of the cholinergic receptor blocker atropine, the α-adrenergic receptor blocker phenoxybenzamine and the β-adrenergic receptor blocker dichloroisoproterenol. The resulting pupil diameter was then measured.

In subsequent experiments, in order to investigate the maturation of the α-adrenoceptors, the cholinergic receptors were inactivated by atropine and the

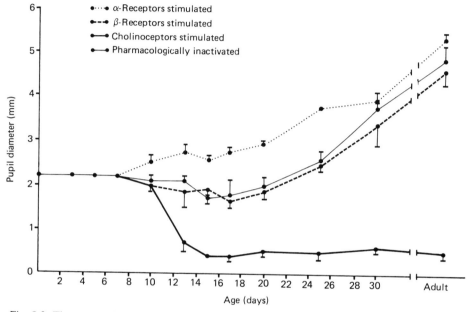

Fig. 8.3. The neonatal development of α- and β-adrenergic and cholinergic receptor responsiveness in the neonatal rat iris, shown against a baseline of pharmacological inactivation. The value for each age group represents the mean of measurements from four animals with the range. (Modified from Davies & Navaratnam, 1979.)

β-adrenergic receptors were blocked by dichloroisoproterenol. The α-adrenergic receptors were then stimulated by the topical application of noradrenaline or the specific α-receptor agonist phenylephrine, and alterations in pupil diameter were noted. Similarly β-adrenergic stimulation was achieved by the application of noradrenaline or the specific β-receptor agonist isoprenaline, after cholinoceptor and α-adrenoceptor blockade. Acetylcholine was used to stimulate cholinoceptors after α- and β-adrenergic receptor blockade.

Prior to the tenth day *post partum*, pupil diameter remains constant at about 2.2 mm and is unaffected by drug treatment or changes in lighting conditions (Fig. 8.3.). On the tenth day of life the inactivated pupil diameter becomes slightly reduced to about 2.1 mm and this is maintained until natural eye-opening occurs on day 13. Before this time, access to the eye was achieved by surgical separation of the eyelids. The inactivated pupil diameter subsequently decreases further to 1.7 mm on day 15 but thereafter it increases to 3.8 mm at 30 days of age and 4.9 mm in the adult. The unresponsiveness of the iris to all stimulation before the tenth day *post partum* indicates that before this time neither the adrenergic nor the cholinergic receptor systems have differentiated sufficiently to mediate a response. The reduction in inactivated pupil diameter which occurs on day ten and the further reduction after natural eye-opening are likely to be due to the development of neuronally independent 'muscle tone' in the iris musculature which is strengthened immediately after eye-opening when the iris responds to light for the first time. However, from the 17th day *post partum* onwards, the steady increase in pupil size is largely a product of the age-related increase in the dimensions of the eye.

From the tenth day *post partum* when the iris first becomes responsive, stimulation of α-adrenergic receptors, after β-receptor and cholinoceptor blockade, results in a dilatation at all times greater than the inactivated pupil diameter of the equivalent age (Fig. 8.3.). Noradrenaline and phenylephrine proved equally effective in eliciting this mydriatic response. Since it appears likely that α-adrenergic receptors may mediate contraction of some sphincter muscle fibres as well as contraction of those in the dilator pupillae (Schaeppi & Koella, 1964*a*), these results indicate that the α-adrenergic mediated contractile system of the dilator is stronger than that in the sphincter and thus masks or overrides its effect at all stages of development.

Stimulation of β-adrenergic receptors with noradrenaline (or isoprenaline which gave identical results) after α-adrenoceptor and cholinoceptor blockade, initially caused a slight reduction in pupil diameter below the inactivated size on the tenth day *post partum* (Fig. 8.3). This oscillates to a slight increase on day 15, but back to less than the inactivated pupil diameter on day 17. From this age onwards, β-adrenergic receptor stimulation results in a pupil diameter smaller than the inactivated diameter. As β-adrenergic receptor systems probably mediate active relaxation of both the sphincter and dilator pupillae (Schaeppi & Koella, 1964*a*, *b*) and are therefore antagonistic in their activity, β-adrenoceptor mediated relaxation of the dilator appears to be the more effective.

The iris musculature first responds to cholinergic receptor stimulation (after α- and β-adrenoceptor blockade) with pupil constriction on the 10th day *post partum* (Fig. 8.3.). This miotic response develops rapidly so that, by the 15th day of life, a pupil diameter of 0.4 mm can be induced and this degree of miosis can be maintained throughout further development. The strength of this response, when compared with the inactivated pupil diameter (Fig. 8.3.), may be explained by the fact that cholinergic receptors probably mediate both contraction of sphincter pupillae and relaxation of dilator pupillae muscle fibres (Schaeppi & Koella, 1964*a*, *b*) and hence these systems act synergistically to produce miosis.

These results indicate that neither the adrenergic nor cholinergic receptor systems in the iris are capable of responding to chemical stimulation before the tenth day *post partum*, just 3 days before eye-opening occurs, even though Lai (1976) and Tervo *et al.* (1978) have shown significant proliferation of adrenergic and cholinergic nerve terminals in the iris by this time. However, the cholinergically mediated miotic response matures rapidly so that by 2 days after normal eye-opening (i.e. day 15) it is apparently functionally mature. On the other hand, the adrenergic responses are slower to mature. The speed of development of the miotic response may have an important protective function since as soon as the normal eye is exposed to light, the pupil can be almost fully constricted and thus the sensitive retina protected from potential damage.

In the same study (Davies & Navaratnam, 1979), the development of functional maturity in the adrenergic terminals in the iris (i.e. their ability to stimulate α-adrenergic receptors) was investigated using amphetamine, which causes the release of endogenous noradrenaline from such terminals (Carlsson, 1966). The cholinergic and β-adrenergic receptors in the irises of a series of neonatal rats were inactivated as described previously. The α-adrenergic receptors were then stimulated by the topical application of amphetamine. When the manifestation of this stimulation due to the release of endogenous noradrenaline was maximal (after 5 min), exogenous noradrenaline was instilled into the eye to determine whether or not further dilatation could be induced. It is evident from Fig. 8.4 that, as would be predicted from the previous

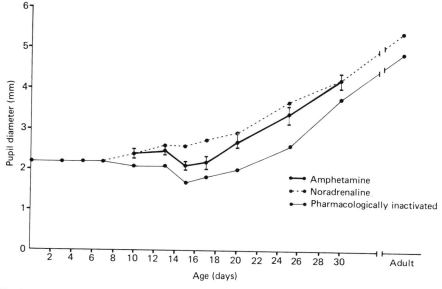

Fig 8.4. The effect of stimulating the α-adrenergic receptors in the neonatal rat iris with endogenous noradrenaline (released by amphetamine) compared with the effect of the administration of exogenous noradrenaline. The value for each age group represents the mean of measurements from four animals with the range. (Modified from Davies & Navaratnam, 1979.)

experiments, amphetamine does not affect pupil diameter until the tenth day *post partum*. At all subsequent ages studied, amphetamine-induced α-adrenergic receptor stimulation results in pupil dilatation. However, when exogenous noradrenaline was applied to the eye after the maximum effect of amphetamine had been achieved, a further dilatation could be produced from the 13th to 25th day *post partum*, with the disparity being greatest between days 15 and 17. In rats aged 30 days and older, the subsequent application of exogenous noradrenaline does not enhance the dilatation produced by amphetamine.

These results therefore suggest that between days 10 and 25 *post partum* there is insufficient noradrenaline present in the developing terminals, or its release mechanisms are immature, thus preventing complete stimulation of the α-adrenergic receptors in the iris. It is also possible that membrane transport mechanisms for the re-uptake of noradrenaline are not fully functional at this stage and, since amphetamine enters the nerve terminal by this route (Iversen, 1967), its effect could be reduced. However, from day 30 onward, amphetamine alone can stimulate the release of sufficient endogenous noradrenaline from adrenergic terminals in the iris to produce maximal dilatation. Thus it would appear that in the neonatal rat iris, the adrenergic receptors (at least the α-adrenoceptors) mature in advance of the capacity of the adrenergic nerve terminals to release sufficient noradrenaline to stimulate them fully. A similar situation has been reported in the case of premature human infants (Lind & Shinebourne, 1970) where mydriasis can be elicited by directly acting sympathomimetic and parasympatholytic agents as early as 28 weeks of gestation. However, the indirectly acting amines tyramine and hydroxyamphetamine were not effective until about 3 weeks before full term, i.e. about 9 weeks after directly acting sympathomimetics can induce pupil dilatation.

The suggestion that the mechanisms for the synthesis and storage of noradrenaline differentiate later than receptor responsiveness is supported by observations on the noradrenaline content of the neonatal and adult rat iris (Davies & Navaratnam, 1979). Prior to the tenth day of life, when receptor responsiveness is first observed in the iris musculature, its noradrenaline content changes very little and remains well below 0.3

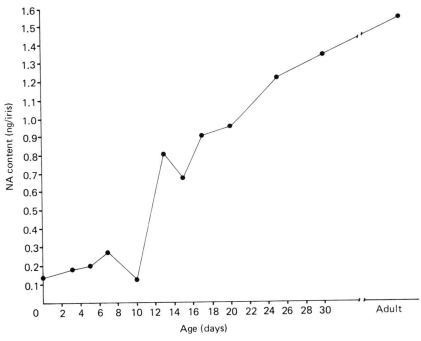

Fig. 8.5. The neonatal increase in the noradrenaline content of the rat iris. The value for each age group represents the mean of measurements of four irises. (Modified from Davies & Navaratnam, 1979.)

ng (Fig. 8.5). However, on day 13 (when normal eye-opening occurs) the noradrenaline content of the iris increases almost three-fold. Thereafter, it increases steadily until it reaches 1.34 ng at 30 days and 1.54 ng in the adult. Thus the noradrenaline content of nerve terminals in the iris increases most markedly just before eye-opening (day 13) when the iris first has to respond to external stimuli. The subsequent increase is steadier, levelling off as maturity is reached, so that by 30 days *post partum* when the application of exogenous noradrenaline cannot induce further pupil dilatation after amphetamine, the iris already contains 87% of the adult transmitter level.

THE DEVELOPMENT OF α-ADRENERGIC RESPONSIVENESS IN THE NEONATAL
RAT IRIS DEPRIVED OF ITS SYMPATHETIC INNERVATION

Since the α-adrenergic receptors in the neonatal rat iris musculature appear to
become responsive in advance of the ability of their adrenergic innervation to
stimulate them fully, it is of interest to know whether these receptors can differentiate
in the absence of their normal innervation or whether an intact innervation is essential

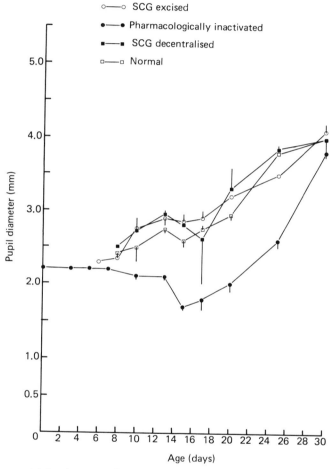

Fig. 8.6. The neonatal development of α-adrenergic responsiveness in the normal rat iris, and in
those whose ipsilateral superior cervical ganglion has been decentralised or extirpated, compared
against a baseline of pharmacological inactivation. The value for each age group represents the
mean of measurements from four animals with the range. (Modified from Davies & Navaratnam,
1981.)

for the development of receptor responsiveness in an effector tissue. With this in view,
Davies & Navaratnam (1981) extirpated or decentralised the superior cervical
ganglion (unilaterally) in two groups of 3-day-old rat pups. The development of
α-adrenergic responsiveness in these animals was then determined in a manner similar
to that described in the previous section and was compared with inactivated irises and
with α-adrenoceptor responsiveness in normal irises at similar stages of development.

Decentralisation of the superior cervical ganglion in the 2–3-day-old rat pup has been shown to prevent the normal neonatal increase in tyrosine hydroxylase activity, [³H] noradrenaline uptake, density and complexity of the innervation and fluorescence intensity in the iris musculature (Black & Mytilineou, 1976a). However, organ growth itself as determined by increase in protein content is not affected. This inhibition of the normal postnatal increase in the density of the iris innervation has

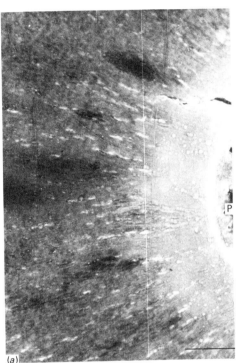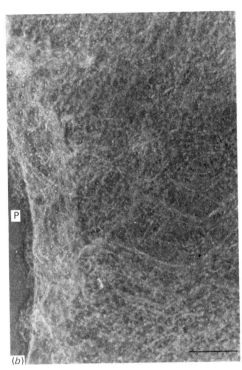

Fig. 8.7. Fluorescence micrographs. (a): The normal adrenergic innervation of the iris of a 30-day-old rat. (b) The iris of a 30-day-old rat after decentralisation of the superior cervical ganglion at 3 days *post partum*. P, pupil. Scale bars represent 200 μm. (Modified from Davies & Navaratnam, 1981.)

also been demonstrated at the ultrastructural level by Lawrence *et al.* (1979), following decentralisation of the 2- or 4-day-old rat superior cervical ganglion.

It can be seen from Fig. 8.6 that the pharmacologically inactivated pupil diameter and α-adrenergic responsiveness in normal irises developed in an almost identical way to that described in the previous section (cf. Fig. 8.3). Surgical decentralisation or extirpation of the superior cervical ganglion at 3 days of age resulted in a mortality of less than 5%. The survivors apparently grew normally in comparison with litter-mates which were used as controls to provide data on inactivated pupil diameter and on the normal development of α-adrenergic responsiveness. However, in 'decentralised' and 'extirpated' animals, eye-opening was delayed for 12–24 hours on the operated side. After eye-opening, the success of the operation was demonstrated by a marked ipsilateral ptosis. Fluorescence histochemical studies on iris 'stretch' preparations also demonstrated the efficacy of the operation. Fig. 8.7 shows the adrenergic terminal innervation of a normal iris at 30 days, at which age its noradrenaline content has been shown to be 87% of the adult value (Davies & Navaratnam, 1979), in comparison with a noradrenaline-depleted, 'decentralised' iris of the same age. The 'decentralised' irises first respond to noradrenaline induced α-adrenergic receptor stimulation (after cholinoceptor and β-adrenergic receptor blockade) by mediating pupil dilatation on the 8th day *post partum* (Fig. 8.6). This dilatation above the inactivated pupil diameter resulted in a pupil diameter of 2.95 mm on day 13, but it decreased slightly over the ensuing 4 days only to increase steadily thereafter, reaching 4.0 mm by 30 days of age. Stimulation of the α-adrenergic receptors in the iris following extirpation of the superior cervical ganglion, at 3 days *post partum*, resulted in an initial pupillary dilatation to 2.75 mm on the tenth day of life (Fig. 8.6). With the exception of a slight transient decrease on day 15, α-adrenoceptor stimulation caused a subsequent steady increase in pupil diameter with age, reaching 4.1 mm by 30 days after birth.

Thus it is evident (Fig. 8.6) that α-adrenergic responsiveness develops similarly in neonatal irises which have been deprived of their sympathetic innervation shortly after birth either by decentralisation or by extirpation of the superior cervical ganglion. Furthermore, the development of α-adrenergic responsiveness in these sympathetically denervated irises is similar to that in the normal iris musculature. In all cases, once a response could be elicited, α-adrenoceptor stimulation results in a pupil diameter greater than that of the pharmacologically inactivated pupil at the same age. If anything, the 'decentralised' and 'extirpated' irises exhibit a slightly greater dilatation after α-adrenergic receptor stimulation than normal irises, until the end of the third week *post partum*. Similarly, it is interesting to note that 'decentralised' irises responded to noradrenaline 2 days earlier (day 8) than normal. Thus neonatal sympathetic denervation may result in iris adrenergic receptor super-sensitivity, as has been demonstrated in the adult rabbit (Colasanti, Chiu & Trotter, 1978).

The possibility exists that the apparently normal development of α-adrenergic responsiveness in 'extirpated' and 'decentralised' animals is due to the fact that sufficient adrenergic innervation may reach the iris and stimulate receptor differentiation before 3 days of age. However, this is unlikely since at 3 days *post partum*, when the operations were performed, Lai (1972*b*) has shown the dilator muscle to be poorly differentiated; the adrenergic neurons in the superior cervical ganglion (whose terminals innervate the iris) are structurally and biochemically immature and they receive virtually no synaptic contacts (Eränkö, 1972*a*, *c*; Davies, 1979). Therefore, the iris musculature is apparently not dependent on the intact sympathetic innervation for normal postnatal growth (Black & Mytilineou, 1976*a*) or for the normal development of α-adrenergic responsiveness.

REGULATION OF THE POSTNATAL DEVELOPMENT OF THE IRIS INNERVATION

The ultrastructural and biochemical differentiation of adrenergic neurons in the superior cervical ganglion, their terminals in the iris and the development of adrenergic responsiveness in the iris appear to be synchronised in the neonatal rat. The majority of adrenergic neurons in the superior cervical ganglion have differentiated to the 'young sympathetic nerve cell' stage by the end of the second week *post partum* (Eränkö, 1972*c*; Davies, 1977) and they appear to have established the mature pattern of synaptic contacts with pre-ganglionic cholinergic nerves. At about the same time, the noradrenaline concentration and tyrosine hydroxylase activity in the ganglion approach adult levels, flourescence intensity nears its maximum and granular fluorescence (which may be an index of functional ability) first appears (Davies, 1977). The pattern of adrenergic nerves in the iris, as visualised by fluorescence histochemistry, appears similar to that in the adult by 14 days *post partum* (Lai, 1976) and the steepest increase in iris noradrenaline content occurs between the 10th and 13th days of life (Davies & Navaratnam, 1979). Moreover, natural eye-opening occurs at this time (day 13) and the iris first becomes responsive to chemical stimulation and light (Davies & Navaratnam, 1979). How is this synchronisation of development achieved?

Black, Hendry & Iversen (1971*b*) provided evidence that trans-synaptic factors regulate the postnatal development of adrenergic neurons in the superior cervical ganglion, with their investigation of the postnatal increase in synaptic number, tyrosine hydroxylase and choline acetyltransferase activity in normal and decentralised mouse superior cervical ganglia. Synapse number remained low and stable in normal ganglia during the first 2 days *post partum* but increased markedly between days 5 and 11 to reach an asymptotic plateau. The developmental curve of increasing choline acetyltransferase activity was found to follow closely that of the increase in synapse number in the superior cervical ganglion. Since Hebb & Waites (1956) have shown choline acetyltransferase (the enzyme catalysing the conversion of acetyl coenzyme A and choline to acetylcholine) to be highly localised to presynaptic cholinergic terminals, this postnatal increase in choline acetyltransferase in the superior cervical ganglion can be considered to reflect the maturation of pre-ganglionic cholinergic terminals. Tyrosine hydroxylase activity rose in two separate phases during neonatal development. The second and major of these phases occurred coincidently with the marked increase in ganglionic synapse number, suggesting that the formation of pre-ganglionic cholinergic synaptic contacts may be necessary for the maturation of tyrosine hydroxylase activity in the post-ganglionic adrenergic neurons. Black, Joh & Reiss (1974) have shown by immunotitration studies that this developmental increase in tyrosine hydroxylase activity, in both the mouse and rat superior cervical ganglion, is due to the induction of new enzyme molecules and not the activation of existing inactive enzyme.

Unilateral decentralisation of the superior cervical ganglion in 5–6-day-old mice (Black *et al.*, 1971*b*) predictably resulted in the reduction of choline acetyltransferase levels in the ganglion to 10% of control levels. Furthermore, the induction of tyrosine hydroxylase activity in adrenergic neurons in the ganglion was also inhibited, failing to increase above the normal 7 day level. Thus decentralisation prevented the normal major increase in tyrosine hydroxylase activity in the superior cervical ganglion during the second week *post partum*, strengthening the hypothesis that the maturation of the adrenergic neurons is dependent on their innervation by normal cholinergic presynaptic endings. Black & Geen (1973) pursued this study further by investigating the effects of long-lasting ganglionic blocking agents on the development of tyrosine hydroxylase activity in the neonatal mouse superior cervical ganglion. Ganglionic blockade prevented the normal induction of tyrosine hydroxylase activity, as was also subsequently shown to be the case in the rat (Black *et al.*, 1974), but did not affect the maturation of choline acetyltransferase activity, indicating that the presynaptic terminals in the ganglion were not damaged.

Thus these results demonstrate that it is blockade of the ganglion *per se* that prevents the normal induction of tyrosine hydroxylase activity and suggest that it is the release of acetylcholine from the developing terminals and the consequent depolarisation of the adrenergic neurons that mediates the trans-synaptic control.

This has been supported by the observation that the incubation *in vitro* of superior cervical ganglia with high potassium (a depolarising agent) concentrations results in elevated tyrosine hydroxylase activity (Mackay & Iversen, 1972). There is also some evidence that acetylcholine is involved in the trans-synaptic regulation of tyrosine hydroxylase activity in the adult rat superior cervical ganglion (Mueller, Thoenen & Axelrod, 1970; Molinoff, Brimijoin & Axelrod, 1972).

The post-synaptic neurons in the mouse superior cervical ganglion have been shown to exert a retrograde trans-synaptic effect over the normal postnatal development of presynaptic cholinergic neurons: Black, Hendry & Iversen (1972*a*) have shown that destruction of the post-synaptic neurons with 6-hydroxydopamine or nerve growth factor antiserum inhibits the neonatal increase in choline acetyltransferase activity in the presynaptic terminals. Nerve growth factor antiserum, which does not affect adult adrenergic neurons, did not alter choline acetyltransferase activity in the adult ganglion. In this case it would seem that morphological contact is the regulating factor since ganglionic blockade (Black & Geen, 1973) does not affect the maturation of choline acetyltranferase in the presynaptic terminals. Thus the cholinergic pre-synaptic neuron and the post-synaptic adrenergic neuron appear to reciprocally regulate each other's neonatal development.

Since orthograde trans-synaptic factors affect the ontogenetic development of adrenergic neurons in the superior cervical ganglion, it would be reasonable to expect that they would also affect the maturation of adrenergic terminals in effector tissue. Black & Mytilineou (1976*a*) have shown this to be the case in the iris. Decentralisation of the 2–3-day-old rat superior cervical ganglion inhibited the normal development of tyrosine hydroxylase activity both in the ganglion itself and in the ipsilateral iris. The uptake of [^{3}H]noradrenaline by the developing adrenergic terminals in the iris was also inhibited by decentralisation. Thus orthograde trans-synaptic factors (probably acetylcholine) exert a regulatory effect both on perikaryon-al maturation in the ganglion and on terminal development in the iris. Lawrence *et al.* (1979) have also demonstrated in a quantitative ultrastructural study that decentralisa-tion of the 2- or 4-day-old superior cervical ganglion inhibits normal terminal proliferation in the rat iris. Since adult levels of tyrosine hydroxylase activity were reached by the 14th day of life in the superior cervical ganglion, but not until day 55 in the iris, Black & Mytilineou (1976*a*) considered there to be a proximo-distal gradient in the maturation of the post-ganglionic neurons innervating the iris.

However, trans-synaptic factors in the superior cervical ganglion are not the only ones regulating the development of the post-ganglionic adrenergic neuron. Dibner & Black (1976) have shown that iridectomy prevents the normal postnatal development of tyrosine hydroxylase activity in these neurons in the rat. The normal neonatal growth and the development of adrenergic sympathetic neurons has been shown to be affected by a specific protein, nerve growth factor (Levi-Montalcini & Angeletti, 1968). It has been suggested that this explains the neuronotrophic performance of sympathetically innervated target organs (Varon & Bunge, 1978). Black, Hendry & Iversen (1972*b*) have shown that neonatal nerve growth factor treatment induces an increase in tyrosine hydroxylase activity in both normal and decentralised mouse superior cervical ganglia. However, this effect was greater in normally innervated ganglia and the difference could not be abolished by treatment of 'decentralised' animals with larger doses of nerve growth factor.

Thus, although nerve growth factor alone can affect the maturation of post-synaptic neurons, the presence of normal presynaptic cholinergic terminals would appear to be a requirement for the maximisation of this effect. Administration of nerve growth factor antiserum, on the other hand, has been demonstrated to impair the development of tyrosine hydroxylase activity in mouse superior cervical ganglia at any time during the first 8 days of life (Hendry & Iversen, 1971). However, if this antiserum is given on day 13 (when Black & Mytilineou (1976a) have shown almost mature levels of tyrosine hydroxylase to be present) or after, it does not affect ganglionic tyrosine hydroxylase activity.

In similar studies on the rat superior cervical ganglion, Thoenen et al. (1972) also found nerve growth factor to have an effect on the induction of tyrosine hydroxylase activity, independent of the integrity of the ganglion's cholinergic input. However, since in their hands decentralisation did not significantly impair the effect of nerve growth factor, they concluded that nerve growth factor is the principal factor regulating the growth and differentiation of the post-synaptic adrenergic neuron and that trans-synaptic factors have only a minor additive effect.

The effect of nerve growth factor on adrenergic terminal maturation in the neonatal iris has been examined by Black & Mytilineou (1976b). They found that, despite the fact that nerve growth factor significantly increased tyrosine hydroxylase activity in both normal and decentralised rat superior cervical ganglia, it only increased tyrosine hydroxylase activity in normally innervated iris terminals and not in those of decentralised neurons. This indicates that trans-synaptic influences are necessary before nerve growth factor can affect the development of the adrenergic innervation of the iris and terminal maturation.

The presence of small amounts of nerve growth factor in the adult rat iris has been demonstrated by means of radio-immunoassay by Johnson et al. (1972), who also demonstrated its release from the iris in organ culture. In vivo, rat superior cervical ganglion transplanted into the anterior chamber of the eye will reinnervate the iris (Olson & Malmfors, 1970) and in vitro a rat iris placed in contact with superior cervical ganglion will be innervated by processes from the ganglion neurons (Silberstein et al., 1971). Supplemental nerve growth factor was found to increase this innervation and nerve growth factor antiserum to reduce it. Thus the iris is capable of producing and releasing nerve growth factor, which in vitro and probably in vivo stimulates its innervation by adrenergic processes. Under what conditions does nerve growth factor normally exert such an effect?

Ebendal et al. (1980) could not detect nerve growth factor activity in freshly excised adult rat iris by bioassay methods, but it was present in cultured iris. Furthermore, when excised donor iris tissue was transplanted into the anterior chamber of a recipient rat eye, after 1 day it was found to contain a similar amount of nerve growth factor to irises cultured for 1 day in vitro. Similar levels of nerve growth factor persisted in the transplants for at least 11 days but after 1 month, when a considerable degree of sympathetic reinnervation had taken place (Olson & Malmfors, 1970), nerve growth factor was no longer detectable. Sympathetic and/or sensory denervation of the adult iris also resulted in significant nerve growth factor activity in the affected iris 10 days after operation. This activity was not detectable just after denervation (2 or 4 days) nor at 1 month, when presumably some reinnervation had occurred.

Thus, the level of nerve growth factor activity may be increased in an adult effector tissue in response to denervation and subsequently decreased upon reinnervation. These findings strongly suggest that nerve growth factor is a neuronotrophic factor which can be produced and released from effector tissue (the iris) in response to denervation in the adult and which attracts reinnervating fibres. It would also appear likely that the neonatal iris, whose physical growth and development of receptor responsiveness occur normally in the absence of and possibly in advance of its innervation (Black & Mytilineou, 1976a; Davies & Navaratnam, 1979, 1981), produces and releases nerve growth factor, thus stimulating sympathetic fibre ingrowth and terminal proliferation. However, this hypothesis remains to be tested directly.

It is evident, therefore, that a number of complexly interlinked ortho- and retrograde trans-synaptic and neuronotrophic factors outlined above (and possibly more yet to be discovered) govern the postnatal development of the sympathetic innervation of the iris, synchronising the development of its constituent parts. Since a parasympathetic neuronotrophic factor has also been identified in the iris (Ebendal *et al.*, 1980) the possibility exists that an equally complex set of factors regulating the development of the parasympathetic innervation of the iris remains to be discovered. The questions therefore arise: Why are such a large number of regulatory factors necessary? Are they hierarchical in nature? Do they have a selective function or are they simply the result of the need for precise synchronisation of development?

REFERENCES

Alphen, G. W. H. M. van, Robinette, S. L. & Macri, F. T. (1964). The adrenergic receptors of the intraocular muscles of the cat. *International Journal of Neuropharmacology*, **2**, 259–72.
Appenzeller, O. (1970). The normal pupil and some pupillary abnormalities. In *The Autonomic Nervous System*, pp. 124–34. Amsterdam & London: North-Holland Publishing Co.
Black, I. B. & Geen, S. C. (1973). Trans-synaptic regulation of adrenergic neuron development: inhibition by ganglionic blockade. *Brain Research*, **63**, 291–302.
Black, I. B., Hendry, I. A. & Iversen, L. L. (1971a) Differences in the regulation of tyrosine hydroxylase and DOPA decarboxylase in sympathetic ganglia and adrenal. *Nature, New Biology*, **231**, 27–9.
Black, I. B., Hendry, I. A. & Iversen, L. L. (1971b) Trans-synaptic regulation of growth and development of adrenergic neurones in a mouse sympathetic ganglion. *Brain Research*, **34**, 229–40.
Black, I. B., Hendry, I. A. & Iversen, L. L. (1972a). The role of post-synaptic neurones in the biochemical maturation of presynaptic cholinergic nerve terminals in a mouse sympathetic ganglion. *Journal of Physiology*, **221**, 149–59.
Black, I. B., Hendry, I. A. & Iversen, L. L. (1972b). Effects of surgical decentralization and nerve growth factor on the maturation of adrenergic neurons in a mouse sympathetic ganglion. *Journal of Neurochemistry*, **19**, 1367–77.
Black, I. B., Joh, T. H. & Reiss, D. J. (1974). Accumulation of tyrosine hydroxylase molecules during growth and development of the superior cervical ganglion. *Brain Research*, **75**, 133–44.
Black, I. B. & Mytilineou, C. (1976a) Trans-synaptic regulation of the development of end organ innervation by sympathetic neurons. *Brain Research*, **101**, 503–21.
Black, I. B. & Mytilineou, C. (1976b). The interaction of nerve growth factor and trans-synaptic regulation in the development of target organ innervation by sympathetic neurons. *Brain Research*, **108**, 199–204.
Burn, J. H. & Rand, M. J. (1958). The action of sympathomimetic amines in animals treated with reserpine. *Journal of Physiology*, **144**, 314–36.
Carlsson, A. (1966). Pharmacological depletion of catecholamine stores. *Pharmacological Reviews*, **18**, 541–9.
Champlain, J. De, Malmfors, T., Olson, L. & Sachs, Ch. (1970). Ontogenesis of peripheral adrenergic neurons in the rat: pre- and postnatal observations. *Acta Physiologica Scandinavica*, **80**, 276–88.
Colasanti, B. K., Chiu, P. & Trotter, R. R. (1978). Adrenergic and cholinergic drug effects on rabbit eyes after sympathetic denervation. *European Journal of Pharmacology*, **47**, 311–18.
Coyle, J. T. & Henry, D. (1973). Catecholamines in fetal and newborn rat brain. *Journal of Neurochemistry*, **21**, 61–7.
Crouch, R. (1936). The efferent fibres of the Edinger-Westphal nucleus. *Journal of Comparative Neurology*, **64**, 365–73.
Cuello, A. C., Hiley, R. & Iversen, L. L. (1973). Use of catechol-*O*-methyltransferase for the radiochemical assay of dopamine. *Journal of Neurochemistry*, **21**, 1337–40.
Davies, D. C. (1977). The differentiation of the neonatal rat superior cervical ganglion. PhD thesis, University of Cambridge.
Davies, D. C. (1978). Neuronal numbers in the superior cervical ganglion of the neonatal rat. *Journal of Anatomy*, **127**, 43–51.

Davies, D. C. (1979). The post-natal differentiation of sympathetic neurons in the rat superior cervical ganglion. *Journal of Anatomy,* **129,** 886.

Davies, D. C. & Navaratnam, V. (1979). Development of adrenoceptive and cholinoceptive responsiveness in the neonatal rat iris. *Experimental Eye Research,* **29,** 203–10.

Davies, D. C. & Navaratnam, V. (1981). Differentiation of α-adrenergic responsiveness in the neonatal rat iris after decentralisation or extirpation of the superior cervical ganglion. *Brain Research,* **213,** 119–26.

Dibner, M. D. & Black, I. B. (1976). The effect of target organ removal on the development of sympathetic neurons. *Brain Research,* **103,** 93–102.

Ebendal, T., Olson, L., Seiger, Å. & Hedlund, K.-O. (1980). Nerve growth factors in the rat iris. *Nature (London),* **286,** 25–8.

Ehinger, B. (1966). Connections between adrenergic nerves and other tissue components in the eye. *Acta Physiologica Scandinavica,* **67,** 57–64.

Ehinger, B. & Falck, B. (1966). Concomitant adrenergic and parasympathetic fibres in the rat iris. *Acta Physiologica Scandinavica,* **67,** 201–7.

Ehinger, B., Falck, B. & Persson, H. (1968). Function of cholinergic nerve fibres in the cat iris dilator. *Acta Physiologica Scandinavica,* **72,** 139–47.

Eränkö, L. (1972a). Postnatal development of histochemically demonstrated catecholamines in the superior cervical ganglion of the rat. *Histochemical Journal,* **4,** 225–36.

Eränkö, L. (1972b). Biochemical and histochemical observations on the postnatal development of cholinesterases in the sympathetic ganglion of the rat. *Histochemical Journal,* **4,** 545–59.

Eränkö, L. (1972c). The ultrastructure of the developing sympathetic nerve cell and the storage of catecholamines. *Brain Research,* **46,** 159–75.

Falck, B. (1962). Observations on the possibilities of the cellular localisation of monamines by a fluorescence method. *Acta Physiologica Scandinavica,* **56,** suppl. 197.

Falck, B., Hillarp, N.-Å., Thieme, G. & Torp, A. (1962). Fluorescence of catecholamines and related compounds condensed with formaldehyde. *Journal of Histochemistry and Cytochemistry,* **10,** 348–54.

Hebb, C. O. & Waites, G. M. H. (1956). Choline acetylase in antero- and retrograde degeneration of a cholinergic nerve. *Journal of Physiology,* **132,** 667–71.

Hendry, I. A. & Iversen, L. L. (1971). Effect of nerve growth factor and its antiserum on tyrosine hydroxylase activity in mouse superior cervical ganglion. *Brain Research,* **29,** 159–62.

Hess, W. R., Koella, W. P. & Szabo, T. (1950). Experimentelle Studien über die antagonische Innervation. *Zeitschrift für die gesamte experimentalle Medizin,* **116,** 431–43.

Hökfelt, T. (1966). Electron microscopic observations on nerve terminals in the intrinsic muscles of the albino rat iris. *Acta Physiologica Scandinavica,* **67,** 255–6.

Hökfelt, T. (1967). Ultrastructural studies on adrenergic nerve terminals in the albino rat iris after pharmacological and experimental treatment. *Acta Physiologica Scandinavica,* **69,** 125–6.

Huhtala, A., Tervo, T., Huikuri, K. T. & Palkama, A. (1976). Effects of denervations on the acetylcholinesterase-containing and fluorescent nerves of the rat iris. *Acta Ophthalmologica,* **54,** 85–98.

Ivens, C., Mottram, D. R., Lever, J. D., Presley, R. & Howells, G. (1973). Studies on the acetylcholinesterase (AChE)-positive and -negative autonomic axons supplying smooth muscle in the normal and 6-hydroxydopamine (6-OHDA) treated rat iris. *Zeitschrift für Zellforschung und mikroskopische Anatomie,* **138,** 211–22.

Iversen, L. L. (1967). *The Uptake and Storage of Noradrenaline in Sympathetic Nerves.* Cambridge University Press.

Johnson, D. G., Silberstein, S., Hanbauer, I. & Kopin, I. J. (1972). The role of nerve growth factor in the ramification of sympathetic nerve fibres in the rat iris in organ culture. *Journal of Neurochemistry,* **19,** 2025–9.

Joseph, D. R. (1921). The inhibitory influence of the cervical sympathetic nerve upon the sphincter muscle of the iris. *American Journal of Physiology,* **55,** 279–80.

Kalina, M. & Wolman, M. (1970). Correlative histochemical and morphological study on the maturation of sensory ganglion cells in the rat. *Histochemie,* **22,** 100–8.

Krnjević, K. & Silver, A. (1966). Acetylcholinesterase in the developing forebrain. *Journal of Anatomy,* **100,** 63–89.

Lai, Y.-L. (1972a). The development of the sphincter muscle in the iris of the albino rat. *Experimental Eye Research,* **14,** 196–202.

Lai, Y.-L. (1972b). The development of the dilator muscle in the iris of the albino rat. *Experimental Eye Research,* **14,** 203–7.

Lai, Y.-L. (1976). Development of the iris innervation in the rat. *Investigative Ophthalmology (and Visual Science),* **15,** 960–6.

Langham, M. E. & Diggs, E. M. (1972). Quantitative studies of the ocular response to norepinephrine. *Experimental Eye Research,* **13,** 161–71.

Lawrence, J. M., Black, I. B., Mytilineou, C., Field, P. M. & Raisman, G. (1979). Decentralization of the superior cervical ganglion in neonates impairs the development of the innervation of the iris. A quantitative ultrastructural study. *Brain Research,* **168,** 13–19.

Levi-Montalcini, R. & Angeletti, P. U. (1968). The nerve growth factor. *Physiological Reviews,* **48,** 534–69.

Levitt, M., Spector, S., Sjoerdsma, A. & Udenfriend, S. (1965). Elucidation of the rate-limiting step in norepinephrine biosynthesis in the perfused guinea pig heart. *Journal of Pharmacology and Experimental Therapeutics*, **148**, 1–8.

Lind, N. A. & Shinebourne, E. (1970). Studies on the development of the autonomic innervation of the human iris. *British Journal of Pharmacology*, **38**, 462P.

Loewenfeld, I. E. (1958). Mechanism of reflex dilation of the pupil. Historical review and experimental analysis. *Documenta Ophthalmologica*, **12**, 185–448.

Mackay, A. V. P. & Iversen, L. L. (1972). Trans-synaptic regulation of tyrosine hydroxylase activity in adrenergic neurones: effect of potassium concentration on cultured sympathetic ganglia. *Naunyn-Schmiedebergs Archiv für experimentelle Pathologie und Pharmakologie*, **272**, 225–9.

Malmfors, T. (1965). The adrenergic innervation of the eye as demonstrated by fluorescence microscopy. *Acta Physiologica Scandinavica*, **65**, 259–67.

Malmfors, T. & Sachs, C. (1965). Direct demonstration of the system of terminals belonging to an individual adrenergic neuron and their distribution in the rat iris. *Acta Physiologica Scandinavica*, **64**, 377–82.

Molinoff, P. B. Brimijoin, S. & Axelrod, J. (1972). Induction of dopamine-β-hydroxylase and tyrosine hydroxylase in rat hearts and sympathetic ganglia. *Journal of Pharmacology and Experimental Therapeutics*, **182**, 116–29.

Mueller, R. A., Thoenen, H. & Axelrod, J. (1970). Inhibition of neuronally induced tyrosine hydroxylase by nicotinic receptor blockade. *European Journal of Pharmacology*, **10**, 51–6.

Niesel, P. (1961). Zur Frage der nervösen Beeinflussung der Aderhautdurchblutung. *Bericht über Versammlung der deutschen ophthalmologischen Gesellschaft (Heidelberg)*, **64**, 86–90.

Nilsson, O. (1964). The relationship between nerves and smooth muscle cells in the rat iris. 1. The dilator muscle. *Zeitschrift für Zellforschung und mikroskopische Anatomie*, **64**, 166–71.

Olson, L. & Malmfors, T. (1970). Growth characteristics of adrenergic nerves in the adult rat. *Acta Physiologica Scandinavica*, **80**, suppl. 348.

Owman, Ch., Sjöberg, N-O. & Swedin, G. (1971). Histochemical and chemical studies on pre- and postnatal development of the different systems of 'short' and 'long' adrenergic neurons in peripheral organs of the rat. *Zeitschrift für Zellforschung und mikroskopische Anatomie*, **116**, 319–41.

Poos, F. (1927). Pharmakologische und physiologische Untersuchungen an den isolierten Irismuskeln. *Archiv für experimentelle Pathogie und Pharmakologie*, **126**, 307–51.

Rüegg, J. C. & Hess, W. R. (1953). Die Wirkung von Adrenalin, Nor-Adrenalin und Acetylcholin auf die isolierten Irismuskeln. *Helvetica Physiologica et Pharmacologica Acta*, **11**, 216–30.

Schaeppi, U. & Koella, W. P. (1964a). Adrenergic innervation of cat iris sphincter. *American Journal of Physiology*, **207**, 273–9.

Schaeppi, U. & Koella, W. P. (1964b). Innervation of cat iris dilator. *American Journal of Physiology*, **207**, 1411–16.

Silberstein, S. D., Johnson, D. G., Jacobowitz, D. M. & Kopin, I. J. (1971). Sympathetic reinnervation of the rat iris in organ culture. *Proceedings of the National Academy of Sciences, USA*, **68**, 1121–4.

Silver, A. (1971). The significance of cholinesterase in the developing nervous system. *Progress in Brain Research*, **34**, 345–55.

Tervo, K., Tervo, T. & Palkama, A. (1978). Pre- and postnatal development of catecholamine-containing and cholinesterase-positive nerves of the rat cornea and iris. *Anatomy and Embryology*, **154**, 253–65.

Thoenen, H., Saner, A., Kettler, R. & Angeletti, P. U. (1972). Nerve growth factor and preganglionic cholinergic nerves: their relative importance to the development of the terminal adrenergic neuron. *Brain Research*, **44**, 593–602.

Tranzer, J. P. & Thoenen, H. (1967). Significance of 'empty vesicles' in post-ganglionic sympathetic nerve terminals. *Experientia*, **23**, 123–4.

Varon, S. S. & Bunge, R. P. (1978). Trophic mechanisms in the peripheral nervous system. *Annual Review of Neuroscience*, **1**, 327–36.

9 Regeneration of axons in the central nervous system

MARTIN BERRY

Anatomy Department, Guy's Hospital Medical School, London SE1 9RT, UK

INTRODUCTION

Current interest in the capacity of axons in the mammalian central nervous system (CNS) to regrow after injury contrasts with a clinical tradition which once held that CNS regeneration was impossible (Spielmeyer, 1922; Ramon y Cajal, 1928; Le Gros Clark, 1942, 1943), and thus unworthy of study. Many research findings have contributed to the modern, more optimistic, attitude which maintains that an understanding of the reasons for the failure of axonal regrowth in mammals might eventually lead to a successful treatment regime for the amelioration of the catastrophic effects of brain damage and spinal cord injury (Berry, 1979; Kiernan, 1979).

Amphibia and fish regenerate their CNS after injury, as do most invertebrates (see Windle, 1955, for reviews). The fundamental phylogenetic causes for such marked variation in reactions to injury by different taxa have never been explained. Regeneration in lower phylogenetic forms is very precise so that original synaptic interrelationships are re-established. Thus there is reason to suppose that functional restitution would return in humans if regeneration could be promoted. One possible explanation for the phylogenetic differences in the response to axotomy is that selection has favoured the perfection of immune surveillance and *pari passu* a reduction in axon-regenerative potential. CNS sequestration by the blood brain barrier (BBB) confers upon this tissue the properties of a foreign antigen with all the attendant hazards of latent autoimmune rejection, of which inhibition of axon growth after damage to the BBB could be but one example (Berry & Riches, 1974; Feringa, Randall & Wendt, 1975). However, much experimental work has failed to support the idea that sensitised lymphocytes, or specific anti-brain antibodies accumulating at the site of CNS injury, are implicated in regenerative failure (Feringa *et al.*, 1976; Willenborg, Staten & Eidelberg, 1977; Mervart & Kiernan, 1978; Heinicke & Kiernan, 1978; Gilad, Gilad & Kopin, 1979; Berry *et al.*, 1979*a,b*).

One encouraging factor that has come to light over the years is that some mammalian CNS axons do regenerate after injury. Thus, successful regeneration is exhibited by neurohypophyseal axons (Stutinsky, Bonvallet & Dell, 1949; Scharrer & Wittenstein, 1952; Beck & Daniel, 1959*a,b*; Rothballer & Skoryna, 1960; Holmes, 1963; Adams, Daniel & Prichard, 1968; Kiernan, 1971), monoaminergic fibres (Björklund *et al.*, 1971; Moore, Björklund & Stenevi, 1971; Björklund, Nobin & Stenevi, 1973), unmyelinated cholinergic fibres (Björklund *et al.*, 1975; Svendgaard, Björklund & Stenevi, 1976), axons in foetal and neonatal brain (Kalil & Reh, 1979), olfactory nerve fibres (Barber, 1981, 1982), retinal axons (McConnell & Berry, 1982*a,b*), and in CNS fibres induced to grow into peripheral nervous system (PNS) grafts (e.g. Benfey & Aguayo, 1982). Accordingly, whilst regrowth in some axons is promoted, in others it is inhibited. This duality of response is intriguing because it clearly demonstrates that growth inhibition or enhancement is selective.

Another example of this is offered by axons at the CNS–PNS interface, where sensory PNS axons readily regenerate as far as the root–cord junction but fail to grow into the CNS. Similarly, motor axons which originate from within the CNS do not grow if injured within the CNS parenchyma but do elongate to re-innervate muscle if injured in a PNS nerve. The selectivity of the axonal injury response has been explained on the basis of autoimmune (Berry & Riches, 1974; Feringa *et al.* 1975), serum (Kiernan, 1978), axon growth inhibitory (Berry, 1982), barrier (Penfield, 1927; Clemente, 1955, 1964; Windle, 1956), growth factor (GF: Berry, 1979) and growth associated protein – GAP – (Levine, Skene & Willard, 1981) hypotheses; but few have stood the test of time (Kiernan, 1979). Selective responsiveness has been investigated as a possible means of repairing damage within the CNS, either by transplanting PNS tissue to bridge the necrotic area (Turbes & Freeman, 1958; Jakoby, Turbes & Freeman, 1960; Perkins, Babbini & Freeman, 1964) or by replacing damaged, potentially regenerative, systems with their foetal or neonatal counterparts (Björklund, Stenevi & Svendgaard, 1976; Björklund & Stenevi, 1979*a,b*; Björklund, Segal & Stenevi, 1979; Björklund *et al.*, 1981).

Other contemporary investigators are exploring the possible role of GFs, in both scarring and axonal growth, as initiators of the production of GAPs (Levine *et al.*, 1981). Successful regrowth appears to depend on the continued production and axonal transport of GAPs (Theiler & McClure, 1978; Benowitz, Shashoua & Yoon, 1981), possibly under the influence of GFs. In this context, regenerative failure could be attributed to the absence or inactivation of GFs (Berry, 1979).

Scarring is an important consideration in the response of the CNS to injury but (like the phenomenon of axonal regeneration) the mechanics of scarring, and the cellular interactions between mesodermal cells and glial cells which ensue, are entirely unknown. Fibroblast growth factors (FGFs) have been isolated from brain tissue (Gospodarowicz, 1974). FGFs are thought to be peptides of myelin basic proteins (MBP: Westall, Lennon & Gospodarowicz, 1978), although more recent work claims that brain FGFs are associated with an acid fraction (Thomas *et al.*, 1980). Of course it is possible that FGFs, whilst promoting scarring, could at the same time inhibit axonal growth in the CNS. This would explain the association between density of scarring and axonal growth failure (Clemente, 1955, 1964; Windle, 1956).

PHYLOGENY

Central axons in fish and Amphibia (Hooker, 1932; Tuge & Hanzawa, 1937; Sperry, 1945; Koppanyi, 1955; Hibbard, 1963; Bernstein, 1967) readily regenerate after injury to re-establish their original connections accurately (Sperry, 1944; Gaze, 1960, 1970; Hibbard & Ornberg, 1976). Reptiles, birds and mammals do not have this capacity for regrowth (Hamburger, 1955). It was thought that the reasons for successful repair in lower vertebrates and invertebrates lay in the properties of the scar (Windle, 1955; Clemente, 1955, 1964) but, more recently, it has been shown that the density and constitution of scar tissue in these lower taxa appear qualitatively identical to those in mammals. For example, in Amphibia, it has been shown that although some fibres may be deflected by collagenous material (Schönheit, 1968), hypertrophic astrocytic scar tissue does not interfere with regeneration (Reier, 1979).

Moreover, Scott & Mathewson (1979) described both the time course of deposition of scar tissue and the nature of the mature cicatrice in *Rana pipiens* as being very similar to that of mammals. In fish, elongating axons grow through scar tissue (Tuge & Hanzawa, 1937; Koppanyi, 1955; Bernstein & Bernstein, 1967) without being deflected. On this evidence it seems likely that, if regeneration could be induced in mammals, the presence of scar tissue would not be counterproductive to the re-formation of severed connections.

GAP-43 (the numbers represent the molecular weight in kilodaltons) is a polypeptide which is transported along axons only during periods of axon growth (Skene & Willard, 1981*a,b,c*). In regenerating optic nerve of the toad (Skene & Willard, 1981*a*) and fish (Benowitz *et al.*, 1981), GAP-43 concentrations increase greatly. As the sprouts invade the tectum and form synapses, GAP-43 levels decline. Levine *et al.* (1981) interpret this finding by proposing that genes regulate axonal growth and that induction of the GAP-43 gene is initiated by signals, originating from either the external or internal environment of the axon, which are then transported by retrograde axonal flow. It is possible that the external signal could be one of a range of growth factors, each of which is specific for a class of neuron. Synaptogenesis in the target signals the repression of GAP-43 production, possibly by employing molecules (supplied by the post-synaptic targets) which are also transported in a retrograde manner. This hypothesis might also explain the accelerated regeneration seen after double lesioning, i.e. when a 'test' lesion is preceded by a 'conditioning' lesion (Brock, 1978; Lanniers & Grafstein, 1980; Edwards, Alpert & Grafstein, 1981). Thus, two stimuli could either doubly induce gene action or modulate repressive feedback systems which control gene expression. The problem of why axons grow after injury in fish and amphibians but not in reptiles, birds and mammals is central to the whole field of axonal regenerative research and will be discussed later in the context of available hypotheses.

ONTOGENY

It is well known that immature animals recover from CNS injury which would cause permanent functional impairment in the adult. The consensus of opinion is that functional recovery in immature animals is attributable to vigorous collateral sprouting of undamaged axons and the production of aberrant pathways (Chambers, 1955; De Meyer, 1967; Sechzer, 1974; Stanfield & Cowan, 1976; Prendergast & Stelzner, 1976*a,b*; Devor, 1976; Leong & Lund, 1973; Baisinger, Lund & Miller, 1977; Castro, 1978*a,b*; D'Amato & Hicks, 1978; Frost & Schneider, 1979; So, 1979; Prendergast & Misantone, 1980). The possibility that recovery might be attributable to enhanced regeneration in immature animals has been investigated many times but with conflicting results. Gerard & Koppanyi (1926) were the first to claim that true regeneration does occur in young rats but this was subsequently disputed by many workers (Hooker & Nicholas, 1927, 1930; Gerard & Grinker, 1931; Feigin, Geller & Wolf, 1951; Freeman, 1955; Hess, 1955, 1957; Stelzner, Ershler & Weber, 1975; Gearhart, Oster-Granite & Guth, 1979; Goldberg & Frank, 1981; Cummings, Bernstein & Stelzner, 1981). Furthermore, although Sugar & Gerard (1940) had reported good regrowth through PNS nerve implants in neonates, Barnard & Carpenter (1949, 1950) repeated the work and found little evidence for regeneration. One reason for the poor response is that young neurons are supersensitive to axotomy so that transneuronal degeneration and cell death occur more readily than in the adult (Brodal, 1940; Lieberman, 1971; Prendergast & Stelzner, 1976*b*; Cox, 1976).

In these studies, designed to investigate regeneration in foetal and neonatal animals, results have been difficult to interpret because of the problem of distinguishing fibres which are actually regenerating from undamaged fibres growing *de novo* through the lesion site (Leong & Lund, 1973; Hicks & D'Amato, 1975; Devor, 1976; Gilson & Stensaas, 1974). Thus, in birds (Clearwaters, 1954) and mammals (Ranson, 1903; Dunn, 1917; Reinis, 1965) many axons have been seen coursing through the scar or deflected by the lesion (De Meyer, 1967; Sechzer, 1974) which were probably not damaged at the time of injury. The first unequivocal demonstration of regeneration in neonates was given by Kalil & Reh (1979). They transected the pyramidal tracts in the hamster at different ages and showed (by injecting radioactive leucine into the motor cortex) that corticospinal axons sprouted above the lesion, decussated and followed an aberrant contralateral path – ultimately to innervate ventral horn cells in an apparently normal manner. Subsequent studies on the normal development of the corticospinal tracts in hamsters have shown that the pathway is established *en masse* soon after birth (Reh & Kalil, 1981, 1982). Myelination commences at day 7 *post partum* and continues at a slow rate until the third week when the number of myelinated fibres increases steeply (Reh & Kalil, 1982).

Berry (1982) has discussed these experimental findings in the context of a hypothesis which proposes that the failure of CNS regeneration in mature animals is associated with the release of a growth inhibitory factor from myelin by proteolysis. The successful axon growth demonstrated by Kalil & Reh (1979) could be correlated with the absence of myelin in the immature hamster.

PERIPHERAL NERVES

Most peripheral nerves have a central component which may course for as great a distance within the CNS as in the PNS. The somata supporting both peripheral and central parts may be either within or outside the CNS. It is a remarkable fact that injury of the axon in the CNS is never associated with regrowth, whilst damage in the PNS is always followed by regeneration. This phenomenon demonstrates two important facts about the regenerative responses of axons. Firstly, neuronal cell bodies have the capacity to support regeneration whether they are housed within or outside the CNS, indicating that the perikarya and nuclei of neurons are not implicated in growth failure. Secondly, these findings strongly suggest that it is the environment of the injured CNS that is not conducive to growth because either it actively inhibits, or is unable to provide the growth factors for GAP production.

A good demonstration of this is seen at the root–cord junction after crushing the dorsal root; axons will regenerate to the CNS boundary but then either stop growing or loop back along the nerve (Lugaro, 1906; Tower, 1931; Ten Cate, 1932; Paskind, 1936; Westbrook & Tower, 1940; Kimmel & Moyer, 1947; Moyer, Kimmel & Winborne, 1953; McCouch, 1955; Gamble, 1976; Stensaas, Burgess & Horch, 1979). Penetration is achieved by a small number of axons but for very short distances only along blood vessels or invading Schwann cells (Tower, 1931; Paskind, 1936; Kimmel & Moyer, 1947; Moyer *et al.*, 1953; Druckman & Mair, 1953; Lampert & Cressman, 1964). Similarly, peripheral nerves embedded into the CNS will not elongate (Le Gros Clark, 1943; Benes, 1968; Kiernan, 1971; Knowles & Berry, 1978) but CNS axons will grow into the graft (Sugar & Gerard, 1940; Brown & McCouch, 1949; Feigin *et al.*, 1951; Sager & Marcovici, 1972; Kao, 1974; Kao *et al.*, 1970; Kao, Chang & Bloodworth, 1977a,b; Chi *et al.*, 1980). Aguayo has used the peripheral nerve grafting technique to demonstrate that intrinsic CNS neurons (those that do not project outside the CNS) are capable of regeneration if they can gain access to the peripheral nerve graft (Aguayo *et al.*, 1979; Aguayo *et al.*, 1982; Benfey & Aguayo, 1982). Moreover, such fibres will grow for distances which are much longer than the length of the CNS projection tract they originally constituted (Richardson, McGuinness & Aguayo, 1980; David & Aguayo, 1981; Benfey & Aguayo,1982). Aguayo's results are a further demonstration that central neurons are capable of regeneration. Conversely, grafts of CNS interposed between the cut ends of a PNS nerve inhibit peripheral nerve outgrowth from the proximal stump (Aguayo *et al.*, 1978; Weinberg & Spencer, 1979). The possible reasons why degenerating central nervous tissue might fail to encourage axon growth is discussed later.

MONOAMINERGIC FIBRES AND UNMYELINATED CHOLINERGIC FIBRES

Monoaminergic (MA) and cholinergic (ChE) axons regenerate into somatic tissue transplanted into the host (Björklund & Stenevi, 1979*a*). MA axons also reconnect (often over long distances) with their innervation fields after terminal degeneration following the administration of the specific MA neurotoxin 6-hydroxydopamine (6-OHDA). MA axons do not regenerate when MA tracts are surgically interrupted, although this latter injury can result in massive paraterminal and/or collateral sprouting (Katzman *et al.*, 1971; Björklund, *et al.*, 1971). For example, Pickel, Krebs & Bloom (1973) and Pickel, Segal & Bloom (1974) demonstrated sprouting of MA fibres, innervating both the hippocampus and cerebellum, after cutting the superior cerebellar peduncle. This was also observed in the cortex and cerebellum after localised cerebral infarction (Robinson, Bloom & Battenberg, 1977).

This phenomenon has subsequently received intense study, from which has evolved the concept of the 'pruning effect', first described in the visual system by Schneider (1970, 1973; see also section 9 on 'Collateral Sprouting', Jonsson & Hallman, 1982, for a recent review). This states that neurons are genetically programmed to elaborate terminal networks of a defined extent, independent of the size of the target area. Thus, if some axon terminals are destroyed, the finite arbor is reconstituted by the formation of new sprouts on intact branches elsewhere in the tree. Pruning also occurs after application of neurotoxins. During development the effect is more florid than in the adult and this could be explained by the fact that collaterals have access to trophic substances released from targets during ontogeny (Iacovitti, Reis & Joh, 1981; Reis, *et al.*, 1981; Schmidt, Kasik & Bhatnagar, 1980; Schmidt, Björklund & Loren, 1981). Release of MA GFs may be limited to the duration of development of the normal innervation fields within a given target. Thus, the critical period for the ontogeny of MA terminal fields is of the same duration as that of the regenerative 'pruning' response and both may be controlled by the same trophic factors (Schmidt *et al.*, 1980, 1981). Sievers & Klemm (1982) have extended this hypothesis to explain the massive cerebellar noradrenaline (NA) hyperinnervation seen in neonates after subcutaneous injection of 6-OHDA. They give evidence that, like axons in many other areas during development, NA fibres normally hyperinnervate their targets. Thus, the exaggerated pruning effect seen in neonates is probably brought about by the cumulative effects of a normal developmental hyperinnervation and the presence of high titres of MA GFs. Iacovitti *et al.* (1981) suggest that another factor, which may be superimposed on the latter two, is the maturity of the axons mediating the response. Thus, cerebellectomy in young animals induces hyperinnervation of brain stem NA fibres, but section of NA tracts to the cerebral hemispheres does not.

Schmidt & Bhatnagar (1979*a–d*) and Schmidt *et al.* (1980) have studied the time course of the neonatal pruning response after high subcutaneous doses of 6-OHDA and found that hyperinnervation of the cerebellum and brain stem occurs maximally soon after birth and, thereafter, declines until it is undetectable by 12 days after birth. Hyperinnervation of the cerebral hemispheres does not occur over this period. Schmidt & Bhatnagar explained these findings by proposing a correlation between differential degrees of developmental advancement of NA terminal arbors in the two sites and the titres of GFs produced, i.e. developing fields receive high, developed fields receive low or zero levels of MA GFs.

Transplants of foetal central and peripheral MA neurons survive and develop stereotyped connections (Stenevi, Björklund & Svendgaard, 1976; Björklund *et al.*, 1976; Björklund *et al.*, 1979). Foetal septum–diagonal band ChE transplants, placed in the septohippocampal ChE pathway after fimbrial lesions have destroyed the ChE input to the hippocampal and dentate gyri, restore the ChE input (Björklund & Stenevi, 1977, 1979*a,b*). Re-innervation from the graft is blocked if the normal ChE innervation remains undisturbed. Similarly, foetal grafts of the locus coeruleus, transplanted into NA denervated hippocampus, re-innervate the hippocampus in a pattern that mimics the normal NA afferents (Björklund *et al.*, 1979). The degree to which such transplants can restore function is remarkable and suggests that not only are the implants capable of precisely re-innervating post-synaptic sites in denervated targets but also that the grafts themselves are precisely re-innervated by appropriate afferent projections (e.g. Björklund & Stenevi, 1979*b*; Perlow *et al.*, 1979; Björklund *et al.*, 1980; Dunnett *et al.*, 1981).

AXONAL REGENERATION IN TISSUE CULTURE

Several workers have severed growing neurites in tissue culture with the intention of observing the behaviour of the proximal and distal stumps (Levi, 1926; Levi & Meyer, 1945; Hughes, 1953; Shaw & Bray, 1977; Bray, Thomas & Shaw, 1978). In all cases the distal stump survives amputation from the cell body. At first the isolated segment retracts but eventually elongates at a normal rate (40–1000 μm h^{-1}) for several hours (Hughes, 1953), but does not exceed its original length (Shaw & Bray, 1977). Depending on the conditions of culture, long segments maintain their polarity and elongate by growth at the original growth cone, but short isolated neurites retract to form a single bead of cytoplasm. Redistribution of material in the bead may be responsible for the consistent finding that two growth cones appear around the surface of the bead which then grow in opposite directions to form a single long neurite with a growth cone at either end. Growth is inhibited, like that in intact fibres, by colchicine and Colcemid (Daniels, 1972), but continues in the presence of cycloheximide and puromycin, indicating that microtubule assembly rather than protein synthesis is occurring at growth cones during elongation. Importantly, the results of Shaw & Bray (1977) show that polymerisation of microtubules is independent of the cell body. Thus, isolated segments grow in the absence of the biosynthetic apparatus housed in the soma. Even when protein synthesis is inactivated, the neurite retains the ability to assemble surface membranes and cytoplasmic tubules and fibrils, but growth ceases when precursor stocks become exhausted. Under normal circumstances the cell body is the source of such building materials.

Growth cones on the proximal stumps quickly re-form (within 10–35 min) after amputation (Bray *et al.*, 1978) and will do so in amino-acid-free media or when cycloheximide or puromycin are added, but do not develop in the presence of colchicine and cytochalasin B. However, with time, antimitotic drugs cause the neurites to collapse, with growth cones appearing along their lengths. These findings show that growth cones can be produced at any point over the surface of the neurite and that changes in the stability of microtubules may in some way control the sitings of the growth cones, possibly by rechannelling materials over the intracytoplasmic transport system. The implications of this work for our understanding of normal axonal growth and regeneration are enormous. Clearly, growth may be inhibited by factors which affect growth cone formation (membrane synthesis, microtubule and microfilament assemblies) or protein synthesis in the soma. Collateral sprouting may be initiated by local disruption or inactivation of microtubule synthesis. The initiation of regeneration and new collateral branches can proceed in the absence of protein synthesis (Bray *et al.*, 1978).

It has been suggested by experiments on neonates, on implanted PNS, and on the MA system that all CNS axons are inherently capable of regeneration after injury but that elongation stops as growth inhibitory substances are released from degenerating CNS by autolysis (Berry, 1982). However, attempts to test this hypothesis by observing the response of amputated neurites in culture over the duration of the abortive response have not been documented. Nonetheless, tissue culture does offer a means of testing the presence and potency of growth inhibitory substances and of discovering their mode of action.

OLFACTORY NERVE FIBRES

Interest in the reaction to injury of the olfactory nerve centres on three unique attributes of the structure. Firstly, it is uncertain whether the nerve is part of the PNS or within the CNS; secondly, the nerve regenerates after injury; and thirdly, the regenerating fibres are able to penetrate the CNS.

When the olfactory nerve is sectioned, or the olfactory epithelium is damaged, the primary olfactory sensory neurons degenerate. However, proliferation by stem cells in the epithelium quickly leads to a reconstitution of primary neurons and to a re-establishment of the nerve (Barber, 1981; Barber & Raisman, 1978). Regenerating olfactory fibres readily enter the olfactory bulb to re-innervate glomeruli and will even penetrate the frontal lobes overlying the cribriform plate in neonates when the bulb has been removed (Graziadei, Levine & Monti Graziadei, 1979). Olfactory fibres appear to be able to induce the formation of glomeruli both in the neonatal cerebral cortex and in layers of the olfactory bulb not normally innervated by them (Graziadei & Samanen, 1980; Barber, 1981).

The difficulty in catagorising the olfactory nerve into PNS or CNS is because glial fibrillar acid protein (GFAP)-positive cells, more similar in appearance to astrocytes than Schwann cells, constitute the sole glial element in the nerve. Moreover, the junction between olfactory nerve and bulb cannot be defined (Barber, 1982). Thus, if the olfactory nerve is within the CNS, it has unique regenerative powers; if within the PNS, it is the only peripheral nerve able to penetrate the adult CNS after injury and re-form central connections. Both phenomena need further investigation because important clues about regenerative failure might thereby be revealed.

Neurohypophyseal axons regenerate after injury (Dellman, 1973) but it is difficult to understand why this should be. Kiernan (1971) thought that pituicytes were a cell type unique to the infundibulum and neurohypophysis and that they encouraged regrowth, rather like Schwann cells in the PNS. However, it was subsequently shown that pituicytes are probably a species of astrocyte, since they contain GFAP-positive fibrils (Suess & Pliska, 1981; Velasco, Roessmann & Gambetti, 1982), and so Kiernan's proposition seems unlikely. On the other hand, Berry & Riches (1974) suggested that, because the tuber cinereum and pituitary stalk are outside the BBB, their constituent proteins are not auto-antigens (like other CNS components) and thus injury would not precipitate autoimmune reactions likely to impair regeneration. However, as already mentioned, there is no evidence that autoimmunity features in the aetiology of CNS regenerative failure (Berry *et al.*, 1979*a,b*). Furthermore scar tissue deposited in the injured infundibulum is similar to that in wounds elsewhere in the CNS (Dellman, 1973) and thus differences in the composition of the scar cannot be invoked to explain the successful growth. Berry (1982) has suggested that the absence of myelin in the hypothalamo-hypophyseal tract could account for regeneration, if autolysis of CNS myelin caused the release of molecules with growth inhibitory potential. This idea is supported both by the findings that growth in other unmyelinated systems is also enhanced (i.e. in the olfactory nerve, retina and immature unmyelinated brain) and by the observation that neurohypophyseal axons do not regenerate into cerebral implants which contain myelinated fibres (Kiernan, 1971).

Although previous reports have maintained that retinal ganglion cell axons exhibit only abortive regeneration (Goldberg, 1976, 1977; Goldberg & Frank, 1979, 1980), a recent quantitative study has unequivocally demonstrated that these retinal axons continue to regrow after injury for at least 100 days (McConnell & Berry, 1982*a,b*). The rate of growth is slow however. In the first 5 days the rate of advancement was $30 \mu\text{m d}^{-1}$ dropping to $3 \mu\text{m d}^{-1}$ thereafter, compared with $1000–2000 \mu\text{m d}^{-1}$ in peripheral nerves and central axons in culture (Hughes, 1953; Shaw & Bray, 1977). One factor contributing to the apparent slow growth was the probable inclusion in the analysis of degenerating or arrested axons after the fifth to tenth day. McConnell & Berry (1982*a,b*) were unable to follow the growth of retinal ganglion cell axons which had gained access to fascicles, so their descriptions were of axons which grew in random directions in areas of the retina deep to the ganglion cell fibre layer. Thus, the normal unidirectional guidance mechanisms operating during the development of ganglion cell axons (Goldberg, 1977; Goldberg & Frank, 1979, 1980) appear either to be absent or ineffective on regenerating fibres.

Random growth by regenerating fibres, like the aberrant growth seen in neonates after injury (see p. 215), demonstrates that guidance mismatching does not inhibit growth as has been suggested (Goldberg & Frank, 1979). The regenerative response of ganglion cell axons in the retina is in marked contrast to their growth failure in the optic nerve after crush or penetrating injuries. However, if the optic nerve is injured near the globe, some optic fibres can loop back into the retina where they continue to grow randomly for long periods (Allcutt & Berry, 1983).

COLLATERAL SPROUTING

Collateral sprouting, and its relevance to regeneration, has been discussed by Berry (1979) and the 'pruning effect' has already been considered with reference to the growth of the MA system (p. 217). Perhaps the important point which both phenomena emphasise is that growth of new fibres does occur in the CNS but outside the area of direct injury, over tracts which have not themselves been damaged. The mode of genesis of collateral sprouts is unknown but does involve the production of growth cones, possibly sited in regions where microtubules are unstable (see p. 218 for discussion of the growth of neurites in tissue culture), but what initiates the latter is unknown. Regulation of sprouting by vacated post-synaptic sites is a possibility and certainly the extent of collateral growth is directly correlated with the severity of denervation (Rubel, Smith & Steward, 1981). Thus, the availability of post-synaptic sites could stimulate sprouting of adjacent axons (Raisman & Field, 1973; Bernstein & Goodman, 1973) since collateral sprouting does not occur in targets where dendritic fields are atrophied (Rubel *et al.*, 1981).

Collateral sprouting is more profuse in young animals than in adults (Guillery, 1972; Schneider, 1973; Stelzner *et al.*, 1975; Prendergast & Stelzner, 1976a,b) and the pruning effect is also exaggerated (Schneider, 1973; Devor, 1976; Devor & Schneider, 1975). The plasticity of young fibre systems undoubtedly accounts for the aberrant fibre growth seen after CNS injury in neonates (De Meyer, 1967; Leong & Lund, 1973; Sechzer, 1974; Castro, 1978b; Cox, 1976; Stanfield & Cowan, 1976; Baisinger *et al.*, 1977; D'Amato & Hicks, 1978; Frost & Schneider, 1979; So, 1979; Bohn & Stelzner, 1979) which further demonstrates that guidance mismatching does not inhibit growth. It is possible, however, that the increased sprouting in neonates may be a mechanism for compensating for fibre and neuron loss, which is greater in the neonate than adult. Thus, Prendergast & Misantone (1980) have suggested that the few axons surviving after injury in infants may branch more than the greater number surviving in adults, perhaps because of the correspondingly greater denervation of targets in the former. Accordingly, the same innervation densities are ultimately established with fewer fibres than in the mature animal. This concept adds an additional dimension to explanations of the 'pruning effect' already considered (p. 217).

SCARRING

It has already been mentioned that early work on regeneration had correlated the density of scarring with regenerative failure. However, it is difficult to see how a physical barrier might stop growth. Indeed, the behaviour of some unmyelinated CNS axons (Sung, 1981) and all PNS fibres is that they are deflected by an obstruction and form neuromatous entanglements. However, Bernstein & Bernstein (1967) provided experimental validation of the hypothesis. They showed that when regenerating axons in the piscine spinal cord are deflected from their growth path by Teflon implants, they form synapses on vacated post-synaptic sites in juxtaposed neuropil (Bernstein & Bernstein, 1969). Synaptogenesis might lead to the observed cessation of growth if molecules passed across these junctions inhibited elongation. In mammals new synapse formation is also seen about the scar in spinal cord lesions (Bernstein & Bernstein, 1971, 1973a,b; Bernstein, Gelderd & Bernstein, 1974; Bernstein, Wells & Bernstein, 1975). However, if such a potent growth inhibitory mechanism is operating after injury, it is difficult to conceive how regeneration is ever possible. For example,

Bernstein & Bernstein (1969) removed the Teflon graft from a group of fish and relesioned the regenerated fibres, which had formed synapses, by transecting the cord more proximally. The cut fibres responded by regenerating through the scar, where the Teflon had been, and re-innervating sites distally, presumably without forming synapses on the multitude of vacated post-synaptic sites *en route* and despite likely perturbations in their forward growth as they entered the scar.

Nonetheless, a correlation does exist between the density of scar tissue and regeneration in neonates, although the relationship is probably non-causal. In young animals collagenous scar tissue does not form in the wound and the glial reaction is weak and transitory (Ranson, 1903; Gerard & Koppanyi, 1926; Brodal, 1940; Becker, 1952; Clearwaters, 1954; Hess, 1956; Reinis, 1965; De Meyer, 1967; Frotscher *et al.*, 1970; Stelzner *et al.*, 1975; Bignami & Dahl, 1976; Prendergast & Stelzner, 1976*a*; Berry & Henry, 1976; Gearhart *et al.*, 1979; Bernstein, Bechard & Stelzner, 1981). In rats little or no collagen is formed in the wound before 8–10 days *post partum* and the organisation of a glia limitans by astrocytes either is not in evidence or is fragmentary (Berry *et al.*, 1983). The site of the original lesion may thus be difficult to detect in a mature animal injured in the neonatal period because, in the absence of scarring, axons and dendrites eventually obliterate the wound. Study of the ontogeny of scarring in the brain may thus lead to an elucidation both of the factors controlling fibroblast accumulation and collagen deposition and of the interrelationship between glia and mesodermal elements which leads to the production of the mature glial-collagen scar. At the same time, such studies may also throw light on a possible relationship between scarring and the failure of axonal regeneration.

Not much is known about the organisation of fibroblasts in brain lesions. They are thought to invade the wound from the connective tissue and muscle surrounding injured CNS tissue (Krikorian, Guth & Donati, 1981) and FGFs, isolated from brain, have been implicated as mitogens (Gospodarowicz, 1974). If FGFs are peptides derived from MBP and released into the wound area by autolysis of CNS myelin (Westall *et al.*, 1978), the absence of myelin in neonates could account for the failure of scar tissue deposition in young animals. If astrocytes were induced and organised to form a glia limitans by fibroblasts, this explanation also provides for the absence (or the fragmentary presence) of basement membrane in immature animals. Further-more, if FGFs also possess axon growth inhibitory potential, then the rationale for the failure of axon growth in the environs of dense glial-collagen scars is also self-evident.

So often such intellectually pleasing solutions are incorrect and the above thesis is no exception. Thomas *et al.* (1980) repeated the work of Gospodarowicz (1974) and confirmed that high titres of FGF activity are found in brain, but suggested that the active molecules are probably derived from an acid protein which contaminated their basic samples. The identity and origin of the acid protein are still a mystery, but presumably a myelin or oligodendrocyte source is still a possibility. We have been studying FGF activity, using the same bioassay system as Gospodarowicz (1974), and have found that FGF activity persists in embryonic and neonatal rats from the 15th day post-conception until the onset of myelination (8–10 days *post partum*) (Berry *et al.*, 1983), periods during which no myelin is present and which precede MBP accumulation in oligodendrocytes during premyelination gliosis (Sternberger *et al.*, 1978). FGF activity is also present in the mutant mice MLD and Shiverer, in which there is a negligible content of MBP (Bourre *et al.*, 1980; Du Povey *et al.*, 1979; Matthieu, *et al.*, 1980; Mikoshiba, Aoki & Tsukada, 1980). FGF titres are also high in the PNS (Berry *et al.*, 1983) where MBP may be present as the P_1 basic protein (Brostoff, Sachs & Di Paolo, 1975).

If the FGFs extracted both from the CNS (of these different animals) and from the PNS are biochemically identical, then MBP seems an unlikely source for this mitogen, since the activity is preserved in embryos and leucodystrophic mice. Oligodendrocytes and astrocytes are also unlikely candidates because of the high level of FGFs in the PNS. The structural entity common to all sites where FGF is found is the axon, so possible autolysis of an axonal protein may yield FGF peptides. It appears, however, that FGFs may not be relevant to scarring since high titres are found in neonatal brain in which a cicatrice does not develop. However, collagen scarring in the immature brain may not proceed in the absence of mature glia. Thus, the appearance of a mature glial-collagen scar at 8–10 days *post partum* in the rat may be related more to the attainment of astrocyte competence in organising fibroblasts than to the presence of FGF. Regenerative capabilities are also unrelated to FGF content of the tissue.

HYPOTHESIS AND CONCLUDING REMARKS

A plenitude of hypotheses exists each one of which purports to explain why the majority of axons in the CNS fail to grow after injury. Kiernan (1979) has sifted through most of them and dismissed all save three; the serum GF, the substrate compatibility, and the GF hypotheses.

The serum GF hypothesis (Kiernan, 1978; Heinicke & Kiernan, 1978) holds that axons of any type will regenerate if their growing tips have access to serum-derived growth promoting proteins. The thesis is fully discussed by Kiernan (1979) but since then more evidence has accrued to support the idea. In peripheral nerves, a zone of increased vascular permeability advances along the distal stump in phase with the advancing front of regenerating fibres (Sparrow & Kiernan, 1981). It is suggested that the growth cones of regenerating peripheral nerves secrete a vasoactive substance, possibly substance P, which encourages the exudation of plasma proteins about young axons. Similarly, in the optic nerves of fish, which also regenerate vigorously, a zone of increased vascular permeability accompanies a spearhead of regenerating axons along the nerve and into the tectum (Kiernan & Contestabile, 1980). Skin, PNS, tendon, thyroid and submandibular autotransplants introduced into the brain do not possess a BBB, and each exhibits a degree of vascularisation, and associated plasma exudation, concomitant with the magnitude of the density of re-innervation (Heinicke, 1980).

Thus, Kiernan and co-workers have substantiated their hypothesis which essentially maintains that GFs are supplied to all axons from the serum and that closure of the BBB soon after injury in reptiles, birds and mammals deprives CNS axons of an essential growth stimulus. Attractive as this hypothesis is, it does not explain the continued slow growth of axons in the retina (McConnell & Berry, 1982*a*,*b*), why all axons do not regenerate in the wake of the increased vascular permeability engendered by growing MA fibres, or why vasoactive substances (effective in the PNS) become effete at the root–cord junction and beyond (within the CNS).

The compatible substrate hypothesis (Kiernan, 1979) proposes that, where growth is successful, the substrate is able to supply essential trophic factors and conversely, where growth fails, a compatible substrate (if present at all) is unable to supply GFs. This thesis implies that, during development, substrate compatibility is ubiquitous, but begs the question relating to specificity for different axon species. Perhaps specificity is implied to account for all cases of successful regeneration in the mammalian CNS. One interesting extension of the hypothesis is that in those adult animals which maintain embryonic properties, like axon guidance and growth, regeneration is possible. Thus, in the regenerating lizard spinal cord (Simpson, 1968; Egar, Simpson & Singer, 1970), regenerating *Triturus* tail (Egar & Singer, 1972; Nordlander & Singer, 1978) and in *Triturus* (Singer, Nordlander & Egar, 1979) and *Xenopus* (Nordlander & Singer, 1982) embryos, spaces (probably formed by glia) later become occupied by axons as though glia form channels through which axons grow and regenerate. Thus, it is possible that, if glia lose their capacity to form channels, regeneration is no longer enhanced, since these same glia may provide signals which direct and promote growth (Simpson, 1968; Nordlander & Singer, 1978; Singer et al., 1979). Similar spaces formed by glia exist in the chick and mammalian embryo (Letourneau, 1975; Egar & Singer, 1977; Silver & Sidman, 1980; Silver, 1980; Karyonek & Goldberg, 1980) which later become filled with axons. However, there is no recapitulation of embryonic status after injury to the adult mammalian CNS (Gearhart et al., 1979).

Of course, substrate compatibility and GF elaboration are related phenomena. The GF hypothesis states that all axon species have unique GFs, like nerve growth factor (NGF) for the MA system. GFs are present in the embryo but either disappear as the animal grows or their potency is masked by some substance released from degenerating CNS. It is possible that the success of MA fibre growth after injury is related to the availability of NGF in CNS. Although medio-dorsal cells in dorsal root ganglia (DRG) respond to NGF soon after formation in chicks (Riopelle & Cameron, 1981), there is no evidence that developing central MA fibres are stimulated by NGF, or fail to develop in the presence of anti-NGF antibody (Björklund, Bjerre & Wiklund, 1975; Konkol et al., 1978; Levi-Montalcini, 1975; Olson & Seiger, 1976; Olson, Ebendal & Seiger, 1979). Nonetheless, NGF may play a trophic role during regeneration of MA fibres in adults (Björklund & Stenevi, 1979a). Small concentrations of NGF are found in mouse CNS (Hendry, 1972; Johnsson, Gordon & Kopin, 1971), embryonic chick and rat brain (Frazier et al., 1974; Greene, 1977; Benowitz & Shashoua, 1979; Riopelle & Cameron, 1981), and in the CNS of fish (Benowitz & Shashoua, 1979). In fish, NGF is probably contained exclusively within astrocytes in periventricular regions and the possibility that NGF (or NGF-like agents) might be contained in glia in birds and mammals is supported by findings that the protein is synthesised in the appropriate glial cultures (Varon, 1975; Ebendal & Jacobson, 1975; Murphy et al., 1977). Moreover, astrocytes in vitro will support NGF-dependent (medio-dorsal DRG) and NGF-independent (ventro-lateral DRGs and nodose ganglion) cells, indicating that the same or different species of astrocyte are elaborating several trophic proteins including NGF (Lindsay, 1979).

It thus seems reasonable to suggest that the success of regeneration in the CNS is related to the availability of specific GFs for different types of axon. Growth might fail if such factors were rendered inactive by substances released from damaged brain tissue or if the products of autolysis competed for specific GF high affinity binding sites. On the basis of these arguments it is difficult, at first sight, to understand why regenerating medio-dorsal NGF-dependent DRG axons fail to penetrate the root–cord junction and yet poisoned MA axons regenerate. One explanation may be that it is degenerating central (oligodendrocyte) myelin which provides the axonal growth inhibitory factors (AGIF: Berry, 1982). Thus, regenerating medio-dorsal DRG axons arrive in the vicinity of high titres of AGIF at the root–cord junction whilst, in the 6-OHDA-treated CNS, no myelin is damaged because this specific neurotoxin affects only MA fibres (which are unmyelinated). As previously mentioned, MA fibres regenerate poorly (if at all) in surgically lesioned CNS where myelinated fibres are also damaged. As Berry (1982) has outlined, the AGIF hypothesis appears to explain much of the phenomenology of CNS regeneration related both to phylogeny and to ontogeny and to all the special cases of successful regeneration in mammals, while also providing ample scope for experimentation.

Work over the past few years has unequivocally demonstrated that CNS neurons are not inherently incapable of growth. Thus, CNS regeneration must either be inhibited by active inhibitory factors released from damaged CNS, or CNS tissue is unable for some reason to produce axonal GFs in adulthood. The possible mechanisms of active inhibition are legion but present technical and experimental expertise offers the means of testing several hypothetical modes of action of AGIF including (*a*) uptake by growth cones with transport to soma and inhibition of GAP production, (*b*) uptake at growth cones and inhibition of microtubule, microfilament and/or membrane assembly, (*c*) competition for GF surface membrane receptors and (*d*) chemical combination with GFs leading to inactivation. The most likely form of AGIF is a peptide released from CNS myelin or oligodendrocytes by autolysis during the post-injury period (Berry, 1982).

REFERENCES

Adams, J. H., Daniel, P. M. & Prichard, M. M. L. (1968). Degeneration and regeneration of hypothalamic nerve fibres in the neurohypophysis after pituitary stalk section in the ferret. *Journal of Comparative Neurology*, **135**, 121–44.

Aguayo, A. J., Bray, G. M., Perkins, C. S. & Duncan, I. D. (1979). Axon-sheath cell interactions in peripheral and central nervous system transplants. *Society of Neuroscience Symposium*, **4**, 361–83.

Aguayo, A. J., David, S., Richardson, P. & Bray, G. M. (1982). Axonal elongation in peripheral and central nervous system transplants. In *Advances in Cellular Neurobiology*, vol. 3, ed. S. Fedoroff & L. Hertz, pp. 215–34. New York: Academic Press.

Aguayo, A. J., Dickson, R., Trecarten, J., Attwell, M., Bray, G. M. & Richardson, P. (1978). Ensheathment and myelination of regenerating PNS fibres by transplanted optic nerve glia. *Neuroscience Letters*, **9**, 97–104.

Allcutt, D. & Berry, M. (1983). Reaction of retinal ganglion cells to optic nerve crush. *Brain Research*, In press.

Baisinger, J., Lund, R. D. & Miller, B. (1977). Aberrant retinothalamic projections resulting from unilateral tectal lesions made in fetal and neonatal rats. *Experimental Neurology*, **54**, 369–82.

Barber, P. C. (1981). Regeneration of vomeronasal nerves into the main olfactory bulb in the mouse. *Brain Research*, **216**, 239–51.

Barber, P. C. (1982). Neurogenesis and regeneration in the primary olfactory pathways of mammals. In *Bibliotheca Anatomica No. 23. Growth and Regeneration of Axons in the Nervous System*, ed. M. Berry, pp. 12–25. Basel: S. Karger.

Barber, P. C. & Raisman, G. (1978). Replacement of receptor neurones after section of the vomeronasal nerves in the adult mouse. *Brain Research*, **147**, 295–313.

Barnard, J. W. & Carpenter, W. (1949). Regeneration in the spinal cord of the rat. *Anatomical Record*, **103**, 422–3.

Barnard, J. W. & Carpenter, W. (1950). Lack of regeneration in the spinal cord of the rat. *Journal of Neurophysiology*, **13**, 223–8.

Beck, E. & Daniel, P. M. (1959*a*). Some changes in the hypothalamus and proximal pituitary stalk after stalk section. *Journal of Physiology*, **146**, 228–48.

Beck, E. & Daniel, P. M. (1959*b*). Changes in the human hypothalamus after pituitary stalk section or hypophysectomy. *Journal of Clinical Pathology*, **12**, 577.

Becker, H. (1952). Zur Faseranatomie des Stamm – und Riechhirns auf Grund von Experimenten aus jugendlichen Tieren. Zugleich ein Beitrag zur Umgestaltung des vor der Reifung Geschadigten Gehirn und zur Agenesiefrage. *Deutsche Zeitschrift für Nervenheilkunde*, **168**, 345–83.

Benes, V. (1968). *Spinal Cord Injury*. London: Baillière, Tindall & Cassell.

Benfey, M. & Aguayo, A. J. (1982). Extensive elongation of axons from rat brain into peripheral nerve grafts. *Nature (London)*, **296**, 150–2.

Benowitz, L. I. & Shashoua, V. E. (1979). Immunoreactive sites for nerve growth factor (NGF) in the goldfish brain. *Brain Research*, **172**, 561–5.

Benowitz, L. I., Shashoua, V. E. & Yoon, M. G. (1981). Specific changes in rapidly transported proteins during regeneration of the goldfish optic nerve. *Journal of Neuroscience*, **1**, 300–7.

Bernstein, D. R., Bechard, D. E. & Stelzner, D. J. (1981). Neuritic growth maintained near the lesion site long after spinal cord transection in the newborn rat. *Neuroscience Letters*, **26**, 55–60.

Bernstein, J. J. (1967). The regenerative capacity of the telencephalon of the goldfish and rat. *Experimental Neurology*, **17**, 44–56.

Bernstein, J. J. & Bernstein, M. E. (1967). Effect of glia–ependymal scar and teflon arrest on the regenerative capacity of goldfish spinal cord. *Experimental Neurology*, **19**, 25–32.

Bernstein, J. J. & Bernstein, M. E. (1969). Ultrastructure of normal regeneration and loss of regenerative capacity following teflon blockade in goldfish spinal cord. *Experimental Neurology*, **24**, 538–57.

Bernstein, J. J. & Bernstein, M. E. (1971). Axonal regeneration and formation of synapses proximal to the site of lesion following hemisection of the rat spinal cord. *Experimental Neurology*, **30**, 336–51.

Bernstein, M. E. & Bernstein, J. J. (1973a). Regeneration of axons and synaptic complex formation rostral to the site of hemisection in the spinal cord of the monkey. *International Journal of Neuroscience*, **5**, 15–36.

Bernstein, J. J. & Bernstein, M. E. (1973b). Neural alteration and reinnervation following axonal regeneration and sprouting in mammalian cord, *Brain, Behaviour and Evolution*, **8**, 135–61.

Bernstein, J. J., Gelderd, J. B. & Bernstein, M. E. (1974). Alteration in neuronal synaptic complement during regeneration and axonal sprouting of rat spinal cord. *Experimental Neurology*, **44**, 470–82.

Bernstein, J. J. & Goodman, D. C. (1973). Neuromorphological plasticity. *Brain, Behaviour and Evolution*, **8**, 1–164.

Bernstein, J. J., Wells, M. R. & Bernstein, M. E. (1975). Dendrites and neuroglia following hemisection of rat spinal cord: effects of puromycin. In *Physiology and Pathology of Dendrites*, ed. G. W. Kreutzberg, pp. 439–52. New York: Raven Press.

Berry, M. (1979). Regeneration in the central nervous system. In *Recent Advances in Neuropathology* vol. 1, ed. W. Thomas Smith & J. B. Cavanagh, pp. 67–111. Edinburgh: Churchill Livingstone.

Berry, M. (1982). Post-injury myelin-breakdown products inhibit axonal growth: An hypothesis to explain the failure of axonal regeneration in the mammalian central nervous system. In *Bibliotheca Anatomica No. 23. Growth and Regeneration of Axons in the Nervous System*, ed. M. Berry, pp. 1–11. Basel: S. Karger.

Berry, M. & Henry, J. (1976). Response of the neonatal central nervous system to injury. *Neuropathology and Applied Neurobiology*, **2**, 377–88.

Berry, M., Knowles, J., Willis, P., Riches, A. C., Morgans, G. P. & Steers, D. (1979a). A reappraisal of the effects of ACTH on the response of the central nervous system to injury. *Journal of Anatomy*, **128**, 859–71.

Berry, M., Maxwell, W., Mathewson, A., McConnell, P., Logan, A., Thomas, G. & Ashurst, D. (1983). Reaction of the central nervous system to injury. *Acta Neurochirurgica*, in press.

Berry, M. & Riches, A. C. (1974). An immunological approach to regeneration in the central nervous system. *British Medical Bulletin*, **30**, 135–40.

Berry, M., Riches, A. C., Knowles, J., Willis, P. & Steers, D. (1979b). Failure of central axonal regeneration after immunosuppressive treatment. *Journal of Anatomy*, **129**, 243–56.

Bignami, A. & Dahl, D. (1976). The astroglial response to stabbing. Immunofluorescence studies with antibodies to astrocyte specific protein (GFA) in mammalian and submammalian vertebrates. *Neuropathology and Applied Neurology*, **2**, 99–110.

Björklund, A., Bjerre, B. & Wiklund, L. (1975). NGF in maintenance and regeneration of adrenergic axons. In *Proceedings of 6th International Congress of Pharmacology, Neurotransmission*, vol. 2, ed. L. Ahtee, pp. 259–74. Oxford: Pergamon Press.

Björklund, A., Dunnett, S. B., Stenevi, V., Lewis, M. E. & Iversen, S. D. (1980). Reinnervation of the denervated striatum by substantia nigra transplants: functional consequences as revealed by pharmacological sensorimotor testing. *Brain Research*, **199**, 307–33.

Björklund, A., Johansson, B., Stenevi, V. & Svendgaard, N.-A. (1975). Reestablishment of functional connections by regenerating adrenergic and cholinergic axons. *Nature (London)*, **253**, 446–8.

Björklund, A., Katzman, R., Stenevi, V. & West, K. A. (1971). Development and growth of axonal sprouts from noradrenaline and 5-hydroxytryptamine neurones in the rat spinal cord. *Brain Research*, **31**, 1–20.

Björklund, A., Noblin, A. & Stenevi, V. (1973). Regeneration of central serotonin neurons after axonal degeneration induced by 5,6-hydroxytryptamine. *Brain Research*, **50**, 214–20.

Björklund, A., Segal, M. & Stenevi, V. (1979). Functional reinnervation of rat hippocampus by locus coeruleus implants. *Brain Research*, **170**, 409–26.

Björklund, A. & Stenevi, V. (1977). Reformation of the severed septohippocampal cholinergic pathway in the adult rat by transplanted septal neurons. *Cell and Tissue Research*, **185**, 289–302.

Björklund, A. & Stenevi, V. (1979a). Regeneration of monoaminergic and cholinergic neurons in the mammalian central nervous system. *Physiological Reviews*, **59**, 62–100.

Björklund, A. & Stenevi, V. (1979b). Reconstruction of the nigrostriatal dopamine pathway by intra-cerebral nigral transplants. *Brain Research*, **177**, 555–60.

Björklund, A., Stenevi, V., Dunnett, S. B. & Iversen, S. D. (1981). Functional reactivation of the deafferented neostriatum by nigral transplants. *Nature (London)*, **289**, 497–9.

Björklund, A., Stenevi, V. & Svendgaard, N.-A. (1976). Growth of transplanted monoaminergic neurones into the adult hippocampus along the perforant path. *Nature (London)*, **262**, 787–91.

Bohn, R. C. & Stelzner, D. J. (1979). Aberrant retino-retinal pathway during early stages of regeneration in adult *Rana pipiens*. *Brain Research*, **160**, 139–44.

Bourre, J. M., Jacque, C., Delassalle, A., Nguyen-Legros, J., Dumont, O., Lachapelle, F., Raoul, M., Alvarez, C. & Baumann, N. (1980). Density profile and basic protein measurement in the myelin range of particulate material from normal developing mouse brain and from neurological mutants (Jimpy, Quaking, Trembler, Shiverer and its mld allele) obtained by zonal centrifugation. *Journal of Neuro-chemistry*, **35**, 458–64.

Bray, D., Thomas, C. & Shaw, G. (1978). Growth cone formation in cultures of sensory neurons. *Proceedings of the National Academy of Sciences, USA*, **75**, 5226–9.

Brock, T. O. (1978). The effect of repeated nerve injury on regenerative repair in the optic nerve of the newt *Triturus viridescens*. *Anatomical Record*, **190**, 349.

Brodal, A., (1940). Modification of the Gudden method for study of cerebral localisation. *Archives of Neurology and Psychiatry*, **43**, 46–58.

Brostoff, S. W., Sachs, H. & Di Paola, C. (1975). The P1 protein of bovine root myelin, partial chemical characterisation. *Journal of Neurochemistry*, **24**, 289–94.

Brown, J. O. & McCouch, G. P. (1949). Abortive regeneration of the transected spinal cord. *Journal of Comparative Neurology*, **87**, 131–7.

Castro, A. J. (1978a). Projections of the superior cerebellar peduncle in rats and the development of new connections in response to neonatal hemicerebellectomy. *Journal of Comparative Neurology*, **178**, 611–28.

Castro, A. J. (1978b). Analysis of corticospinal and rubrospinal projections after neonatal pyramidotomy in rats. *Brain Research*, **144**, 155–8.

Chambers, W. W. (1955). Structural regeneration in mammalian central nervous system in relation to age. In *Regeneration in the Central Nervous System*, ed. W. F. Windle, pp. 135–46. Springfield, Illinois: Charles C. Thomas.

Chi, N. N., Bignami, A., Bich, N. T. & Dahl, D. (1980). Autologous sciatic nerve grafts to the rat spinal cord: Immunofluorescence studies with neurofilament and gliofilament (GFA) antisera. *Experimental Neurology*, **68**, 568–80.

Clark, W. E. Le Gros (1942). The problem of neuronal regeneration in the central nervous system. I. The influence of spinal ganglia and nerve fragments grafted in the brain. *Journal of Anatomy*, **77**, 20–48.

Clark, W. E. Le Gros (1943). The problem of neuronal regeneration in the central nervous system. II. The insertion of peripheral nerve stumps into the brain. *Journal of Anatomy*, **77**, 251–9.

Clearwaters, K. P. (1954). Regeneration of the spinal cord of the chick. *Journal of Comparative Neurology*, **101**, 317–29.

Clemente, C. D. (1955). Structural regeneration in the mammalian central nervous system and the role of neuroglia and connective tissue. In *Regeneration in the Central Nervous System*, ed. W. F. Windle, pp. 147–61. Springfield, Illinois: Charles C. Thomas.

Clemente, C. D. (1964). Regeneration in the vertebrate central nervous system. *International Review of Biology*, **6**, 257–301.

Cox, V. S. (1976). Ultrastructure of the axon reaction in the immature rat thalamus. *Journal of Neuropathology and Experimental Neurology*, **35**, 191–203.

Cummings, J. P., Bernstein, D. R. & Stelzner, D. J. (1981). Further evidence that sparing of function after spinal cord transection in the neonatal rat is not due to axonal generation or regeneration. *Experimental Neurology*, **74**, 615–20.

D'Amato, C. J. & Hicks, S. P. (1978). Normal development and post-traumatic plasticity of corticospinal neurons in rats. *Experimental Neurology*, **60**, 557–69.

Daniels, M. P. (1972). Colchicine inhibition of nerve fibre formation *in vitro*. *Journal of Cell Biology*, **53**, 164–76.

David, S. & Aguayo, A. J. (1981). Axonal elongation into peripheral nervous system bridges after central nervous system injury in adult rats. *Science*, **214**, 931–3.

Dellman, H.-D. (1973). Degeneration and regeneration of neurosectory systems. *International Review of Cytology*, **36**, 215–315.

De Meyer, W. E. (1967). Development of axonal pathway after neurosurgical lesions in the septum of the fetal rat: fornix ventralis, corpus callosum and anterior commissure. In *Biological and Environmental Determinants of Early Development*, ed. J. I. Nurnberge, pp. 269–80. Baltimore: Williams and Wilkins.

Devor, M. (1976). Neuroplasticity on the rearrrangement of olfactory tract fibres after neonatal transection on hamsters. *Journal of Comparative Neurology*, **166**, 49–72.

Devor, M. & Schneider, G. E. (1975). Neuroanatomical plasticity: the principle of conservation of total axonal arborization. In *Aspects of Neural Plasticity*, ed. F. Vital-Durand & M. Jeannrod, pp. 191–201. Paris: INSERM.

Druckman, R. & Mair, W. G. P. (1953). Aberrant regenerating nerve fibres in injury to the spinal cord. *Brain*, **76**, 448–54.

Dunn, E. H. (1917). Primary and secondary findings in a series of attempts to transplant cerebral cortex in the albino rat. *Journal of Comparative Neurology*, **27**, 565–82.

Dunnett, S. B., Björklund, A., Stenevi, V. & Iversen, S. D. (1981). Behavioural recovery following transplantation of substantia nigra in rats subjected to 6-OHDA lesions of the nigrostriatal pathway. II. Bilateral lesions. *Brain Research*, **229**, 457–70.

Du Povey, P., Jacque, C., Bourre, J. M., Cesselin, F., Privat, A. & Baumann, N. (1979). Immunochemical studies of myelin basic protein in shiverer mouse devoid of major dense line of myelin. *Neuroscience Letters*, **12**, 113–18.

Ebendal, T. & Jacobson, C. A. (1975). Human glial cells stimulating outgrowth of axons in cultured chick embryo ganglia. *Zoon*, **3**, 169–72.

Edwards, D. L., Alpert, R. M. & Grafstein, B. (1981). Recovery of vision in regeneration of goldfish optic axons: enhancement of axonal outgrowth by a conditioning lesion. *Experimental Neurology*, **72**, 672–86.

Egar, M., Simpson, S. B. & Singer, M. (1970). The growth and differentiation of the regenerating spinal cord of the lizard, *Anolis carolineus*. *Journal of Morphology*, **131**, 131–52.

Egar, M. & Singer, M. (1972). The role of ependyma in spinal cord regeneration in a Urodele, *Triturus*. *Experimental Neurology*, **37**, 422–30.

Egar, M. & Singer, M. (1977). Interependyma channels and cell death in normal development of chick hindbrain. *Anatomical Record*, **187**, 573–4.

Feigin, I., Geller, E. H. & Wolf, A. (1951). Absence of regeneration in the spinal cord of the young rat. *Journal of Neuropathology and Experimental Neurology*, **10**, 420–5.

Feringa, E. R., Kinning, W. K., Britten, A. G. & Vahesing, H. L. (1976). Recovery in rats after spinal cord injury. *Neurology*, **26**, 839–43.

Feringa, E. R., Randall, D. J. & Wendt, J. S. (1975). Spinal cord regeneration in rats after immunosuppressive treatment. Theoretical consideration and histologic results. *Archives of Neurology*, **32**, 676–83.

Frazier, W. A., Boyd, L. F., Pulliam, M. W., Szutowicz, A. & Bradshaw, A. E. A. (1974). Properties and specificity of binding sites for ^{125}I-nerve growth factor in embryonic heart and brain. *Journal of Biological Chemistry*, **249**, 5918–23.

Freeman, I. W. (1955). Functional recovery in spinal rats. In *Regeneration in the Central Nervous System*, ed. W. F. Windle, pp. 195–207. Springfield, Illinois: Charles C. Thomas.

Frost, D. O. & Schneider, G. E. (1979). Plasticity of the retinotectal projections after partial lesions of the retina in newborn Syrian hamsters. *Journal of Comparative Neurology*, **185**, 517–68.

Frotscher, M., Buch, E., Mannsfeld, B. & Wenzel, J. (1970). Zur Regeneration des Cortex cerebri nach Replantation eines Cortexabschnittes bei *Rattus norvegicus*. *Journal für Hirnforschung*, **12**, 123–33.

Gamble, H. J. (1976). Spinal and cranial nerve roots. In *The Peripheral Nerve*, ed. J. Landon, p. 330. London: Chapman & Hall.

Gaze, R. M. (1960). Regeneration of the optic nerve in amphibia. *International Review of Neurology*, **2**, 1–40.

Gaze, R. M. (1970). *The Formation of Nerve Connections*. London & New York: Academic Press.

Gearhart, J., Oster-Granite, M. L. & Guth, L. (1979). Histological and functional changes after transection of the spinal cord of fetal and neonatal mice. *Experimental Neurology*, **66**, 1–15.

Gerard, R. W. & Grinker, R. R. (1931). Regenerative possibilities of the central nervous system. *Archives of Neurology and Psychiatry*, **26**, 469–84.

Gerard, R. W. & Koppanyi, T. (1926). Studies on spinal cord regeneration in the rat. *American Journal of Physiology*, **76**, 214–42.

Gilad, G. M., Gilad, V. H. & Kopin, I. J. (1979). Reaction of the mutant mouse nude to axonal injuries to the central nervous system. *Experimental Neurology*, **65**, 87–98.

Gilson, B. C. & Stensaas, L. J. (1974). Early axonal chewing following lesions of the dorsal columns in rats. *Cell and Tissue Research*, **149**, 1–20.

Goldberg, S. (1976). Central nervous system regeneration and ophthalmology. *Survey of Ophthalmology*, **20**, 261–72.

Goldberg, S. (1977). Unidirectional, bidirectional and random growth of embryonic optic axons. *Experimental Eye Research*, **25**, 399–404.

Goldberg, S. & Frank, B. (1979). The guidance of optic axons in the developing and adult mouse retina. *Anatomical Record*, **193**, 763–74.

Goldberg, S. & Frank, B. (1980). Will central nervous systems in the adult mammal regenerate after bypassing a lesion? A study in the mouse and chick visual system. *Experimental Neurology*, **70**, 675–89.

Goldberg, S. & Frank, B. (1981). Do young axons regenerate better than old axons? *Experimental Neurology*, **74**, 245–59.

Gospodarowicz, D. (1974). Localisation of a fibroblast growth factor and its effect alone and with hydrocortisone on 3T3 cell growth. *Nature (London)*, **249**, 123–7.

Graziadei, P. P. C., Levine, R. R. & Monti Graziadei, G. A. (1979). Plasticity of connections of the olfactory sensory neuron: regeneration into the forebrain following bulbectomy in the neonatal mouse. *Neuroscience*, **4**, 713–27.

Graziadei, P. P. C. & Samanen, D. W. (1980). Ectopic glomerular structures in the olfactory bulb of neonatal and adult mice. *Brain Research*, **187**, 467–72.

Greene, L. A. (1977). A convenient and sensitive quantitative bioassay for nerve growth factor NGF activity employing a clonal pheochromocytoma cell line. *Brain Research*, **133**, 350–3.

Guillery, R. W. (1972). Experiments to determine whether retino-geniculate axons can form trans-laminar collateral sprouts in the dorsal lateral geniculate nucleus of the cat. *Journal of Comparative Neurology*, **146**, 407–20.

Hamburger, V. (1955). Regeneration in the central nervous system of reptiles and of birds. In *Regeneration in the Central Nervous System*, ed. W. F. Windle, pp. 47–53. Springfield, Illinois: Charles C. Thomas.

Heinicke, E. A. (1980). Vascular permeability and axonal regeneration in tissues autotransplanted into the brain. *Acta Neuropathologica*, **49**, 177–85.

Heinicke, E. A. & Kiernan, J. A. (1978). Vascular permeability and axonal regeneration in skin autotransplanted into the brain. *Journal of Anatomy*, **125**, 409–20.

Hendry, I. A. (1972). Developmental changes in tissue and plasma concentrations of the biologically active species of nerve growth factor in the mouse by using a two-site radioimmunoassay. *Biochemical Journal*, **128**, 1265–72.

Hess, A. (1955). Discussion of failure of regeneration in the mammalian fetus. In *Regeneration in the Central Nervous System*. ed. W. F. Windle, pp. 176–8. Springfield, Illinois: Charles C. Thomas.

Hess, A. (1956). Reactions of mammalian fetal spinal cord, spinal ganglia and brain to injury. *Journal of Experimental Zoology*, **132**, 349–74.

Hess, A. (1957). The experimental embryology of the foetal nervous system. *Biological Reviews*, ·**32**, 231–60.

Hibbard, E. (1963). Regeneration in the severed spinal cord of chordate larvae of *Petromyzon marinus*. *Experimental Neurology*, **7**, 175–85.

Hibbard, E. & Ornberg, R. L. (1976). Restoration of vision in genetically eyeless axolotls (*Ambystoma mexicanum*). *Experimental Neurology*, **50**, 113–23.

Hicks, S. P. & D'Amato, C. J. (1975). Motor-sensory cortex–corticospinal system and developing locomotion and placing in rats. *American Journal of Anatomy*, **143**, 1–42.

Holmes, R. L. (1963). Regeneration of hypothalamo-neurohypophyseal nerve fibres after pituitary stalk section. *Journal of Anatomy*, **97**, 310.

Hooker, D. (1932). Spinal cord regeneration in the young rainbow fish, *Lebistes reticulatus*. *Journal of Comparative Neurology*, **56**, 277–97.

Hooker, D. & Nicholas, J. S. (1927). The effect of injury to the spinal cord of rats in prenatal stages. *American Journal of Physiology*, **81**, 503.

Hooker, D. & Nicholas, J. S. (1930). Spinal cord section in rat fetuses. *Journal of Comparative Neurology*, **50**, 413–67.

Hughes, A. (1953). The growth of embryonic neurites. A study on cultures of chick neural tissues. *Journal of Anatomy*, **87**, 150–62.

Iacovitti, L., Reis, D. J. & Joh, T. H. (1981). Reactive proliferation of brain stem noradrenergic nerves following neonatal cerebellectomy in rats: role of target maturation on neuronal response to injury during development. *Developmental Brain Research*, **1**, 3–24.

Jakoby, R. K., Turbes, C. C. & Freeman, L. W. (1960). The problem of neuronal regeneration in the central nervous system. I. The insertion of centrally connected peripheral nerve stumps into the spinal cord. *Journal of Neurosurgery*, **17**, 385–93.

Johnsson, D. G., Gordon, R. & Kopin, I. J. (1971). A sensitive radioimmunoassay for 75 nerve growth factor antigens in serum and tissue. *Journal of Neurochemistry*, **18**, 2355–62.

Jonsson, G. & Hallman, H. (1982). Response of central monoamine neurons following an early neurotoxic lesion. In *Bibliotheca Anatomica. No. 23. Growth and Regeneration of Axons in the Nervous System*, ed. M. Berry, pp. 76–92. Basel: S. Karger.

Kalil, D. & Reh, T. (1979). Regrowth of severed axons in the neonatal central nervous system: establishment of normal connections. *Science*, **205**, 1158–61.

Kao, C. C. (1974). Comparison of healing process in transected spinal cords grafted with autogenous brain tissue, sciatic nerve and nodose ganglion. *Experimental Neurology*, **44**, 424–39.

Kao, C. C., Chang, L. W. & Bloodworth, J. M. B. (1977a). Electron microscopic observations of the mechanisms of terminal club formation in transected spinal cord axons. *Journal of Neuropathology and Experimental Neurology*, **36**, 140–56.

Kao, C. C., Chang, L. W. & Bloodworth, J. M. B. (1977b). Axonal regeneration across transected mammalian spinal cord. An electron microscopic study of delay microsurgical nerve grafting. *Experimental Neurology*, **54**, 591–615.

Kao, C. C., Shimizu, Y., Perkins, L. C. & Freeman, L. W. (1970). Experimental use of cultured cerebellar cortical tissue to inhibit the collagenous scar following spinal cord transection. *Journal of Neurosurgery*, **33**, 127–39.

Karyonek, S. R. & Goldberg, S. (1980). Preneural pathways in the embryonic chick retina. *Society of Neuroscience Abstracts*, **6**, 488.

Katzman, R., Björklund, A., Owman, C. H., Stenevi, V. & West, K. A. (1971). Evidence for regenerative axon sprouting in central catecholamine neurons in the rat mesencephalon following electrolytic lesions. *Brain Research*, **25**, 579–96.

Kiernan, J. A. (1971). Pituicytes and the regenerative properties of neurosecretory and other axons in the rat. *Journal of Anatomy*, **109**, 97–114.

Kiernan, J. A. (1978). An explanation of axonal regeneration in peripheral nerves and its failure in the central nervous system. *Medical Hypotheses*, **4**, 15–26.

Kiernan, J. A. (1979). Hypotheses concerned with axonal regeneration in the mammalian nervous system. *Biological Reviews*, **54**, 155–97.

Kiernan, J. A. & Contestabile, A. (1980). Vascular permeability associated with axonal regeneration in the optic system of goldfish. *Acta Neuropathologica*, **51**, 39–45.

Kimmel, D. L. & Moyer, E. K. (1947). Dorsal roots following anastomosis of the central stumps. *Journal of Comparative Neurology*, **87**, 289–319.

Knowles, J. F. & Berry, M. (1978). Effects of deoxycorticosterone acetate on regeneration of axons in the mammalian central nervous system. *Experimental Neurology*, **62**, 1–15.

Konkol, R. J., Mailman, R. B., Bendeich, E. G., Garrison, A. M., Mueller, R. A. & Breese, G. R. (1978). Evaluation of the effects of nerve growth factor and anti-nerve growth factor on the development of central catecholamine-containing neurons. *Brain Research*, **144**, 277–85.

Koppanyi, T. (1955). Regeneration in the central nervous system of fishes. In *Regeneration in the Central Nervous System*, ed. W. F. Windle, pp. 3–19. Springfield, Illinois: Charles C. Thomas.

Krikorian, J. G., Guth, L. & Donati, E. J. (1981). Origin of the connective tissue scar in the transected rat spinal cord. *Experimental Neurology*, **72**, 698–707.

Lampert, P. & Cressman, M. (1964). Axonal regeneration in the dorsal columns of the spinal cord of adult rats – an electron microscopic study. *Laboratory Investigation*, **13**, 825–39.

Lanniers, H. N. & Grafstein, B. (1980). Effect of a conditioning lesion on regeneration of goldfish optic axons: ultrastructural evidence of enhanced outgrowth and pinocytosis. *Brain Research*, **196**, 547–53.

Leong, S. K. & Lund, R. D. (1973). Anomalous bilateral corticofugal pathways in albino rats after neonatal lesions. *Brain Research*, **62**, 218–221.

Letourneau, D. C. (1975). Cell-to-substratum adhesion and guidance of axonal elongation. *Developmental Biology*, **44**, 92–101.

Levi, G. (1926). Ricerche sperimentali soora elementi nervosi sviluppati 'in vitro'. *Archiv für experimentalen Zellforschung*. **2**, 244–72.

Levi, G. & Meyer, H. (1945). Reactive, regressive and regenerative processes of neurons cultivated *in vitro* and injured with the micromanipulator. *Journal of Experimental Zoology*, **99**, 141–81.

Levi-Montalcini, R. (1975). Milestones, answered questions and current studies on nerve growth factor. In *Proceedings of 6th International Congress of Pharmacology, Neurotransmission*, vol. 2, ed. A. Ahtee, pp. 221–30. Oxford: Pergamon Press.

Levine, J., Skene, P. & Willard, M. (1981). GAPs and fodin. Novel axonally transported proteins. *Trends in Neurosciences*, **4**, 273–6.

Lieberman, A. R. (1971). The axon reaction: a review of the principal features of perikaryal responses to axon injury. *International Review of Neurobiology*, **14**, 49–124.

Lindsay, R. M. (1979). Adult rat brain astrocytes support survival of both NGF-dependent and NGF-insensitive neurones. *Nature (London)*, **282**, 80–2.

Lugaro, E. (1906). Sulla presenta rigenerazione autogena delle radici posteriori. *Revisti di patologia nervosa e mentale*, **11**, 337–40.

McConnell, P. & Berry, M. (1982a). Regeneration of axons in the mouse retina after injury. In *Bibliotheca Anatomica No. 23. Growth and Regeneration of Axons in the Nervous System*, ed. M. Berry, pp. 26–37. Basel: S. Karger.

McConnell, P. & Berry, M. (1982b). Regeneration of ganglion cell axons in the adult mouse retina. *Brain Research*, **241**, 362–5.

McCouch, G. P. (1955). Comments on regeneration of functional connections. In *Regeneration in the Central Nervous System*, ed. W. F. Windle, pp. 171–5. Springfield, Illinois: Charles C. Thomas.

Matthieu, J.-M., Ginalski, H., Friede, R. L. & Cohen, S. R. (1980). Low myelin basic protein levels and normal myelin in peripheral nerves of myelin deficient mice (MLD). *Neuroscience*, **5**, 2315–20.

Mervart, M. & Kiernan, J. A. (1978). Axonal regeneration in experimental allergic peripheral neuritis. *Acta Neuropathologica*, **41**, 197–200.

Mikoshiba, K., Aoki, E. & Tsukada, Y. (1980). 2^1–3^1–cyclic nucleotide 3^1–phosphohydrolase activity in the central nervous system of a myelin deficient mutant (Shiverer). *Brain Research*, **192**, 195–204.

Moore, R. Y., Björklund, A. & Stenevi, V. (1971). Plastic changes in the adrenergic innervation of the rat septal area in response to denervation. *Brain Research*, **33**, 13–35.

Moyer, E. K., Kimmel, D. L. & Winborne, L. W. (1953). Regeneration of sensory nerve roots in young and in senile rats. *Journal of Comparative Neurology*, **98**, 283–308.

Murphy, R. A., Oger, J., Saide, J. D., Blanchard, M. H., Arnason, B. G. W., Hogan, C., Pantazis, N. J. & Young, M. (1977). Secretion of nerve growth factor by central nervous system glioma cells in culture. *Journal of Cell Biology*, **72**, 769–73.

Nordlander, R. H. & Singer, M. (1978). The role of ependyma in regeneration of the spinal cord in the Urodele amphibian tail. *Journal of Comparative Neurology*, **180**, 349–74.

Nordlander, R. H. & Singer, M. (1982). Spaces precede axons in *Xenopus* embryonic spinal cord. *Experimental Neurology*, **75**, 221–8.

Olson, L., Ebendal, T. & Seiger, A. (1979). NGF and anti-NGF: evidence against effects of fiber growth in locus coeruleus from cultures in perinatal CNS tissues. *Developmental Neuroscience*, **2**, 160–76.

Olson, L. & Seiger, A. (1976). Locus coeruleus: fibre growth regulation *in oculo*. *Medical Biology*, **54**, 142–5.

Paskind, H. A. (1936). Regeneration of posterior root fibres in cat. *Archives of Neurology and Psychiatry*, **36**, 1077–84.

Penfield, W. (1927). The mechanism of cicatrical contraction in the brain. *Brain*, **50**, 499–517.

Perkins, L., Babbini, A. & Freeman, L. W. (1964). Distal–proximal nerve implants in spinal cord transection. *Neurology*, **14**, 949–54.

Perlow, M. J., Freed, W. J., Hoffer, B. J., Seiger, A., Olson, L. & Wyatt, R. J. (1979). Brain grafts reduce motor abnormalities produced by destruction of nigrostriated dopamine system. *Science*, **204**, 643–7.

Pickel, V. M., Krebs, H. & Bloom, F. E. (1973). Proliferation of norepinephrine-containing axons in rat cerebellar cortex after peduncle lesions. *Brain Research*, **59**, 169–79.

Pickel, V. M., Segal, M. & Bloom, F. E. (1974). Axonal proliferation following lesions of cerebellar peduncles. A combined fluorescence microscopic and radioautographic study. *Journal of Comparative Neurology*, **155**, 43–60.

Prendergast, J. & Misantone, L. J. (1980). Sprouting by tracts descending from the midbrain to the spinal cord: the result of thoracic funiculotomy in the newborn, 21-day-old, and adult rat. *Experimental Neurology*, **69**, 458–80.

Prendergast, J. & Stelzner, D. J. (1976a). Increases in collateral axonal growth rostral to a thoracic hemisection in neonatal and weanling rat. *Journal of Comparative Neurology*, **166**, 145–62.

Prendergast, J. & Stelzner, D. J. (1976b). Changes in the magnocellular portion of the red nucleus following thoracic hemisection in the neonatal and adult rat. *Journal of Comparative Neurology*, **166**, 163–72.

Raisman, G. & Field, P. M. (1973). A quantitative investigation of the development of collateral reinnervation after partial deafferentation of the septal nuclei. *Brain Research*, **50**, 241–64.

Ramon y Cajal, S. (1928). *Degeneration and Regeneration in the Nervous System*. London: Oxford University Press.

Ranson, S. W. (1903). On the medullated nerve fibres crossing the site of lesions in the brain of the white rat. *Journal of Comparative Neurology*, **13**, 185–207.

Reh, T. & Kalil, K. (1981). Development of the pyramidal tract in the hamster. I. A light microscopic study. *Journal of Comparative Neurology*, **200**, 55–67.

Reh, T. & Kalil, K. (1982). Development of the pyramidal tract in the hamster. II. An electron microscopic study. *Journal of Comparative Neurology*, **205**, 77–88.

Reier, P. J. (1979). Penetration of grafted astrocytic scars by regenerating optic nerve axons in *Xenopus* tadpoles. *Brain Research*, **164**, 61–8.

Reinis, S. (1965). Contribution to the problem of the regeneration of nerve fibres in the central nervous system after operative damage in the early postnatal period. *Acta Anatomica*, **60**, 165–80.

Reis, D. J., Ross, R. A., Iacovitti, L., Gilad, G. & Joh, T. H. (1981). Changes in neurotransmitter synthesising enzymes during regenerative, compensatory and collateral sprouting of central catecholamine neurons in adult and developing rats. In *Lesion-induced Plasticity in Sensorimotor Systems*, ed. J. Flodar and W. Precht. pp. 87–102. Berlin: Springer.

Richardson, P. M., McGuiness, V. M. & Aguayo, A. J. (1980). Axons from CNS neurones regenerate into PNS grafts. *Nature (London)*, **284**, 264–5.

Riopelle, R. J. & Cameron, D. A. (1981). Neurite growth promoting factors of embryonic chick – ontogeny, regional distribution, and characteristics. *Journal of Neurobiology*, **12**, 175–86.

Robinson, R. G., Bloom, F. E. & Battenberg, E. L. F. (1977). A fluorescent histochemical study of changes in noradrenergic neurons following experimental cerebral infarction in the rat. *Brain Research*, **132**, 259–72.

Rothballer, A. B. & Skoryna, S. C. (1960). Morphological effects of pituitary stalk section in the dog, with particular reference to neurosecretory material. *Anatomical Record*, **136**, 5–25.

Rubel, E. W., Smith, Z. D. J. & Steward, O. (1981). Sprouting in the avian brainstem auditory pathway: dependence on dendritic integrity. *Journal of Comparative Neurology*, **203**, 397–414.

Sager, O. & Marcovici, G. (1972). Regeneration in the central nervous system. *Review of Roumanian Neurology*, **9**, 23–9.

Scharrer, E. A. & Wittenstein, G. J. (1952). The effect of the interruption of the hypothalamo-hypophyseal neurosecretory pathway in the dog. *Anatomical Record*, **112**, 387.

Schmidt, R. H. & Bhatnagar, R. K. (1979a). Regional development of norepinephrine, dopamine-β-hydroxylase and tyrosine hydroxylase in the rat brain subsequent to neonatal treatment with subcutaneous 6-hydroxydopamine. *Brain Research*, **166**, 293–308.

Schmidt, R. H. & Bhatnagar, R. K. (1979b). Assessment of the effects of neonatal subcutaneous 6-hydroxydopamine on noradrenergic and dopaminergic innervation of the cerebral cortex. *Brain Research*, **166**, 309–19.

Schmidt, R. H. & Bhatnagar, R. K. (1979c). Distribution of hypertrophied locus coeruleus projections to adult cerebellum after neonatal 6-hydroxydopamine. *Brain Research*, **172**, 23–33.

Schmidt, R. H. & Bhatnagar, R. K. (1979d). Critical periods for noradrenergic regeneration in rat brain regions following neonatal subcutaneous 6-hydroxydopamine. *Life Science*, **25**, 1641–50.

Schmidt, R. H., Björklund, A. & Loren, I. (1981). Neuron–target interactions in the development of central catecholamine systems. In *Development of the Nervous System*, ed. D. R. Garrod & J. D. Feldman, pp. 85–106. Cambridge University Press.

Schmidt, R. H., Kasik, S. A. & Bhatnagar, R. K. (1980). Regenerative critical periods for locus coeruleus in postnatal rat pups following intracisternal 6–hydroxydopamine: a model for noradrenergic development. *Brain Research*, **191**, 173–90.

Schneider, G. E. (1970). Mechanisms of functional recovery following lesions of visual cortex or superior colliculus in neonate and adult hamsters. *Brain, Behavior and Evolution*, **3**, 295–323.

Schneider, G. E. (1973). Early lesions of superior colliculus: factors affecting the formation of abnormal retinal projections. *Brain, Behavior and Evolution*, **8**, 73–109.

Schönheit, B. (1968). Weitere Centersuchungen zur Regeneration des Riickenmorphia bei *Rana esculenta* L. und *Rana temporaria* L. *Zeitschrift für microskopische–anatomische Forschung*, **78**, 557–96.

Scott, T. M. & Mathewson, A. J. (1979). Scar formation during regeneration of the central nervous system. *Journal of Anatomy*, **129**, 222–3.

Sechzer, J. A. (1974). Axonal regeneration or generation after corpus callosum section in the neonatal rat. *Experimental Neurology*, **45**, 186–8.

Shaw, G. & Bray, D. (1977). Movement and extension of isolated growth cones. *Experimental Cell Research*, **104**, 55–62.

Sievers, J. & Klemm, H. P. (1982). Locus coeruleus–cerebellum: interaction during development. In *Bibliotheca Anatomica No. 23. Growth and Regeneration of Axons in the Nervous System*, ed. M. Berry, pp. 56–75. Basel: S. Karger.

Silver, J. (1980). Mechanism of axon guidance during the formation of central nervous system commissures. *Society of Neuroscience Abstracts*, **6**, 484.

Silver, J. & Sidman, R. L. (1980). A mechanism for the guidance and topographic patterns of retinal ganglion cell axons. *Journal of Comparative Neurology*, **189**, 101–11.

Simpson, S. B. (1968). Morphology of the regenerated spinal cord in the lizard, *Anolis carolinensis*. *Journal of Comparative Neurology*, **134**, 193–210.

Singer, M., Nordlander, R. H. & Egar. M. (1979). Axonal guidance during embryogenesis and regeneration in the spinal cord of the newt: the blueprint hypothesis of neuronal pathway patterning. *Journal of Comparative Neurology*, **185**, 1–22.

Skene, J. H. P. & Willard, M. (1981a). Changes in axonally transported proteins during axon regeneration in toad retinal ganglion cells. *Journal of Cell Biology*, **89**, 86–95.

Skene, J. H. P. & Willard, M. (1981b). Axonally transported proteins associated with axon growth in rabbit central and peripheral nervous systems. *Journal of Cell Biology*, **89**, 96–103.

Skene, J. H. P. & Willard, M. (1981c). Characteristics of growth-associated proteins during axon regeneration in toad retinal ganglion cells. *J. Neuroscience*, **1**, 419–26.

So, K.-F. (1979). Development of abnormal recrossing retino-tectal projections after superior colliculus lesions in newborn Syrian hamsters. *Journal of Comparative Neurology*, **186**, 241–58.

Sparrow, J. R. & Kiernan, J. A. (1981). Endoneurial vascular permeability in degenerating and regenerating peripheral nerves. *Acta Neuropathologica*, **53**, 181–8.

Sperry, R. W. (1944). Optic nerve regeneration with return of vision in anurans. *Journal of Neurophysiology*, **7**, 57–69.

Sperry, R. W. (1945). Restoration of vision after crossing of optic nerves and after contralateral transplantation of the eye. *Journal of Neurophysiology*, **8**, 15–28.

Spielmeyer, W. (1922). *Histopathologie der Nervous System*, Berlin: Springer.

Stanfield, B. & Cowan, W. M. (1976). Evidence for a change in the retinohypothalamic projection in the rat following early removal of one eye. *Brain Research*, **104**, 129–36.

Stelzner, D. J., Ershler, W. B. & Weber, E. D. (1975). Effects of spinal transection in neonatal and weanling rats: survival of function. *Experimental Neurology*, **46**, 156–77.

Stenevi, V., Björklund, A. & Svendgaard, N.-A. (1976). Transplantation of central and peripheral monoamine neurons to the adult rat brain: techniques and conditions for survival. *Brain Research*, **114**, 1–20.

Stensaas, L. J., Burgess, P. R. & Horch, K. W. (1979). Regenerating dorsal root axons are blocked by spinal cord astrocytes. *Society of Neuroscience Abstracts*, **5**, 684.

Sternberger, N. H., Itoyama, Y., Kies, M. & Webster, D. DeF. (1978). Immunocytochemical method to identify basic protein in myelin forming oligodendrocytes of newborn rat CNS. *Journal of Neurocytology*, **7**, 251–63.

Sternberger, N. H., Quarles, R. H., Itoyama, Y. & Webster, H. DeF. (1978). Myelin-associated glycoprotein demonstrated immunocytochemically in myelin and myelin-forming cells of developing rat. *Proceedings of the National Academy of Sciences, USA*, **76**, 1510–14.

Stutinsky, F., Bonvallet, M. & Dell, P. (1949). Les modifications hypophysaires au cours du diabete insipide expérimentale chez le chien. *American Journal of Endocrinology*, **10**, 505–17.

Suess, V. & Pliska, V. (1981). Identification of the pituicytes as astroglial cells by indirect immunofluorescence-staining for the glial fibrillar acidic proteins. *Brain Research*, **221**, 27–33.

Sugar, O. & Gerard, R. W. (1940). Spinal cord regeneration in the rat. *Journal of Neurophysiology*, **3**, 1–19.

Sung, J. H. (1981). Tangled masses of regenerated central nerve fibres (non-myelinated central neuromas) in the central nervous system. *Journal of Neuropathology and Experimental Neurology*, **40**, 645–57.

Svendgaard, N.-A., Björklund, A. & Stenevi, V. (1976). Regeneration of central cholinergic neurones in the adult brain. *Brain Research*, **102**, 1–22.

Ten Cate, J. (1932). Befunde nach der experimentellen Isolierung eines Ruchenmarlssabschnittes. *Archives néerlandaises de physiologie de l'homme et des animaux*. **17**, 149–238.

Theiler, R. F. & McClure, W. O. (1978). Rapid axoplasmic transport of proteins in regenerating sensory nerve fibers. *Journal of Neurochemistry*, **31**, 433–47.

Thomas, K. A., Riley, M. C., Lemmon, S. K., Baglan, N. C. & Bradshaw, R. A. (1980). Brain fibroblast growth factor. Nonidentity with myelin basic protein fragments. *Journal of Biological Chemistry*, **255**, 5517–20.

Tower, S. S. (1931). A search for trophic influences of posterior spinal roots on skeletal muscle, with a note on the nerve fibres found in the proximal stumps of the roots after excision of the root ganglion. *Brain*, **54**, 99–110.

Tuge, H. & Hanzawa, S. (1937). Physiological and morphological regeneration of the sectioned spinal cord in adult teleosts. *Journal of Comparative Neurology*, **67**, 343–65.

Turbes, C. C. & Freeman, L. W. (1958). Peripheral nerve–spinal cord anastomosis for experimental cord transection. *Neurology*, **8**, 857–61.

Varon, S. (1975). Nerve growth factor and its mode of action. *Experimental Neurology*, **48**, 75–92.

Velasco, M. E., Roessmann, V. & P. Gambetti, (1982). The presence of glial fibrillary acidic protein in the human pituitary gland. *Journal of Neuropathology and Experimental Neurology*, **41**, 150–63.

Weinberg, E. L. & Spencer, P. S. (1979). Studies on the control of myelinogenesis. 3. Signalling of oligodendrocyte myelination by regenerating peripheral axons. *Brain Research*, **162**, 273–9.

Westall, F. C., Lennon, V. A. & Gospodarowicz, D. (1978). Brain-derived fibroblast growth factor: identity with a fragment of the basic protein of myelin. *Proceedings of the National Academy of Sciences, USA*, **75**, 4675–8.

Westbrook, W. H. L. Jr & Tower, S. S. (1940). An analysis of the problem of emergent fibers in the posterior spinal root, dealing with the rate of growth of extraneous fibers into the roots after ganglionectomy. *Journal of Comparative Neurology*, **72**, 383–97.

Willenborg, D. O., Staten, E. A. & Eidelberg, E. (1977). Studies on cell-mediated hypersensitivity to neural antigens after experimental spinal cord injury. *Experimental Neurology*, **54**, 383–92.

Windle, W. F. (1955). *Regeneration in the Nervous System*. Springfield, Illinois: Charles C. Thomas.

Windle, W. F. (1956). Regeneration of axons in the vertebrate central nervous system. *Physiological Reviews*, **36**, 427–40.

10 The neuroendocrine anatomy of the limbic system: a discussion with special reference to steroid responsive neurons, neuropeptides and monoaminergic systems

B. J. EVERITT, J. HERBERT and E. B. KEVERNE

Department of Anatomy, University of Cambridge, Downing Street, Cambridge CB2 3DY, UK

INTRODUCTION

The two-way interaction between neurons and endocrine systems has focussed attention on the nature of the controls exerted by the one on the other. Our knowledge of the structure and connections of the limbic system, long known to be particularly closely concerned with such neuroendocrine function, has recently been supplemented by the discovery of chemically identified neural pathways within this part of the brain. In this chapter we discuss three such systems which seem, on present evidence, to represent by their interaction a new understanding of neuroendocrinology. This is not intended as an exhaustive review but, rather, as a discussion of the principles by which these systems (the steroid binding neurons, the neuropeptide-containing pathways and the monoaminergic systems) are distributed and some of the ways in which they interact in a neuroendocrine context.

GONADAL HORMONES AND THE BRAIN

There is no questioning the fact that gonadal steroids exert powerful effects on the brain. In the adult female, oestrogens promote sexual behaviour, influence luteinising hormone releasing hormone (LHRH) release, increase locomotor activity and decrease feeding behaviour. Each of these aspects has been scrutinised independently, an approach which has resulted in assigning separate functions to the different steroid-hormone-concentrating parts of the brain. This has usually been accomplished by direct implantation of minute amounts of steroid hormone in, or by electrolytic lesions to, those areas of the brain which concentrate steroid hormones (as identified by autoradiography). Hence, the preoptic area and ventromedial hypothalamus have been shown to be important in sexual behaviour (Christensen & Clemens, 1974; Davis, McEwen & Pfaff, 1979); this same area and the mediobasal hypothalamus regulate gonadotrophin release (Hayashi & Gorski, 1974); the corticomedial amygdala is important for certain olfactory effects (Scalia & Winans, 1975); while the ventromedial nucleus of the hypothalamus is thought to be important in feeding behaviour (Grossman, 1975). Such fractionation of function with respect to the steroid concentrating neurons is fragmentary and simplistic. This has become evident as a result of the double labelling of neurons by autoradiography and retrograde fluorescent-dye tracing. Such techniques have shown that certain hypothalamic nuclei contain a mixed population of steroid concentrating neurons whose terminals are distributed to several different parts of the brain (Morrell & Pfaff, 1982). An alternative approach, therefore, to understanding the significance of the distribution of steroid concentrating neurons in the brain is to consider them as part of a functionally unified system. Since there is no restriction to the passage of unbound steroid hormones from the vascular to the cerebral compartment, high affinity oestradiol binding neurons will be activated in all parts of the brain simultaneously. Therefore, this system may be viewed as functioning to integrate a number of the strategies that an animal adopts within the context of a given behaviour and, in the case of gonadal steroids, it is appropriate to consider sexual behaviour.

The distribution of steroid binding neurons

The uptake of sex hormones into the cells of the brain has been shown autoradiographically by use of radio-labelled steroid hormones (reviewed in: Stumpf, 1975; Pfaff & Conrad, 1978). The neuroanatomical distribution of these cells includes various components of the limbic forebrain, the preoptic area, hypothalamus and mesencephalic regions deep to the tectum. Although radioactive steroid hormones are located in weakly labelled neurons sparsely scattered throughout the brain, including the cortex, heavy labelling of a large percentage of cells occurs particularly in the septal and preoptic regions. The region of most dense labelling can be found in the medial preoptic nucleus and in the periventricular preoptic nucleus. Closely related to this, many cells in the anterior hypothalamus, particularly around the third ventricle, take up gonadal steroid hormone. The suprachiasmatic nucleus is, however, only lightly labelled, in contrast to the arcuate nucleus which is intensely labelled. Labelling also occurs throughout the ventromedial nucleus, particularly its ventro-lateral segment. Only a few cells in the dorsomedial nucleus accumulate gonadal steroids, while the ventral premammillary nucleus contains high numbers of labelled cells throughout its extent (Pfaff & Keiner, 1973; Stumpf, Sar & Keefer, 1975). Hence, even within the hypothalamus, the steroid concentrating neurons are restricted in their distribution to areas concerned primarily with sexual and neuroendocrine-related functions.

Other areas of the limbic brain which have been demonstrated autoradiographically to take up oestradiol and testosterone include the medial and cortical amygdaloid nuclei (Sheridan, 1979), the septum and the olfactory tubercle (Stumpf & Sar, 1975). These areas have in common an important role in olfactory processing. The septum not only receives an olfactory input but also has a population of LHRH neurons which projects to the olfactory and accessory olfactory bulbs (Jennes & Stumpf, 1980), while the cortical and medial amygdaloid nuclei receive sensory information from these structures before relaying it on to the bed-nucleus of stria terminalis, itself an area which takes up steroid hormones (Sheridan, 1979). Since olfactory cues play an important role in both sexual attraction and neuroendocrine function, and since endocrine status is important for determining sexual odour preferences, one can envisage how steroidal activation of this diffuse population of neurons switches the animal into a sensory mode directed primarily towards sexual objects.

Correlation between monoamines and steroid binding neurons

There is a dual morphological relationship between the noradrenergic neurons and sex steroids, a relationship unique to this group of aminergic neurons. Those noradrenergic neurons which project to areas containing sex steroid concentrating neurons (olfactory tubercle, septum, hypothalamus, corticomedial amygdala), themselves take up oestradiol (Jennes & Stumpf, 1975; Heritage, Grant & Stumpf, 1977), while the density of receptors in the areas to which they project is influenced by steroid hormones (Wilkinson *et al.*, 1979). About 50–80% of the catecholamine neurons in the noradrenergic cell groups A1 (lateral tegmentum), A2 (solitary tract) and in the vicinity of the lateral lemniscus (A7) take up oestradiol, while relatively few (25%) of the noradrenergic neurons of the locus coeruleus – which project primarily to the cortex – accumulate oestradiol (Heritage *et al.*, 1981). In contrast, neither the cell bodies of dopamine neurons in the midbrain (A8, A9, A10), nor their terminals are associated with sex hormones. However, some of the dopaminergic neurons in the arcuate nucleus and periventricular nucleus which are involved in neuroendocrine regulation of the pituitary (LH and prolactin) do concentrate gonadal steroid hormones. Hence, the neurons of the ascending aminergic projections are quite different from each other with respect to their ability to accumulate gonadal steroids. In particular, it is a sub-group of the noradrenergic neurons, those that ascend in the ventral bundle, which are primarily associated with gonadal hormones both at their terminals and their cell bodies.

It should, therefore, come as no surprise that this same group of noradrenergic neurons is particularly concerned with reproductive neuroendocrinology. For example, destruction of the ventral noradrenergic bundle, which supplies principally the limbic system, interferes with the behavioural response of oestrous female rats to male rats. Such females can no longer respond to the sensory stimulus given them by a mounting male, and fail to show lordosis in response. Even if they were to mate, the neuroendocrine system no longer responds in the normal way to the stimulus of copulation by inducing a period of pseudopregnancy (Hansen, Stanfield & Everitt, 1981). Similar findings followed from experiments on neuroendocrine responses to olfactory stimuli in a different context. Female mice, in whom the noradrenergic input to the olfactory bulbs had been removed, 'blocked' their pregnancy not only to a strange male, but to their own mate as well. Evidently they failed to respond to (and hence 'remember') the olfactory stimulus given by him during copulation and which normally prevents them from inhibiting 'his' pregnancy (Keverne & Riva, 1982). These experiments show that sensory information associated with particularly important episodes in an animal's reproductive life is not processed normally in the absence of noradrenaline.

Binding of sex steroids by receptors in the brain

A pattern common to all steroid target tissues, including the brain, is the entry of steroid hormones into the cell where they become tightly and specifically bound to cytoplasmic proteins. The steroid receptor complex is translated to the cell nucleus, and here it stays for a period of several hours, in association with the DNA, to promote transcription. The mRNA formed will subsequently be translated in its turn, and specific protein formation will then alter cell structure and function (O'Malley & Means, 1974).

The distribution of oestradiol receptors correlates positively with the pattern of uptake demonstrated in autoradiography. Oestrogen receptors in the adult rat brain are confined mainly to the hypothalamus, the amygdaloid nucleus and the preoptic area (McGinnis *et al.*, 1982). The concentration of oestradiol receptors in the hypothalamus of the rat fluctuates with the oestrous cycle, being lowest at pro-oestrus; this may reflect an increase in nuclear translocation due to high endogenous titres of oestrogen at this time of the cycle (McEwen *et al.*, 1979).

The testosterone binding in the hypothalamus of male rats appears to have a lower affinity for androgen than does the analogous system in the female for oestrogen.

Limited capacity binding of testosterone occurs only to a small degree in the nuclear fractions of cells obtained from the preoptic–hypothalamic area and amygdala, and from the cytoplasmic fraction of these areas in castrated rats. However, the concentration and kinetics of uptake do not differ from the cortex. Either there are fewer androgen than oestrogen binding sites in the mammalian brain, or the binding of androgen is weaker than that of oestrogen. Studies on whole tissue of steroid hormone competition have revealed that unlabelled oestradiol competes more effectively with radioactive oestradiol for hypothalamic binding sites than cold testosterone does with radioactive testosterone (McEwen & Pfaff, 1970). In the same brain regions, oestradiol is as effective in competing with radioactive testosterone for receptors as is testosterone itself. In contrast, testosterone does not compete effectively against [³H]oestradiol. Some of these effects may be due to metabolism of testosterone to oestradiol. Certainly, studies both *in vivo* and *in vitro* illustrate that binding of oestradiol is not significantly affected by cold testosterone, while binding of testosterone is significantly displaced by cold oestradiol. It therefore comes as no surprise to find that oestradiol has the ability to replace testosterone centrally in inducing sexual behaviour of castrated rats, providing peripheral target tissues remain activated (Pfaff, 1970).

Progesterone binding in the brain is of limited capacity and high affinity. It is highly progestin specific, and not readily displaced by testosterone or oestradiol. Throughout much of the rat brain, progestin receptor levels appear to be unaffected by oestradiol. This is not the case in the preoptic–hypothalamic area in which oestradiol treatment produces a large increase in progestin receptors in 4 days. After oestrogen treatment, progestin receptor concentrations rise in the mediobasal hypothalamus and in the preoptic area to levels more than three-fold greater than in other brain regions (Blaustein & Feder, 1979). However, not all oestrogen sensitive neurons are programmed to form progestin receptors (e.g. corticomedial amygdala) and not all progestin receptors are influenced by oestradiol (e.g. cortex and midbrain) (McGinnis *et al.*, 1981).

It is important to note that oestradiol induces progestin receptor synthesis in those areas of the brain which mediate female reproductive behaviour. Moreover, the time course of induction and decay of mating behaviour is similar to that of inducible progestin receptors. After 48 hours of oestrogen stimulation the number of inducible progestin receptors in the preoptic–hypothalamic area of the brain is maximal, as is sexual receptivity, while the converse applies 48 hours after oestradiol withdrawal. Recently it has been found that continuous exposure to oestradiol is not essential either for sexual behaviour or for increase of progestin receptors. A discontinuous exposure to oestradiol, in two 1-hour periods spaced 14 hours apart, is sufficient to elevate cytosol receptors and sexual receptivity in the female rat (Parsons *et al.*, 1981).

Metabolism of sex steroids in the brain

In order to establish that a steroid hormone activates a behavioural or neuroendocrine mechanism, it is not sufficient simply to demonstrate a target area for that hormone within the brain. It is also essential to show that the hormone can reach this area in sufficient quantities to saturate the receptors. This may require an investigation of the relative affinity or changing affinity of the receptors for the hormone. It is also important to further examine the fate of that steroid after cytoplasmic binding, especially the processes which initiate conversion to active or inactive metabolites.

The conversion of testosterone to oestradiol may play an important role in the fate of testosterone in the brain, and conceivably in the developmental effects of this hormone on the undifferentiated brain. As much as 80% of nuclear bound radioactivity in the brain 2 hours after a single injection of [³H]testosterone in 5-day-old male or female rats is [³H]oestradiol (Lieberburg & McEwen, 1975). In the adult male dove, no circulating oestrogen can be detected in the blood plasma of the male, and yet oestrogen has specific effects on male nest-orientated courtship patterns. The area of the brain responsible for this behaviour, the preoptic area, has a rich aromatase system which converts testosterone to oestradiol, and in which the aromatase enzyme is itself induced by high levels of testosterone (Steimer & Hutchison, 1981).

In addition to aromatisation, testosterone is converted within the mammalian brain to a number of 5-α reduced metabolites, of which dihydrotestosterone (DHT) is the principal (Massa *et al.*, 1972). The pattern of conversion to DHT differs according to the brain areas and in the male rat is highest in the midbrain, hypothalamus and thalamus. Thus, conversion of testosterone to DHT as an inactive metabolite could theoretically decrease the concentration of testosterone available to bind to the nuclear fraction or that available for aromatisation to oestradiol. Hence, although brain tissues may take up and bind testosterone, the amount available for behavioural or differentiative effects could be reduced by activating the 5α-reductase enzyme as opposed to the aromatase enzyme.

Local effects of steroid in the brain

Although steroid hormones are actively taken up by specific areas of the brain, in order to relate this to function it is necessary to demonstrate that the application of these hormones in the form of implants to these areas of the brain can influence components of reproductive activity. Although the septum, the preoptic area and the hypothalamus take up oestradiol, it is only when oestradiol is implanted into the ventromedial hypothalamus of ovariectomised females that sexual behaviour is elicited. The question arises therefore as to what the significance might be of the uptake of oestradiol into these other areas (septum, preoptic area) and into the corticomedial amygdala, the arcuate nucleus, the mesencephalic central grey and noradrenergic cell groups of the pons and medulla. One plausible answer is that steroid uptake into these other regions of the brain engages neural mechanisms which are functionally related to reproductive activity. Such functions will include enhancement of sensory stimuli relevant to sexual behaviour, enhancement of motor patterns (e.g. lordosis) relevant to sexual behaviour and co-ordination of sexual behaviour with neuroendocrine mechanisms that are essential to reproductive success and pregnancy. The sex steroids do not have this capacity in themselves, and therefore part of their function can be seen in terms of recruiting a wide range of neural systems (noradrenaline and 5-hydroxytryptamine in the brain stem, dopamine in arcuate and periventricular nuclei, LHRH in septal–preoptic area), while still other neural systems may interact to modulate the action of steroid hormones (e.g. prolactin and opiate peptides).

NEUROENDOCRINE PEPTIDES

Neuroendocrine peptides form part of the wider peptidergic systems of the brain which have recently been recognised and which have attracted a great deal of interest. They also play an essential part in the function of the pituitary, either by regulating its action or, in some cases, by acting themselves as peripheral hormones in their own right. We shall not attempt an exhaustive catalogue of these substances, but select four for discussion. Each of these, as will be explained later, represents a different class of peptide according to the classification proposed in this paper. Thus we shall seek to demonstrate some of the principles underlying the distribution and functions of these compounds.

Methods of study

Two principal techniques have been used to study the presence and distribution of neuroendocrine peptides within the brain. The first relies upon the now well known methods of immunohistochemistry, which both help to identify the peptide and also allow its distribution to be directly studied. The principal problems with this method lie with its specificity and sensitivity. The production of antibodies is improving rapidly, allowing greater selectivity with respect to the compounds against which they are directed. However, recognition of the multiple processing of peptides within a given pathway (or in different pathways), together with the existence of precursor peptides which may or may not react with the antibody itself, still limits these techniques. Sensitivity becomes a problem when, for example, intraneuronal concentrations are being studied; these may be orders of magnitude lower than those in terminals.

The second technique relies upon removal of small parts of the brain (usually by the punch technique) followed by radioimmunoassay of the peptide concerned. This technique loses the fine anatomical definition offered by the first, since the accuracy and size of the punch technique determine the level of analysis possible. However, such examinations *in vitro* do allow contemporary methods of separation and identification (for example by high performance liquid chromatography) to be applied to the peptides under study, thus rendering their identification that much more secure. Some combination of the two techniques or coalescence of the results derived from both should yield comprehensive information about the distribution of these neuroendocrine peptides. To this has to be added a further area of study, not considered here, which concerns the distribution and nature of the receptors responding to these compounds.

The four neuroendocrine peptides to be considered are: LHRH, β-endorphin, oxytocin, and prolactin. All of them, with the probable exception of prolactin, are found within the neural systems of the brain (where they may act as neurotransmitters) and are released into the circulation. A closer examination shows that resemblance between them ends at this point, and we shall use known differences to try to bring some order to the present confusion surrounding the classification of these neuropeptides. It is important to point out that we have ignored or neglected instances where the same peptides may be found in peripheral structures. For example, LHRH (or a compound like it) is known to be present in the gonads; oxytocin has been found to be released also from the ovary; many other peptides (e.g. enkephalin, substance P, and somatostatin), not the subject of detailed consideration in this paper, are also found in peripheral organs. Nevertheless, it is our belief that the system we shall propose does have general validity.

Classifying the neuroendocrine peptides

The neuropeptides are classified according to the way in which they are arranged relative to the central nervous system and the periphery. As will become apparent, there are clear indications that these differences have functional as well as systematic importance.

Type 1 peptides are represented by LHRH. They are distributed in a well-defined system of pathways (considered in more detail below) originating in cell bodies lying in the rostral basal forebrain. The terminals of such systems are, in general, to be found in two sites: (*a*) in synaptic approximation to nuclear groups in various parts of the diencephalon and brain stem (for example, the amygdala, the olfactory bulb, the habenula and the midbrain); (*b*) as terminals in the external layer of the median eminence, from here to be discharged into the portal system and conveyed to the anterior pituitary. Whether the intracerebral and portal venous terminal systems arise from the same cell bodies is not known. A wide variety of other small peptides acting upon the anterior pituitary falls into the same category as LHRH; these include somatostatin, vasoactive intestinal peptide (VIP) and corticotrophin releasing factor (CRF).

Type 2 peptides are closely related to type 1 and are represented by oxytocin (and vasopressin). These peptides have a distribution within the brain which in many cases is rather similar to type 1 peptides (at least as far as their terminal areas are concerned). However, the peripherally projecting axons are not limited to releasing their hormone directly into the portal system and hence have more than a localised action on the anterior pituitary. Oxytocin, for example, is released into the blood stream and therefore has effects upon target sites at a considerable distance. The difference between these two classes of peptides lies therefore in the nature of their peripheral mode of release and action.

Type 3 peptides, which include β-endorphin, have a different arrangement. There is a central system in which groups of cell bodies containing the peptide are distributed to wide areas of the brain, again principally limbic areas, diencephalic regions and those within the brain stem. However, there is no peripheral projection from these neurons but, instead, the same peptide is found in cells of the anterior pituitary from which it is released into the peripheral circulation. Adrenocorticotrophic hormone (ACTH), as might be expected from its common genesis with β-endorphin, shares this characteristic. Thus, like type 2 peptides, there is both a peripheral and a central component; the important difference is that for type 3 peptides each component arises from distinct cellular populations. This implies that the central and peripheral systems could act, on occasion, independently of each other.

The three systems so far described share a common characteristic in that a peptide released into the peripheral compartment has great difficulty in entering the central one. Irrespective of whether the central and peripheral components can act in concert, it seems that there are mechanisms which separate the effects of the peptides on receptors lying within the brain from those lying in peripheral structures.

Type 4 peptides are those which are released from the anterior pituitary and for which the presence of an intracranial component seems to be open to question. The peptides themselves (e.g. prolactin and LH) have considerably larger molecular weights than those hitherto considered. They are released from the anterior pituitary under conditions which may reflect the activity of centrally acting peptides such as those already considered in earlier categories. However, they differ from the former in that they can enter the brain from the peripheral vascular system, and thus act as peripherally derived neuropeptides. The criteria on which the classification of this group of peptides depend, however, would be jeopardised if (as some preliminary observations indicate) there are neural systems in the brain which make both prolactin and LH. Should this be the case, then type 4 neuropeptides will become more closely related to type 3, the distinction being in the relative permeability of the blood–brain barrier to the two groups.

We now consider in more detail the distribution and action of each of the four chosen peptides in order to illustrate this scheme of classification.

LHRH

Cell bodies. There has been considerable controversy over the location and numbers of LHRH-containing neurons. Earlier studies showed very few, and those that were observed seemed to lie within the mediobasal hypothalamus in the region of the arcuate nucleus (Zimmerman *et al.*, 1974) or within the anterior hypothalamus (Barry, Dubois & Poulain, 1973). More recent studies, using more sensitive techniques or animals treated with colchicine (which prevents the transport of LHRH from cell bodies to axons) have considerably modified these earlier views. It is now generally agreed that a scattered population of LHRH neurons lies in the rostral part of the hypothalamus and preoptic area in basal forebrain (Naik, 1976). These cell bodies are not restricted to any anatomically recognised nuclear group. The medial preoptic area is one major source (Jennes & Stumpf, 1980; King *et al.*, 1982), particularly the medial preoptic nucleus adjoining the third ventricle (Silverman, 1976). Most authors also report cell bodies lying more laterally, in the lateral preoptic area or the lateral hypothalamic area (King *et al.*, 1982). LHRH neurons are consistently found in the medial septum and in the area of the diagonal band including the bed-nucleus of the stria terminalis (BNST) (Setalo *et al.*, 1976; Silverman, 1976; Ibata *et al.*, 1979) and in some cases they extend as far forward as the anterior olfactory nucleus (Jennes & Stumpf, 1980). Whilst there is no disagreement that the suprachiasmatic nucleus contains many LHRH terminals, some authors also find cell bodies within this nucleus (Barry *et al.*, 1973; Silverman, 1976) whilst others do not (e.g. Hoffman & Gibbs, 1982). A major focus of disagreement, however, is whether or not LHRH neurons can be found within the arcuate nucleus, a point of importance considering this area's role in the negative feedback control of the anterior pituitary. Whilst earlier studies (Silverman, 1976) suggested these exist, there seems to be an increasing consensus from later ones that the arcuate nucleus does not, in fact, contain LHRH cell bodies (Merchenthaler *et al.*, 1980; Kawano & Daikoku, 1981). Some of the neurons previously considered to be LHRH-positive might have been misidentified. Merchenthaler & coworkers (1980) suggest that at least one antibody ('Sorrentino F') cross-reacts with ACTH and hence would be visible in the arcuate nucleus. Leonardelli & Tramu (1979) point out that anti-β-endorphin antibodies stain some LHRH neurons, though failing to confirm that antibodies against $ACTH_{17-39}$ show cross-reactivity. Nevertheless they consider that LHRH neurons are to be found within the arcuate nucleus.

Projections. There is beginning to be general agreement over the projection of the fibres from these cell bodies. There are, it seems, four main areas of projection:

(*a*) There is a recently described pathway directed anteriorly and entering the olfactory bulbs (Jennes & Stumpf, 1980).

(*b*) There is a comparatively rich innervation of the intralimbic areas surrounding those in which lie most of the LHRH neurons. Thus, the preoptic area, the septum and the vascular organ of the lamina terminalis (OVLT) all contain LHRH-positive terminals. This projection also includes fibres which enter the amygdala (Phillips *et al.*, 1980) particularly the corticomedial nuclei.

(c) Like many other peptidergic pathways originating from the basal forebrain, LHRH-positive fibres can be traced down to the brain stem. Such fibres can travel caudally through the hypothalamus, either close to the ventricles or through the medial forebrain bundle, supplying the mediobasal hypothalamus, including the arcuate, ventromedial, and dorsomedial nuclei. Some run on through the hypothalamus into the brain stem. An important component of this projection is that to the median eminence, considered more fully in the next category. The second path to the brain stem runs through the stria medullaris, thence to the habenulae, on through the fasciculus retroflexus towards the interpeduncular nucleus, thus entering the mesencephalon (Barry *et al.*, 1973; Silverman, 1976; Jennes & Stumpf, 1980). It terminates chiefly in the midbrain raphe and the central grey. Barry *et al.* (1973) point to the similarity between this pathway and that followed by the oxytocin containing fibres.

(d) The earliest studies on LHRH showed a massive projection to the median eminence, and this has been confirmed in more recent investigations. The idea that median eminence projections come largely from cell bodies within the arcuate nucleus (Silverman, 1976) has failed to win universal support in more recent studies (Ibata *et al.*, 1979; Hoffman & Gibbs, 1982). The majority of immunohistochemical studies point to a particularly high concentration of LHRH terminals in the lateral part of the external layer of the median eminence (Barry *et al.*, 1973). This is particularly interesting with reference to the disposition of dopamine in this structure, bearing in mind the close relationship often postulated between dopamine and LHRH release.

Oxytocin

Cell bodies. Of the two *posterior* pituitary peptides, more attention has been directed towards vasopressin than oxytocin. Whilst it may be legitimate to apply conclusions inferred from studying one to the other, there are clear differences in the patterns of release of oxytocin and vasopressin under physiological conditions (Poulain & Wakerley, 1982) which argue against too easy an extrapolation. There is also the problem that, in some studies, immunohistochemical procedures have been directed against the carrier peptide neurophysin, rather than oxytocin. Antibodies against neurophysins will not only stain cells that manufacture the oxytocin precursor, but (unless particular precautions are taken) vasopressin-containing cells as well. Unlike LHRH, most oxytocin-positive cells have been found within anatomically discrete nuclei. The supraoptic, paraventricular and (more recently) suprachiasmatic nuclei all contain neurophysin-positive cell bodies (Sofroniew & Glasmann, 1981), though those in the last named group may be vasopressin-containing. Immunochemically identified cells may also be found in parts of the medial septum, which is particularly interesting since electrophysiological experiments (Poulain, Lebrun & Vincent, 1981) as well as anatomical studies (Powell & Rorie, 1969) suggest an interaction between this part of the brain and the magnocellular nuclei.

Projections. Fibres from both oxytocin- and vasopressin-containing cell bodies innervate areas rather similar to those receiving input from LHRH neurons. Thus, there is a considerable terminal field located in the septum and OVLT and projections as far as the amygdala (but see Thomson, 1982). The second major projection follows the route to the brain stem also taken by LHRH-containing fibres (Buijs, 1978). Thus some fibres run along the side of the third ventricle to reach the brain stem, whereas others take a more indirect route via the stria medullaris and the habenula (Sofroniew & Glasmann, 1981; Swanson & Kuypers, 1980). A third large projection is to the median eminence and to the posterior pituitary. It is becoming apparent that it might be important to distinguish between these two areas of termination, first demonstrated by Zimmerman and colleagues (Hillman *et al.*, 1977).

Recently Swanson & Kuypers (1980) have suggested that the cellular architecture of the paraventricular nucleus may reflect the terminal areas to which its neurons project. They draw attention to the fact that this nucleus is made up of three magnocellular and five parvocellular parts. The magnocellular divisions, they suggest, project to the posterior pituitary and there is little or no evidence for branches of this system joining the projection of the parvocellular cells. It is the latter that give rise to the extensive intracerebral projections which, taking the course already described, innervate areas of the brain stem, including the dorsal vagal complex, parabrachial nucleus, locus coeruleus, and dorsal raphe, and extend down to the spinal cord. Terminals in the median eminence may come from the parvocellular, rather than the magnocellular, divisions of the nucleus.

β-Endorphin

Cell bodies. A major problem in identifying β-endorphin cell bodies stems from the recent knowledge that the brain contains at least two other systems of opiate-containing neurons: the enkephalins and the dynorphins (Corbett *et al.*, 1982). Furthermore, it is now equally well known that β-endorphins arise from a precursor (pro-opiomelanocortin) from which originate other peptides, including ACTH and melanocyte stimulating hormone (α-MSH) (Eipper & Mains, 1980). When one speaks, therefore, of β-endorphin-positive systems, it is highly likely that the same systems will contain not only the precursor molecule but also these other peptides. A question of considerable interest concerns the processing of these precursor molecules into their descendent peptides, and whether this varies in different parts of the system, or under different conditions (Al-Noalmi *et al.*, 1982; Zakarian & Smyth, 1982). It must be understood that, in the account which follows, these provisos will apply to neurons or terminal areas which are characterised as containing β-endorphin.

There has been some success in distinguishing β-endorphin from other opiates. Whilst it is probably too early to be confident in the case of dynorphin, the development of relatively specific antisera has demonstrated that the enkephalinergic pathways are distinct from those containing β-endorphin, since their distribution and the kind of neurons they occupy are substantially different (Dupont *et al.*, 1980). There is general agreement amongst workers using immuno-histochemical methods that neurons containing β-endorphin are found within and adjacent to the arcuate nucleus in the ventromedial hypothalamus; this is supported by experiments in which this peptide is reduced by lesioning the structure (Krieger *et al.*, 1979). Thus, like oxytocin, but distinct from LHRH, there is some correspondence between the cytological classification of the hypothalamic nuclei and this chemically identifiable system of neurons. However, β-endorphin-containing neurons are also found just lateral to the arcuate nucleus (Finley, Lindstrom & Petrusz, 1981) as well as in the arcuate nucleus itself (Sofroniew, 1979). As pointed out above, the same neurons are positive for ACTH and lipotrophin (β-LPH) as well as the 16 K precursor (pro-opiomelanocortin) (Stengaard-Pederson & Larsson, 1981; de Kloet, Palkovits & Mezey, 1981). There is also some evidence that β-endorphin cell bodies can be found in the magnocellular nuclei. Watkins (1980) describes cells in both the supraoptic and paraventricular nuclei as positive for antisera raised against $ACTH_{1-39}$ (not $ACTH_{1-24}$) though this staining was abolished by previous absorption with neurophysin, thus raising questions about its specificity (see also Larsson, 1980). Arcuate nucleus neurons have also been found to contain β-LPH and ACTH (Nilaver *et al.*, 1979). It is perhaps relevant here to recall that the same nucleus has been demonstrated histochemically to contain dopamine- and LH-containing neurons (Hostetter, Gallo & Brownfield, 1981) and is well known to be able to take up and bind oestradiol using specific cytoplasmic receptors.

Projections. As do the other two peptides already considered, β-endorphin neurons form an extensive plexus of fibres in the region near their origin, as well as projecting to more distant parts of the brain. Within the hypothalamus, fibres are found surrounding the arcuate nucleus itself as well as the dorso- and ventromedial nuclei (Nilaver *et al.*, 1979), and extend more anteriorly into the bed-nucleus of the stria terminalis, nucleus accumbens and the lateral septum (Sofroniew, 1979; Finley *et al.*, 1981). In common with the oxytocin and LHRH systems, there is a prominent projection to the amygdala, in particular to the medial, basomedial and central nuclei (Finley *et al.*, 1981).

The projection of β-endorphin-containing neurons to the midbrain also compares closely with the two peptides already discussed. The periaqueductal grey and reticular formation of the pons are areas of particularly dense innervation; the anatomical similarities of these pathways to the vasopressinergic pathways projecting from the suprachiasmatic nucleus have been pointed out by Sofroniew (1979). The pathway via the habenula, characteristic for the oxytocin and LHRH systems, should be particularly noted.

Studies using radioimmunoassay have, in general, confirmed these findings with the added advantage of specificity referred to above. Such studies (including one in man) confirm the high concentration of β-endorphin in the arcuate nucleus, lesser amounts in the magnocellular groups in the hypothalamus, the medial preoptic/anterior hypothalamus and the periaqueductal grey (Wilkes *et al.*, 1980; Dorsa, Majumdar & Chapman, 1981). There are lesser amounts in the bed-nucleus of the stria terminalis, the septum and the amygdala (though the high quantities in the medial part might have been diluted by the much lower amounts found in the lateral nuclei) and, noticeably, no detectable levels of β-endorphin in the cerebral cortex. Reports on the levels present in the median eminence, which also receives a β-endorphin-containing innervation from the arcuate nucleus, are inconsistent between authors using this technique. Some investigators (Dupont *et al.*, 1980) find high levels in this structure; others (Wilkes *et al.*, 1980) find rather less, and, most recently (Dorsa *et al.*, 1981), levels reported in the median eminence were actually lower than those in both the anterior hypothalamus and the periaqueductal grey. Nevertheless, the general pattern of these studies and of those using histological immunofluorescence seems consistent.

It is well established that β-endorphin is released from cells of the anterior pituitary into the peripheral circulation (Guillemin *et al.*, 1977).

Prolactin

There are two reports which suggest that prolactin-containing cell bodies or fibres can be found within the brain. An initial report claimed to have demonstrated a periventricular plexus of prolactin-containing fibres (Fuxe *et al.*, 1977) and, more recently, both scattered fibres and cell bodies have been described within the hypothalamus (Toubeau *et al.*, 1979). However, the greatest caution must be attached to this kind of finding particularly when dealing with peptides as large as prolactin.

Whether or not there really is a prolactin-containing system of neurons within the brain remains, for the moment, open to debate.

Interactions between peripheral and central compartments

The thesis advanced in this paper is that different neuropeptides concerned with neuroendocrine function can be distinguished by their distributions in either the central or the peripheral compartment. Two important functional considerations follow from this: (a) whether both the central and peripheral components of some systems may be activated simultaneously as part of a co-ordinated neuroendocrine response; and (b) whether the receptors to such neuropeptides in the brain can be exposed to peptide derived not only from central neural terminals but also from the peripheral circulation. As will now be demonstrated, each of our four model peptides shows distinct differences in these properties.

LHRH

Whether or not LHRH is simultaneously released centrally and into the portal system is important when one comes to consider the possible functions of this neuroendocrine peptide. The effects upon the anterior pituitary of LHRH released into the portal vessels do not need detailed documentation here, as they are now extremely well known. A pulse of LHRH releases a corresponding pulse of gonado-trophin from the pituitary, though it is still undecided whether this decapeptide has its principal action upon LH or whether both LH and follicle stimulating hormone (FSH) are activated by the same peptide (Fink, 1979). The essential function of LHRH is to regulate the oestrous cycle in females and gonadal function in males, and to modulate periodic reproductive phenomena, such as the annual breeding season.

A second, and more contentious, issue is whether LHRH has any behavioural effect. An increasing number of studies seems to show that injecting LHRH peripherally, or into the cerebral ventricles, or into the periaqueductal grey, increases the display of sexual behaviour, an effect particularly demonstrable in the female rat (Beyer et al., 1982; Tennent, Smith & Dorsa, 1982). LHRH seems to have an action comparable, in some respects, to that normally exerted by progesterone in that an ineffective dose of oestradiol is made effective by adding the peptide. Conversely, LHRH antibodies or antagonists injected into the brain have been shown to reduce the display of lordosis behaviour in female rats (Sirinathsinghji et al., 1983).

It is clearly possible, on these grounds, to postulate co-ordinated central and peripheral actions of LHRH. The first would play some role in the timing of sexual behaviour which, in many animals, is limited to the period during which the animal is fertile; the second would ensure fertility by timing ovulation to coincide with displays of sexual activity. Since LHRH is ejected from the hypothalamus directly into the portal system, transfer into the brain from the peripheral compartment is less important than is the case for some other neuroendocrine peptides. Under normal conditions, the amount of LHRH reaching the peripheral blood from this source may be too small to have any effect upon the brain itself, even if the peptide could cross the blood–brain barrier in effective quantities.

Oxytocin

Oxytocin presents a substantially different picture. There are adequate levels in the peripheral plasma to act upon peripheral target tissues and hence, possibly, upon brain itself. As with LHRH, there is evidence of both a central and a peripheral action for oxytocin, which may be co-ordinated. Oxytocin plays a well known role in milk ejection, and a more contentious one in the initiation of uterine contractions during parturition. Both these processes are closely associated temporally with the display of maternal behaviour. It is therefore interesting to note that oxytocin injected directly into the lateral ventricles has been claimed to initiate maternal activity in nulliparous rats (Pedersen & Prange, 1979; Pedersen et al., 1982), animals notoriously difficult to persuade to show this behaviour by other hormonal treatments (Rosenblatt, Siegel & Mayer, 1979). In view of these apparently co-ordinated central and peripheral roles, it is therefore of considerable interest to find that neither oxytocin nor its companion peptide vasopressin can cross the blood–brain barrier with any facility (Jones & Robinson, 1982; Wang et al., 1982). Both compounds are found in the cerebrospinal fluid (CSF), but there is no correlation with levels in blood; infusions of oxytocin or vasopressin peripherally do not result in appreciable changes in levels in the CSF. It seems clear, therefore, that even if the magnocellular and parvocellular systems releasing oxytocin work in concert, they do so only to the extent that they may both be regulated by the same central mechanisms. There is little evidence that peripherally derived oxytocin can act upon the brain which thus, it seems, remains the preserve of centrally released oxytocin.

β-Endorphin

β-Endorphin presents differences both from LHRH and from oxytocin. As already described, separate populations of cells release β-endorphin either centrally (from the arcuate nucleus) or peripherally (from the anterior pituitary). There has, as yet, been no coherent account of what either central or peripheral β-endorphin may do under physiological circumstances, though many neuroendocrine effects of the peptide have been described. As with oxytocin, recent evidence suggests that the peripheral and central compartments do not communicate directly (Foley et al., 1979; Nakao et al., 1980). β-endorphin derived from the plasma does not cross into the brain (Mohs et al., 1982), though small modifications to the molecule, making it more lipophilic, can induce such a transfer to take place (Kastin, Jemison & Coy, 1980). It therefore seems unlikely that the central receptors to β-endorphin in the limbic system and brain stem will be affected by peptide derived from the vascular compartment. The best documented effect of β-endorphin on the anterior pituitary is prolactin release. This reliably follows an injection of the peptide into the ventricles and has also been found to occur after intravenous injection (Catlin et al., 1980; Wehrenberg et al., 1981). It seems agreed that β-endorphin does not act directly upon the anterior pituitary to regulate prolactin, but only indirectly via the hypothalamus (Wardlaw et al., 1980). This might, at first sight, be taken as evidence for interaction between the peripheral and central compartments. However, it must be recalled that the external layer of the median eminence, in which many interactions concerning the function of the anterior pituitary occur, is outside the blood–brain barrier. It is therefore highly feasible that peripherally administered β-endorphin can act upon axon terminals in this structure which, in turn, regulate substances (including dopamine) entering the portal system and hence the secretion of prolactin (Gudelsky & Porter, 1979). The fact that β-endorphin in the peripheral and central compartments is produced from different cells suggests (though it does not prove) that co-ordinated secretion between the two compartments is much less likely than is the case for oxytocin or LHRH.

Prolactin

Though one cannot yet be persuaded that prolactin is produced centrally, there is no doubt that it is secreted in large quantities from the anterior pituitary. The peptide differs from the other three in being much larger (molecular weight about 22 000) and also, more importantly for the purposes of this discussion, in that it enters the brain relatively easily (Martensz & Herbert, 1982). Levels of prolactin in the CSF are about 10–20% of those in plasma. Furthermore, these levels rise and fall as do those in the blood. Prolactin derived either from the animal's own pituitary, or from an injection into the peripheral venous system, seems to reach the CSF equally easily. This entrance, however, is not as free as with some other hormones, for example lipid-soluble steroids. Whereas the latter enter the brain extremely rapidly, and can be detected in high levels within a few minutes of being given peripherally, prolactin enters the CSF slowly, so that after a peripheral injection, levels within the brain will still be rising 90 minutes later even though those in the plasma are falling towards their initial levels. Secondly, though prolactin in the blood exists in at least two forms ('big' and monomeric), only the monomeric form is found in the CSF. Such observations suggest, but do not prove, that some selective mechanism is acting to regulate the entry of prolactin into the brain.

Prolactin serves as an external neuropeptide operating upon the brain from the vascular compartment and should therefore be considered in conjunction with the other three. The only clue concerning the site of action of prolactin in the brain must be indirect: either the demonstration of localised biochemical changes within the brain, or the existence of a population of receptors. It is now well known that prolactin injected either peripherally or centrally can alter dopamine turnover in the hypothalamus and modulate sexual behaviour (Bailey & Herbert, 1982) and prolactin secretion (Herbert & Martensz, 1983). Very recently, a population of high affinity receptors for prolactin has been demonstrated within the hypothalamus (Di Carlo & Muccioli, 1981). Further work is needed before we can define those parts of the brain which may be directly responsive to prolactin. Whether some other peptides derived from the anterior pituitary, for example LH and growth hormone, behave in a manner comparable to prolactin is still undecided, though the present evidence suggests that prolactin may enter the brain with ease (Dubey *et al.*, 1983).

THE MONOAMINES

The cerebral monoamines (MA) – noradrenaline (NA), dopamine (DA) and 5-hydroxytryptamine (5HT) – have long been suggested to be of importance in neuroendocrine integration. Following the early discovery of their high concentration in the hypothalamus, many psychopharmacological experiments, using drugs which alter catechol- or indolaminergic activity in the brain, have revealed major effects on circulating levels of anterior and posterior pituitary hormones and on hormone-dependent behaviours. Despite this volume of pharmacological data, little progress has been made in defining the subsets of aminergic systems which might regulate these neuroendocrine processes. In this section we will summarise briefly the neuro-anatomical distribution of NA-, DA- and 5HT-containing neurons, focus attention on several hypothalamic and limbic structures in order to highlight their relationship to the peptidergic systems and steroid-hormone-sensitive parts of the brain, and make some assessment of their interactions in neuroendocrine events.

Dopamine

The majority of DA neurons are localised in the midbrain tegmentum, where they form two crescentic masses within the substantia nigra pars compacta which join around the interpeduncular nucleus in the midline to form a continuous band of cells with a precise topographical distribution to the forebrain (Dahlström & Fuxe, 1964; Moore & Bloom, 1978). Numerous DA neurons also extend dorsally throughout the mesencephalic raphe nuclei and then separate, rostrally, around the enlarging aqueduct to form a large periventricular group of neurons throughout the anterior–posterior extent of the hypothalamus (Hökfelt *et al.*, 1976). These neurons are found extending from the base of the third ventricle, so encompassing the arcuate nucleus group, to its top, reaching laterally as an expansion in the paraventricular nucleus. The more laterally placed DA neurons of the substantia nigra also appear to extend rostrally to form a large group in the zona incerta (Lindvall & Björklund, 1978).

The projections of DA neurons are well known and all ascending axons run initially within the medial forebrain bundle (Lindvall & Björklund, 1978; Moore & Bloom, 1978). They include the nigrostriatal and mesostriatal (from A10) pathways which innervate the striatal complex, including the nucleus accumbens septi (Ungerstedt, 1971). The more medial mesencephalic DA neurons (mesolimbic projections) also innervate the septal nuclei and amygdala, particularly the central nucleus, as well as the medial frontal, entorhinal and anterior cingulate cortices (mesocortical projections). Little is known of the destinations of axons arising from periventricular DA neurons except those lying within the arcuate nucleus; these project to the median eminence to end in close association with the primary portal capillary plexus (tubero-infundibular DA neurons; Fuxe & Hökfelt, 1969). Those DA neurons lying in the zona incerta project intrahypothalamically both to the median eminence region and, in larger number, to the medial anterior hypothalamic and preoptic areas, including the OVLT (incerto-hypothalamic system).

Noradrenaline

The most widely studied system of NA neurons is that situated in the pontine locus coeruleus, from which axons pass both caudally to the spinal cord (where they innervate neurons in dorsal, intermediolateral and ventral horns) and rostrally (branching widely within the brain stem to innervate, predominantly, sensory nuclei of cranial nerves) (Ungerstedt, 1971; Lindvall & Björklund, 1978; Moore & Bloom, 1979). Ascending axons form three pathways, the most important of which is the dorsal noradrenergic bundle (DNAB) which courses through the mesencephalon ventral and lateral to the periaqueductal grey and eventually joins the median forebrain bundle (MFB) at the level of the mamillary nuclei. The two smaller projections run within the central tegmental tract to join the MFB in the rostral midbrain (Lindvall & Björklund, 1978; Moore & Bloom, 1979). The terminal fields of axons arising from the locus coeruleus are many and diverse. In the diencephalon, there is some termination in periventricular hypothalamic and thalamic nuclei and also the anterior hypothalamic and preoptic areas; the telencephalon, the striatal complex, nucleus accumbens, amygdala and septal nuclei all receive coeruleal afferents (Lindvall & Björklund, 1978). Much of this innervation pattern is overlapped to some extent by lateral tegmental NA neurons. However, the hippocampus and entire cerebral cortex receive their NA innervation solely from the locus coeruleus as does the cerebellar cortex.

The lateral tegmental NA cell groups are found in the medullary reticular formation (Dahlström & Fuxe, 1964; Lindvall & Björklund, 1978). They lie in the region of the lateral reticular nucleus (A1) and anterior from this position around the dorsal accessory inferior olive (A3) and the emerging seventh cranial nerve (A5) (Lindvall & Björklund, 1978). Dorsally in the medulla, in the dorsal vagal complex and nucleus of the solitary tract, lies cell group A2 (Lindvall & Björklund, 1978). Ascending projections run first through the central tegmental tract, as the so-called ventral noradrenergic bundle (VNAB), to join the MFB (Ungerstedt, 1971). The cerebral cortex and hippocampus do not receive a lateral tegmental NA innervation, emphasising the sub-cortical, particularly diencephalic, termination of these neurons. Thus, the entire hypothalamus receives a rich NA innervation, in particular paraventricular, supraoptic and dorsomedial nuclei (Lindvall & Björklund, 1978). In the telencephalon, the septal nuclei and amygdala receive a prominent NA innervation arising in part from lateral tegmental cell groups.

5-Hydroxytryptamine

Neurons containing 5HT are largely restricted to the midline raphe nuclei of the medulla, pons and midbrain (Dahlström & Fuxe, 1964). In general, the medullary cell groups B1–B4 (largely in the nuclei raphe obscurus and magnus) project within the brain stem and caudally, down the spinal cord, to innervate neurons in dorsal and ventral horns and the intermediolateral cell column (Steinbusch, 1981). Ascending projections arise largely from mesencephalic 5HT neurons in the nucleus raphe dorsalis (B7), nucleus centralis superior (B8) and within the ventral medial lemniscus (B9) with a small contribution from positive cell groups (B5 and B6) (Azmitia, 1978; Steinbusch, 1981).

The axons course rostrally in the MFB and, like NA projections, are distributed widely in the diencephalon and telencephalon as a result of their repeated branching. Within the diencephalon, the suprachiasmatic nuclei receive the densest innervation but there are also abundant 5HT terminals in the median eminence, anterior hypothalamic and preoptic areas and mamillary nuclei. The periventricular, medial thalamic, ventromedial and lateral geniculate nuclei in the thalamus are also characterised by a very dense 5HT innervation (Steinbusch, 1981). In the telencephalon, it has been found that the septal nuclei, amygdala, striatum, the entire cortical mantle and hippocampus receive prominent inputs (Steinbusch, 1981) in a manner very similar to that described previously for NA. Clearly, projections of NA neurons from the locus coeruleus and 5HT neurons from the mesencephalic raphe together form part of the non-specific afferents to the cortex from the brain stem reticular formation.

NEUROENDOCRINE FUNCTIONS AND THE CATECHOLAMINES

Dopamine

Interest in neuroendocrine function of monoamine neurons settles quite naturally on the hypothalamus. The earliest histofluorescence studies (Fuxe & Hökfelt, 1969) focussed attention on the arcuate nucleus DA neurons in particular, since their axons project directly to the external layer of the median eminence around the portal capillary plexus (the tubero-infundibular DA, or TIDA, system). The precise role of this system in regulating anterior pituitary function is still far from clear, but early pharmacological and neurochemical studies emphasised that DA manipulations had profound effects on prolactin and LH secretion (Fuxe *et al.*, 1976). Since then it has become clear that DA secreted directly into portal blood, primarily from the more medial DA terminals in the external layer (Fuxe *et al.*, 1976) can regulate prolactin secretion and that DA is a most important prolactin inhibitory factor (PIF). Further, the TIDA system of neurons is the final common path through which neurally mediated (e.g. Keverne, 1982) and prolactin feedback events, which alter secretion, are largely channelled (Yen & Jaffe, 1978).

This humoral function of the TIDA system would appear to be consistent with the observation that these neurons lack a high affinity, specific re-uptake system (Annunziato *et al.*, 1980), which, unfortunately, also renders these neurons resistant to the neurotoxic effects of 6-hydroxydopamine (6-OHDA), a widely used neurotoxin for catecholamines.

The situation regarding the control of LH secretion is more complex. There is considerable overlap in the lateral portion of the median eminence with LHRH immunoreactive terminals (Fuxe *et al.*, 1976), a region where axo-axonic contacts between DA axons and other axons have been identified elecronmicroscopically (Fuxe & Hökfelt, 1969). Thus, the anatomical conditions seem right for neural interaction between DA and LHRH neurons, which may regulate the latter's secretion, although local, humoral interactions between DA and LHRH terminals in the pericapillary space also seem likely. Neuropharmacological and neurochemical studies *in vivo* strongly indicate that DA exerts an inhibitory influence on LH (hence LHRH) secretion (e.g. Fuxe *et al.* 1976; Yen & Jaffe, 1978; Löfstrom & Bäckström 1981; Wuttke *et al.*, 1981) but studies *in vitro* have shown that DA added to the culture medium induces release of LHRH from the hypothalamus (Rotsztejn *et al.*, 1978). This discrepancy has yet to be resolved. The observation that many DA-containing perikarya in the arcuate nucleus take up and bind oestradiol (E_2) (Heritage *et al.*, 1977) has reinforced the view that at least part of the negative feedback action of E_2 on LH secretion is mediated by a direct action on TIDA neurons – although the speed of the negative feedback effect of E_2 (onset within 30 minutes, maximal in 2–4 hours) is not entirely consistent with a genomic action of the steroid (see also McEwen *et al.*, 1981).

The problem of assessing compartmentalisation in the intrahypothalamic DA system has not been addressed adequately. Thus it is not clear whether a subset of these DA neurons elaborates PIF and functions as a humoral system regulating prolactin while another regulates LH secretion. The fact that high levels of prolactin may be associated with either low or high circulating levels of LH (e.g. during late pro-oestrus/oestrus in the rat: see Fink, 1979), suggests this DA system does not function simply as a whole. It has recently become clear, however, that the arcuate nucleus DA neurons projecting to the median eminence are not an isolated group but are associated with an extensive periventricular hypothalamic population of DA neurons, many of which also project to the portal capillaries (Fuxe & Hökfelt, 1969). Thus, division of these neurons into subsets associated with specific releasing/inhibiting hormones or an action on the pituitary itself may become apparent on the basis of their terminal distribution in the median eminence (see Fuxe *et al.*, 1976).

Noradrenaline

The noradrenergic innervation of the hypothalamus has long been implicated in the regulation of gonadotrophin secretion (e.g. Markee, Sawyer & Hollinshead, 1948); more recently this has included prolactin secretion as well (see Höhn & Wuttke,

1978). There is general agreement that increased noradrenergic activity induced by, for example, intraventricular or intrahypothalamic NA infusions (Gallo, 1982; Parvizi & Ellendorff, 1982) is associated with enhanced LH secretion. Conversely, measurements of NA turnover during pro-oestrus (Löfström & Bäckström, 1981; Wuttke et al., 1981) or following LH-secretion-inducing oestradiol treatment in ovariectomised rats (Löfstrom et al., 1977; Crowley, 1982) reveals a surprisingly clear correlation between increased NA turnover in the medial preoptic area, in the arcuate nucleus, in the median eminence or in all three, and increased plasma levels of LH. It is not altogether clear, therefore, at which site oestradiol and NA mechanisms interact, if they do, to bring about this change in LH (and presumably LHRH) secretion, since all three sites contain E_2 receptors. Furthermore, E_2 has been reported to increase NA receptor number in the preoptic area (Andersson et al., 1981). The NA innervation of the hypothalamus arises largely from cell groups A1 and A2 in the lateral medulla (Ungerstedt, 1971) so it is somewhat surprising, therefore, that lesions to the VNAB are not associated with disrupted oestrous cycles in female rats (Martinovic & McCann, 1977; Nicholson et al., 1978; Clifton & Sawyer, 1979; Hancke & Wuttke, 1979; Hansen, Stanfield & Everitt, 1981). Such observations add to the problem of assigning a function to the oestradiol sensitivity of medullary NA neurons (see Stumpf & Sar, 1981) although a role in feedback regulation of LHRH secretion cannot be ruled out in the light of so much correlative data.

The relationship between preoptic area NA turnover and prolactin secretion (Wuttke et al., 1981, Crowley, 1982) has been explored comparatively little. However, lesions of the VNAB which markedly attenuate the female rat's lordotic response to tactile stimuli from the male, also prevent cervical stimulation during pro-oestrus from inducing pseudopregnancy (Hansen et al., 1981, and see above). It is an assumption, but a reasonable one, that failure of appropriate prolactin secretion in VNAB-lesioned rats underlies this result, although whether such an effect is mediated via the preoptic area (a site important in regulating prolactin secretion – Neill, 1980) is unclear at present. Local injection of 6-OHDA into hypothalamic terminal regions has occasionally been attempted but is fraught with difficulties – for example, it is virtually impossible to prevent extensive DA depletion in the same area, while short-term recovery through the local sprouting of undamaged axons is difficult both to assess and to control (see Robbins & Everitt, 1982).

The paraventricular (PVN) and supraoptic (SO) nuclei have long been known to have a rich NA innervation (Ungerstedt, 1971; Lindvall & Björklund, 1978) although its detailed analysis has occurred only recently (Swanson & Mogenson, 1981). Thus, the magnocellular division of both PVN and SO receive their NA innervation entirely from cell groups A1 and A2 (nucleus of solitary tract) in the medulla and only those regions containing vasopressin neurons (i.e. posterior lateral PVN, ventral SO) appear to be in receipt of these afferents, although the exact disposition of oxytocin neuron densities has not been thoroughly studied (Swanson & Mogenson, 1981). Such precise compartmentalisation of this NA input argues strongly for a role in modulating vasopressin secretion, particularly in response to visceral afferent cues, since the glossopharyngeal and vagus nerves provide the major input to this system (Lightman, Everitt & Todd, unpublished). Recently, it has been demonstrated that haemorrhage, a potent stimulus to vasopressin secretion which depends on visceral afferent discharge, has a markedly reduced ability to induce vasopressin secretion in rats bearing lesions to the VNAB or DNAB (a number of lateral tegmental NA neurons run within the latter). At present, there is little evidence to suggest oxytocin secretion is affected by NA neuron lesions (Bridges, Clifton & Sawyer, 1982) but this possibility has not been explored fully.

Within the parvocellular division of PVN, there are many neurons containing somatostatin (Swanson & Mogenson, 1981) and corticotrophin releasing factor (Olschowka *et al.*, 1982) which probably project to the external layer of the median eminence. This division of PVN is also in receipt of a rich NA innervation (from locus coeruleus and medullary NA groups; Swanson & Mogenson, 1981), and there is some pharmacological evidence linking NA to the secretion of ACTH and somatostatin (e.g. Andersson *et al.*, 1981; Torres *et al.*, 1982), but the precise relationship between them has not been studied in detail.

MONOAMINES, STEROIDS AND PEPTIDES: SOME CORRELATED NEUROENDOCRINE EFFECTS

The preoptic and anterior hypothalamic areas, together with the ventromedial nucleus, in female rodents at least, are critically involved in the effects of hormones on sexual behaviour (Davidson, 1966; Rubin & Barfield, 1980). These areas, as we have seen, receive moderate-to-dense inputs from NA-, DA- and 5HT-containing neurons in the brain stem. In addition LHRH-containing neurons in the preoptic area have been implicated not only in the control of LH secretion, but in the regulation of sexual behaviour as well (Tennent *et al.*, 1982; Sirinathsinghji *et al.*, 1983) and are seen to be responsive to circulating oestradiol and testosterone levels (Shivers *et al.*, 1983). While manipulating monoamines has potent effects on sexual behaviour in male and female mammals (Everitt, 1978), it is far from clear whether the important site of action of monoamines on sexual behaviour in any way involves hypothalamic mechanisms. Thus, enhancing DA activity somewhat facilitates sexual activity in males and proceptivity in females, respectively; a more dramatic depression of behaviour follows reduction of DA activity. These effects seem largely explicable in terms of altered striatal function (Everitt *et al.*, 1975a; Caggiula *et al.*, 1979; Robbins & Everitt, 1982). On the other hand, no one has yet manipulated DA directly in the preoptic–anterior hypothalamic areas, which are in receipt of zona incerta DA afferents, and studied either sexual behaviour or the secretion of LH by the anterior pituitary. Similarly, while VNAB lesions impair lordotic responses in female rats (Hansen *et al.*, 1981), the effect seems most parsimoniously attributed to disturbed somato-sensory processing (Hansen *et al.*, 1981; Herbert, 1983) which may not involve hypothalamic mechanisms at all. Nevertheless, intrahypothalamic administration of adrenergic drugs does influence sexual activity in female rats (Zemlan *et al.*, 1978). The prolongation of ejaculation latencies and the post-ejaculatory refractory period which follows lesions to the DNAB (Hansen *et al.*, 1982) have been attributed to loss of spinal rather than preoptic NA, since infusions of 6-OHDA into the cervical or lumbar cord result in very similar behavioural consequences (Hansen & Ross, 1983; Everitt & Hansen, 1983).

Serotonin has long been associated with the control of sexual behaviour (Meyerson & Malmnäs, 1978). Meyerson and co-workers continue to present evidence that progesterone induces 'heat' in female rats by removing an inhibitory influence of 5HT systems on a hypothalamic substrate regulating sexual behaviour (Sietnieks & Meyerson, 1982). Progesterone clearly elicits lordosis after implantation in the preoptic–anterior hypothalamic areas (Rodriguez-Sierra & Komisaruk, 1982), pargyline (a monoamine oxidase inhibitor which causes increased 5HT levels) inhibits lordosis when placed in the hypothalamus (Luine & Fischette, 1982) while oestradiol significantly increases the density of 5HT receptors in the preoptic and anterior hypothalamic areas (Biegon et al., 1982). Furthermore, lesions to the hypothalamic 5HT input by injecting 5,7-dihydroxytryptamine into the midbrain greatly increases sexual activity in oestrogen-treated female (Everitt et al., 1975b) and castrated male (Larsson et al., 1978) rats. Despite some evidence to the contrary (Bradshaw, Erskine & Baum, 1982) this is an impressive array of data suggesting hypothalamic steroid–5HT interactions.

It may prove possible to integrate these data with those concerning a circadian rhythm in the behavioural sensitivity to steroids (oestradiol) in females at least. Thus, ovariectomised female rats bearing E_2 implants only display 'heat' during the dark phase of the day–night cycle (Södersten & Hansen, 1977). Lesions of the suprachiasmatic nuclei (SCN) abolish this rhythm and result in continuous high levels of receptivity (Hansen, Södersten & Srebro, 1978). The SCN receive, as we have seen, the most profuse 5HT input of any diencephalic or telencephalic structure (Steinbusch, 1981) and lesions of 5HT neurons in the brain stem result in elevated levels of sexual receptivity (Everitt et al., 1975b). Although SCN neurons appear not to be addressed directly by steroids, they clearly have a major influence on steroid sensitivity of the hypothalamus (in the regulation of LH secretion as well – Weigand & Terasawa, 1982). The relationships between day length, oestradiol and 5HT within the SCN have not yet been studied directly. It is also worth noting in passing that there is a noradrenergic input to this structure and levels of this amine show a pronounced circadian rhythm, and are responsive to environmental sensory cues.

The septal nuclei which have a poorly defined neuroendocrine function are perhaps not unrelated to this debate. The lateral nuclei, particularly their ventral parts, bind E_2; the same area receives a dense 5HT innervation (Köhler, Chan-Palay & Steinbusch, 1982) and is in receipt of a vasopressin-containing projection from the SCN (Swanson & Mogenson, 1981; Köhler et al., 1982). Septal lesions markedly enhance the female rat's behavioural response to E_2 (see Lisk & MacGregor, 1982) which may reflect one aspect of the complex septal hyperactivity syndrome – and E_2 increases the density of 5HT receptors in the lateral septum (Biegon et al., 1982). Vasopressin infusion in the lateral ventricle inhibits lordosis induced by E_2 and progesterone (Södersten et al., 1983). The latter authors argue that activity in the SCN is responsible for terminating 'heat' by reducing neural (hypothalamic septal) sensitivity to E_2 – hence the effects of SCN or septal lesions – and that this effect of SCN activity is mediated by vasopressin neurons projecting to the lateral septum. All the ingredients of an intriguing steroid–peptide–amine interaction are present, but again they await direct and detailed study.

No review of anatomical neuroendocrinology would be complete without mentioning the amygdala, although it should be stated at the outset that little is known of its role in regulating anterior pituitary secretion or sexual and aggressive behaviours (Herbert, 1983). As we have described, cortical and medial nuclei of the amygdala receive primarily NA afferents from both coeruleal and medullary cell groups (Lindvall & Björklund, 1978) and these would seem most likely to interact directly with E_2-dependent functions of these olfactory-related structures. The lateral and basal nuclei of the amygdala are in receipt primarily of 5HT afferents from dorsal and medial raphe nuclei (Steinbusch, 1981). This group of amygdaloid nuclei primarily receives cortical afferents and projects to the central nucleus as well as septal nuclei. Thus, these 5HT inputs may play an important role in the transmission of sensory information from cortex to limbic brain. Lesions of this zone of the amygdala produce aberrant social, sexual, aggressive and ingestive behaviours in cats and monkeys (Kluver–Bucy Syndrome), and more detailed investigation of serotoninergic mechanisms at this site is clearly warranted. Recently, the central nucleus of the amygdala has been identified as the principal site for the convergence and origin of numerous peptidergic systems ultimately projecting from the amygdala via the stria terminalis (Roberts *et al.*, 1982). The dense DA innervation of the central nucleus arising from the ventral tegmental area (VTA; Lindvall & Björklund, 1978) is clearly strategically placed to influence this major amygdaloid outflow which is directed, at least in part, to the hypothalamus. Local DA manipulations of the amygdala have been few, but changes in hunger- and thirst-motivated behaviour have been reported (Lenärd & Hahn, 1982) as well as changes in sexual behaviour (D. J. S. Sirinathsinghji, personal communication). The use of selective methods to manipulate aminergic, peptidergic and steroidal components of the amygdala (as well as the parts of the limbic system) will surely yield valuable information which may help reveal the function of this key area of the brain.

The work of our laboratory is supported principally by an MRC programme grant, together with project grants from the MRC and ARC.

REFERENCES

Al-Noalmi, M. C., Biggins, J. A., Edwardson, J. A., McDermott, J. R. & Smith, A. I. (1982). Corticotrophin-related peptides in the intermediate lobe of the rodent pituitary gland: characterization by high performance liquid chromatography and radioimmunoassay. *Regulatory Peptides*, **3**, 351–9.

Andersson, K., Fuxe, K., Eneroth, P., Blake, C. A., Agnati, L. F. & Gustafsson, J. A. (1981). Effects of androgenic and adrenocortical steroids on hypothalamic and preoptic catecholamine nerve terminals and on the secretion of anterior pituitary hormones. In *Steroid Hormone Regulation of the Brain*, ed. K. Fuxe, J. A. Gustafsson & L. Wetterberg, pp. 117–33. Oxford: Pergamon.

Annunziato, L., Leblanc, P., Kordon, C. & Weiner, R. J. (1980). Differences in the kinetics of dopamine uptake in synaptosome preparations of the median eminence relative to other dopaminergic innervated brain regions. *Neuroendocrinology*, **31**, 316–20.

Azmitia, E. C. (1978). The serotonin-producing neurons of the midbrain median and dorsal raphe nuclei. In *Handbook of Psychophrenology*, vol. 9, ed. L. C. Iversen, S. D. Iversen & S. H. Snyder, pp. 233–314. New York: Plenum.

Bailey, D. J. & Herbert, J. (1982). Impaired copulatory behaviour of male rats with hyperprolactinaemia induced by domperidone or pituitary grafts. *Neuroendocrinology*, **35**, 186–93.

Barry, J., Dubois, M. P. & Poulain, P. (1973). LRF-producing cells of the mammalian hypothalamus: a fluorescent antibody study. *Zeitschrift für Zellforschung*, **148**, 351–66.

Beyer, C., Gomora, P., Canchola, E. & Sandoral, Y. (1982). Pharmacological evidence that LHRH action on lordosis behaviour is modulated through a rise in c-AMP, *Hormones and Behaviour*, **16**, 107–12.

Biegon, A., Fischette, C. T., Rainbow, T. C. & McEwen, B. S. (1982). Serotonin receptor modulation by estrogen in discrete brain nuclei. *Neuroendocrinology*, **35**, 287–91.

Blaustein, J. D. & Feder, H. H. (1979). Cytoplasmic progestin-receptors in guinea pig brain: characteristics and relationship to the induction of sexual behaviour. *Brain Research*, **169**, 481–97.

Bradshaw, W. G., Erskine, M. S. & Baum, M. J. (1982). Dissociation of the effects of gonadal steroids on brain serotonin metabolism and sexual behaviour in the male rat. *Neuroendocrinology*, **34**, 38–45.

Bridges, R. S., Clifton, D. K. & Sawyer, C. H. (1982). Postpartum luteinizing hormone release and maternal behaviour in the rat after late-gestational depletion of hypothalamic norepinephrine. *Neuroendocrinology*, **34**, 286–91.

Buijs, R. M. (1978). Intra- and extrahypothalamic vasopressin and oxytocin pathways in the rat. *Cell and Tissue Research*, **192**, 423–35.

Caggiula, A. R., Herndon, J. G., Scanlon, R., Greenstone, D., Bradshaw, W. & Sharp, D. (1979). Dissociation of active from immobility components of sexual behaviour in female rats by central 6-hydroxydopamine: implications for CA involvement in sexual behaviour and sensimotor responsiveness. *Brain Research*, **172**, 505–20.

Catlin, D. H., Poland, R. E., Gorelick, D. A., Gerner, R. H., Hui, K. K., Rubin, R. T. & Li, C. H. (1980). Intravenous infusion of β-endorphin increases serum prolactin, but not growth hormone or cortisol, in depressed subjects and withdrawing methadone addicts. *Journal of Clinical Endocrinology and Metabolism*, **50**, 1021–5.

Christensen, L. W. & Clemens, L. G. (1974). Intrahypothalamic implants of testosterone or estradiol and resumption of masculine sexual behaviour in long term castrated rats. *Endocrinology*, **95**, 984–90.

Clifton, D. K. & Sawyer, C. H. (1979). LH release and ovulation in the rat following depletion of hypothalamic norepinephrine: chronic vs. acute effects. *Neuroendocrinology*, **78**, 442–9.

Corbett, A. D., Paterson, S. J., McKnight, A. T., Magnan, J. & Kosterlitz, H. W. (1982). Dynorphin$_{1-8}$ and dynorphin$_{1-9}$ are ligands for the κ-subtype of opiate receptor. *Nature (London)*, **299**, 79–81.

Crowley, W. R. (1982). Effects of ovarian hormones on norepinephrine and dopamine turnover in individual hypothalamic and extrahypothalamic nuclei. *Neuroendocrinology*, **34**, 381–6.

Dahlström, A. & Fuxe, K. (1964). Evidence for the existence of monoamine-containing neurons in the central nervous system. I. Demonstration of monoamines in the cell bodies of brain stem neurons. *Acta Physiologica Scandinavica* (Suppl. 232), 1–55.

Davidson, J. M. (1966). Activation of the male rat's sexual behaviour by intracerebral implantation of androgen. *Endocrinology*, **79**, 783–94.

Davis, P. G., McEwen, B. & Pfaff, D. W. (1979). Localised behavioural effects of tritiated oestradiol in the ventromedial hypothalamus. *Endocrinology*, **104**, 898–903.

de Kloet, E. R., Palkovits, M. & Mezey, E. (1981). Opiocortin peptides: localization, source and avenues of transport. *Pharmacology and Therapeutics*, **12**, 321–51.

Di Carlo, R. & Muccioli, G. (1981). Changes in prolactin binding sites in the rabbit hypothalamus induced by physiological and pharmacological variations of prolactin serum levels. *Brain Research*, **230**, 445–50.

Dorsa, D. M., Majumdar, L. A. & Chapman, M. B. (1981). Regional distribution of gamma- and beta-endorphin-like peptides in the pituitary and brain of the rat. *Peptides* **2** (Suppl. 1), 71–7.

Dubey, A. K., Herbert, J., Martensz, N. D., Beckford, N. & Jones, M. T. (1983). Differential penetration of anterior pituitary peptides into the CSF of rhesus monkeys. *Life Sciences* (in press).

Dupont, A., Lepine, J., Langelier, P., Merand, Y., Rouleau, D., Vaudry, H. Gros, C. & Barden, N. (1980). Differential distribution of β-endorphin and enkephalins in rat and bovine brain. *Regulatory Peptides*, **1**, 43–52.

Eipper, B. A. & Mains, R. E. (1980). Structure and biosynthesis of pro-adrenocorticotropin/endorphin and related peptides. *Endocrine Reviews*, **1**, 1–27.

Everitt, B. J. (1978). A neuroanatomical approach to the study of monoamines and sexual behaviour. In *Biological Determinants of Sexual Behaviour*, ed. J. B. Hutchison, pp. 555–74. Chichester: Wiley.

Everitt, B. J., Fuxe, K., Hökfelt, T. & Jonsson, G. (1975a). Role of monoamines in the control by hormones of sexual receptivity in the female rat. *Journal of Comparative and Physiological Psychology*, **89**, 556–72.

Everitt, B. J., Fuxe, K. & Jonsson, G. (1975b). The effects of 5,7-dihydroxytryptamine lesions of ascending 5-hydroxytryptamine pathways on the sexual and aggressive behaviour of female rats. *Journal de Pharmacologie (Paris)*, **6**, 25–32.

Everitt, B. J. & Hansen, S. (1983). Catecholamines and hypothalamic hormone-dependent mechanisms in the control of sexual behaviour. In *Psychopharmacology of Sexual Disorders*, ed. D. Wheatley. Oxford University Press (in press).

Fink, G. (1979). Neuroendocrine control of gonadotrophin secretion. *British Medical Bulletin*, **35**, 155–60.

Finley, J. C. W., Lindstrom, P. & Petrusz, P. (1981). Immunocytochemical localization of β-endorphin-containing neurons in the rat brain. *Neuroendocrinology*, **33**, 28–42.

Foley, K. M., Kourides, I. A., Inturrisi, C. E., Kaiko, R. F., Zaroulis, C. G., Posner, J. B., Houde, R. W. & Li, C. H. (1979). β-endorphin: analgesic and hormonal effects in humans. *Proceedings of the National Academy of Sciences, USA*, **76**, 5377–81.

Fuxe, K. & Hökfelt, T. (1969). Catecholamines in the hypothalamus and in the pituitary gland. In *Frontiers in Neuroendocrinology 1969*, ed. W. F. Ganong & L. Martini, pp. 47–96. New York: Academic Press.

Fuxe, K., Hökfelt, T., Eneroth, P., Gustafsson, J. A. & Skett, P. (1977). Prolactin-like immunoreactivity: localisation in nerve terminals of the hypothalamus. *Science*, **196**, 899–910.

Fuxe, K., Hökfelt, T., Löfström, A., Johansson, O., Agnati, L., Everitt, B. J., Goldstein, M., Jeffcoate, S., White, N., Eneroth, P., Gustaffson, J. & Skett, P. (1976). On the role of neurotransmitters and hypothalamic hormones and their interaction in hypothalamic and extrahypothalamic control of pituitary function and sexual behaviour. In *Subcellular Mechanisms in Reproductive Neuroendocrinology*, ed. F. Naftolin, K. J. Ryan & J. Davis, pp. 193–246. Amsterdam: Elsevier.

Gallo, R. V. (1982). Luteinizing hormone secretion during continuous or pulsatile infusion of norepinephrine: central nervous desensitisation to constant norepinephrine input. *Neuroendocrinology*, **35**, 380–7.

Grossman, S. P. (1975). Role of the hypothalamus in the regulation of food and water intake. *Psychological Reviews*, **82**, 200–24.

Gudelsky, G. A. & Porter, J. C. (1979). Morphine and opioid induced inhibition of the release of dopamine from tuberoinfundibular neurons. *Life Sciences*, **25**, 1697–9.

Guillemin, R., Vargo, T., Rossier, J., Minick, S., Ling, N., Rivier, C., Vale, W. O. & Bloom, F. (1977). β-endorphin and adrenocorticotropin are secreted concomitantly by the pituitary gland. *Science*, **197**, 1367–9.

Hancke, J. L. & Wuttke, W. (1979). Effect of chemical lesions of the ventral noradrenergic bundle or of medial preoptic area on preovulatory LH release in rats. *Brain Research*, **35**, 127–34.

Hansen, S., Köhler, C. & Ross, S. B. (1982). On the role of the dorsal mesencephalic tegmentum in the control of sexual behaviour in the male rat: effects of electrolytic lesions, ibotenic acid and DSP4. *Brain Research*, **240**, 311–20.

Hansen, S. & Ross, S. (1983). Role of descending monoaminergic neurons in the control of sexual behaviour: effects of intrathecal infusion of 6-hydroxydopamine and 5,7-dihydroxytryptamine. *Neuroscience Letters* (in press).

Hansen, S., Södersten, P. & Srebro, B. (1978). A daily rhythm in the behavioural sensitivity of the female rat to oestradiol. *Journal of Endocrinology*, **77**, 381–8.

Hansen, S., Stanfield, E. J. & Everitt, B. J. (1981). The effects of lesions of lateral tegmental noradrenergic neurons on components of sexual behaviour and pseudopregnancy in female rats. *Neuroscience*, **6**, 1105–17.

Hayashi, S. & Gorski, R. A. (1974). Critical exposure time for androgenisation by intracranial crystals of testosterone propionate in neonatal female rats. *Endocrinology*, **94**, 1161–7.

Herbert, J. (1983). Behaviour and the limbic system, with special reference to sexual and aggressive interactions. In: *The Limbic System*, ed. M. Trimble. Chichester: Wiley. (In press.)

Herbert, J. & Martensz, N. D. (1983). The effects of intraventricular prolactin infusions on pituitary responsiveness to thyrotropin releasing hormone, 5-hydroxytryptophan or morphine in rhesus monkeys. *Brain Research*, **258**, 251–62.

Heritage, A. S., Grant, L. D. & Stumpf, W. E. (1977). [³H]estradiol in catecholamine neurons of the rat brain stem: combined localisations by autoradiography and formaldehyde-induced fluorescence. *Journal of Comparative Neurology*, **176**, 607–30.

Heritage, A. S., Stumpf, W. E., Sar, M. & Grant, L. D. (1981). [³H]dihydrotestosterone in catecholamine neurons of rat brain stem: combined localisation by autoradiography and formaldehyde induced fluorescence. *Journal of Comparative Neurology*, **200**, 289–307.

Hillman, M. A., Recht, L. D., Rosario, S. L., Seit, S. M., Robinson, A. G. & Zimmerman, E. A. (1977). The effects of adrenalectomy and glucocortical replacement on vasopressin and vasopressin–neurophysin in the zona externa of the rat. *Endocrinology*, **101**, 42–9.

Hoffman, G. E. & Gibbs, P. (1982). LHRH pathways in the rat brain: 'deafferentation' spares a sub-chiasmatic LHRH projection to the median eminence. *Neuroscience*, **7**, 1979–93.

Höhn, K. H. & Wuttke, W. O. (1978). Changes in catecholamine turnover in the anterior part of the mediobasal hypothalamus and the medial preoptic area in response to hyperprolactinaemia in ovariectomized rats. *Brain Research*, **156**, 241–52.

Hökfelt, T., Johansson, O., Fuxe, K., Goldstein, M. & Park, D. (1976). Immunohistochemical studies on the localisation and distribution of monoamine neuron systems in the rat brain. I. Tyrosine hydroxylase in the mes- and diencephalon. *Medical Biology*, **54**, 427–53.

Hostetter, G., Gallo, R. V. & Brownfield, M. S. (1981). Presence of immunoreactive luteinizing hormone in the rat forebrain. *Neuroendocrinology*, **33**, 241–5.

Ibata, Y., Watanabe, K., Kinoshita, H., Kubo, S. & Sano, Y. (1979). The location of LH-RH neurons in the rat hypothalamus and their pathways to the median eminence. *Cell and Tissue Research*, **198**, 381–95.

Jennes, L. & Stumpf, W. E. (1975). Hormone uptake sites in relationship to CNS biogenic amine systems. In *Anatomical Neuroendocrinology*, ed. W. E. Stumpf & L. D. Grant, pp. 445–64. Basle: Karger.

Jennes, L. & Stumpf, W. E. (1980) LHRH-systems in the brain of the golden hamster. *Cell and Tissue Research*, **209**, 239–56.

Jones, P. M. & Robinson, I. C. A. F. (1982). Differential clearance of neurophysin and neurohypophysial peptides from the cerebrospinal fluid in conscious guinea pigs. *Neuroendocrinology*, **34**, 297–302.

Kastin, A. J., Jemison, M. T. & Coy, D. H. (1980). Analgesia after peripheral administration of enkephalin and endorphin analogues. *Pharmacology, Biochemistry and Behaviour*, **11**, 713–16.

Kawano, H. & Daikoku, S. (1981). Immunohistochemical demonstration of LHRH neurons and their pathways in the rat hypothalamus. *Neuroendocrinology*, **32**, 179–86.

Keverne, E. B. (1982). The accessory olfactory system and its role in pheromonally mediated changes in prolactin. In *Olfaction and Endocrine Regulation*, ed. W. Breipohl, pp. 127–40. London: IRL Press.

Keverne, E. B. & Riva, C. de la (1982). Pheromones in mice: reciprocal interactions between the nose and brain. *Nature (London)*, **296**, 148–50.

King, J. C., Tobet, S. A., Snavely, F. L. & Arimura, A. A. (1982). LHRH immunopositive cells and their projections to the median eminence and organum vasculosum of the lamina terminalis. *Journal of Comparative Neurology*, **209**, 287–300.

Köhler, C., Chan-Palay, V. & Steinbusch, H. (1982). The distribution and origin of serotonin-containing fibres in the septal area: a combined immunohistochemical and fluorescent retrograde tracing study in the rat. *Journal of Comparative Neurology*, **209**, 91–111.

Krieger, D. T., Liotta, A. S., Nicholsen, G. & Kizer, J. S. (1979). Brain ACTH and endorphin reduced in rats with monosodium glutamate-induced arcuate nuclear lesions. *Nature (London)*, **278**, 562–3.

Larsson, K., Everitt, B. J., Fuxe, K. & Södersten, P. (1978). Sexual behaviour in male rats after intracerebral injection of 5,7-dihydroxytryptamine. *Brain Research*, **141**, 293–303.

Larsson, L.-I. (1980). ACTH-like and opioid peptides in gut and brain. *Biomedical Research (Suppl.)*, **1**, 79–83.

Lenärd, L. & Hahn, Z. (1982). Amygdalar noradrenergic and dopaminergic mechanisms in the regulation of hunger- and thirst-motivated behaviour. *Brain Research*, **233**, 115–32.

Leonardelli, V. & Tramu, G. (1979). Immunoreactivity for β-endorphin in LH-RH neurons of the fetal human hypothalamus. *Cell and Tissue Research*, **203**, 201–7.

Lieberburg, I. & McEwen, B. (1975). Estradiol 17β: a metabolite of testosterone recovered in cell nuclei from limbic areas of neonatal rat brains. *Brain Research*, **85**, 165–70.

Lindvall, O. & Björklund, A. (1978). Organisation of catecholamine neurons in the rat cental nervous system. In *Handbook of Psychophrenology*, vol. 9, ed. L. L. Iversen, S. D. Iversen & S. H. Snyder, pp. 139–232. New York: Plenum.

Lisk, R. D. & MacGregor, L. (1982). Subproestrous estrogen levels facilitate lordosis following septal or cingulate lesions. *Neuroendocrinology*, **35**, 313–20.

Löfström, A. & Bäckström, T. (1981). Plasma steroid-catecholamine relationships in limbic and related areas of the brain. In *Steroid Hormone Regulation of the Brain*, ed. K. Fuxe, J. A. Gustafsson & L. Wetterberg, pp. 147–60. Oxford: Pergamon.

Löfström, A., Eneroth, P., Gustafsson, J. A. & Skett, P. (1977). Effects of estradiol benzoate on catecholamine levels and turnover in discrete areas of the median eminence and the limbic forebrain, and on serum LH, FSH and prolactin concentration in the ovariectomized female rat. *Endocrinology*, **101**, 1559–69.

Luine, V. N. & Fischette, C. T. (1982). Inhibition of lordosis behaviour by intrahypothalamic implants of pargyline. *Neuroendocrinology*, **34**, 237–44.

McEwen, B. S., Biegon, A., Rainbow, T., Paden, C., Snyder, L. & DeGroff, V. (1981). The interaction of estrogen with intracellular receptors and with putative neurotransmitter receptors: implication for the mechanism of activation of sexual behaviour and ovulation. In *Steroid Hormone Regulation of the Brain*, ed. K. Fuxe, J. A. Gustafsson & L. Wetterberg, pp. 15–30. Oxford: Pergamon.

McEwen, B. S., Davis, P. G., Parsons, B. & Pfaff, D. W. (1979). The brain as a target for steroid hormone action. *Annual Review of Neuroscience*, **2**, 65–112.

McEwen, B. S. & Pfaff, D. W. (1970). Factors influencing sex hormone uptake by rat brain regions. *Brain Research*, **21**, 1–16.

McGinnis, M. Y., Krey, L. C., MacLusky, N. J. & McEwen, B. S. (1981). Characterisation of steroid receptor levels in intact and ovariectomised oestrogen treated rats. *Neuroendocrinology*, **33**, 155–61.

Markee, J. E., Sawyer, C. H. & Hollinshead, W. H. (1948). Adrenergic control of the release of luteinizing hormone from the hypophysis of the rabbit. *Recent Progress in Hormone Research*, **2**, 117–31.

Martensz, N. D. & Herbert, J. (1982). Relationship between prolactin in the serum and cerebrospinal fluid of ovariectomised female rhesus monkeys. *Neuroscience*, **7**, 2801–12.

Martinovic, J. V. & McCann, S. M. (1977). Effects of lesions in the ventral noradrenergic tract produced by microinjection of 6-hydroxydopamine on gonadotropin release in the rat. *Endocrinology*, **100**, 1206–13.

Massa, R., Stupnicka, E., Kniewald, Z. & Martini, L. (1972). The transformation of testosterone into dihydrotestosterone by the brain and anterior pituitary. *Journal of Steroid Biochemistry*, **3**, 385–99.

Merchenthaler, I., Kovacs, G., Lovasz, G. & Setalo, G. (1980). The preoptic–infundibular LHRH tract of the rat. *Brain Research*, **198**, 63–74.

Meyerson, B. & Malmnäs, C.-O. (1978). Brain monoamines and sexual behaviour. In *Biological Determinants of Sexual Behaviour*, ed. J. B. Hutchison, pp. 521–54. Chichester: Wiley.

Mohs, R. C., Davis, B. M., Rosenberg, G. S., Davis, K. L. & Krieger, D. T. (1982). Naloxone does not affect pain sensitivity, mood or cognition in patients with high levels of beta-endorphin in plasma. *Life Sciences*, **30**, 1827–33.

Moore, R. T. & Bloom, F. E. (1978). Central catecholamine neuron symptoms: anatomy and physiology of the dopamine systems. *Annual Review of Neuroscience*, **1**, 129–70.

Moore, R. T. & Bloom, F. E. (1979). Central catecholamine neuron symptoms: anatomy and physiology of the norepinephrine and epinephrine systems. *Annual Review of Neuroscience*, **2**, 113–68.

Morrell, J. I. & Pfaff, D. W. (1982). Characterisation of estrogen-concentrating hypothalamic neurons by their axonal projections. *Science*, **217**, 1273–5.

Naik, D. V. (1976). Immunohistochemical localisation of LHRH neurons in the mammalian hypothalamus. In *Neuroendocrine Regulation of Fertility*, ed. T. C. Anand Kumar, pp. 80–91. Basel: Karger.

Nakao, K., Nakai, Y., Oki, S., Matsubara, S., Konishi, T., Nishitani, H. & Imura, H. (1980). Immunoreactive β-endorphin in human cerebrospinal fluid. *Journal of Clinical Endocrinology and Metabolism*, **50**, 230–3.

Neill, J. (1980). Neuroendocrine regulation of prolactin secretion. In *Frontiers in Neuroendocrinology*, ed. L. Martini & W. F. Ganong, vol. 6, pp. 129–55. New York: Raven.

Nicholson, G., Treeley, G., Humm, J., Youngblood, W. & Kizer, J. S. (1978). Lack of effect of noradrenergic denervation of the hypothalamus and medial preoptic area on the feedback regulation of gonadotropin secretion in the oestrous cycle of the rat. *Endocrinology*, **103**, 559–66.

Nilaver, G., Zimmerman, E. A., Defenini, R., Llotta, A. S., Krieger, D. T. & Brownstein, M. J. (1979). Adrenocorticotropin and β-lipotropin in the hypothalamus. *Journal of Cell Biology*, **81**, 50–8.

Olschowka, J. A., O'Donohue, T. L., Mueller, G. P. & Jacobowitz, D. M. (1982). Hypothalamic and extrahypothalamic distribution of CRF-like immunoreactive neurons in the rat brain. *Neuroendocrinology*, **35**, 305–8.

O'Malley, B. W. & Means, A. R. (1974). Female steroid hormones and target cell nuclei. *Science*, **183**, 610–20.

Parsons, B., Rainbow, T. C., Pfaff, D. W. & McEwen, B. S. (1981). Oestradiol, sexual receptivity and cytosol progestin receptors in rat hypothalamus. *Nature (London)*, **292**, 58–9.

Parvizi, N. & Ellendorff, F. (1982). Further evidence on dual effects of norepinephrine on LH secretion. *Neuroendocrinology*, **35**, 48–55.

Pedersen, C. A., Ascher, J. A., Monroe, Y. L. & Prange, A. J. Jr. (1982). Oxytocin induces maternal behavior in virgin female rats. *Science*, **216**, 648–9.

Pedersen, C. A. & Prange, A. J., Jr. (1979). Induction of maternal behavior in virgin rats after intracerebroventricular administration of oxytocin. *Proceedings of the National Academy of Sciences, USA*, **76**, 6661–5.

Pfaff, D. (1970). Nature of sex hormone effects on rat sex behaviour: specificity of effects and individual patterns of response. *Journal of Comparative and Physiological Psychology*, **73**, 349–58.

Pfaff, D. W. & Conrad, L. C. A. (1978). Hypothalamic neuroanatomy: steroid hormone binding and patterns of axonal projections. *International Review of Cytology*, **54**, 425–65.

Pfaff, D. W. & Keiner, M. (1973). Atlas of oestradiol-concentrating cells in the central nervous system of the female rat. *Journal of Comparative Neurology*, **151**, 121–58.

Phillips, H. S., Hostetter, G., Kerdelhue, B. & Kozlowski, G. P. (1980). Immunocytochemical localization of LHRH in central olfactory pathways of hamster. *Brain Research*, **193**, 574–9.

Poulain, D. A., Lebrun, C. J. & Vincent J. D. (1981). Electrophysiological evidence for connections between septal neurones and the supraoptic nucleus of the hypothalamus of the rat. *Experimental Brain Research*, **42**, 260–8.

Poulain, D. A. & Wakerley, J. B. (1982). Electrophysiology of hypothalamic magnocellular neurons secreting oxytocin and vasopressin. *Neuroscience*, **7**, 773–808.

Powell, E. W. & Rorie, D. K. (1969). Septal projections to nuclei functioning in oxytocin release. *American Journal of Anatomy*, **120**, 605–10.

Robbins, T. W. & Everitt, B. J. (1982). Function studies of central catecholamine neurons. *International Review of Neurobiology*, **23**, 303–65.

Roberts, E. W., Woodhouse, P. C., Polak, J. M. & Crow, J. (1982). Distribution of neuropeptides in the limbic system of the rat: the amygdaloid complex. *Neuroscience*, **7**, 99–131.

Rodriguez-Sierra, J. F. & Komisaruk, B. R. (1982). Common hypothalamic sites for activation of sexual receptivity in female rats by LHRH, PGE$_2$ and progesterone. *Neuroendocrinology*, **35**, 363–9.

Rosenblatt, J. S., Siegel, H. I. & Mayer, A. D. (1979). Progress in the study of maternal behaviour in the rat: hormonal, non-hormonal, sensory and developmental aspects. *Advances in the Study of Behaviour*, **10**, 225–311.

Rotsztejn, W. H., Drouva, S. V., Pattou, E. & Kordon, C. (1978). Effect of morphine on the basal and the dopamine-induced release of LHRH from the mediobasal hypothalamic fragments *in vitro*. *European Journal of Pharmacology*, **50**, 285–6.

Rubin, B. S. & Barfield, R. J. (1980). Priming of estrous responsiveness by implants of 17β-estradiol in the ventromedial hypothalamic nucleus of female rats. *Endocrinology*, **106**, 504–9.

Scalia, F. & Winans, S. S. (1975). The differential projection of the olfactory bulb and accessory olfactory bulb in mammals. *Journal of Comparative Neurology*, **161**, 31–56.

Setalo, G., Vigh, S., Schally, A. V., Arimura, A. & Flerko, B. (1976). Immunohistological study of the origin of LH-RH-containing nerve fibers of the rat hypothalamus. *Brain Research*, **103**, 597–602.

Sheridan, P. J. (1979). The nucleus interstitialis striae terminalis and the nucleus amygdaloideus medialis: prime targets for androgen in the rat brain. *Endocrinology*, **104**, 130–6.

Shivers, B. D., Harlan, R. E., Morell, J. I. & Pfaff, D. W. (1983). Immunocytochemical localisation of luteinizing hormone releasing hormone in male and female rat brains: quantitative studies on the effects of gonadal steroids. *Neuroendocrinology*, **36**, 1–12.

Sietnieks, A. & Meyerson, B. J. (1982). Enhancement by progesterone or 5-hydroxytryptophan inhibition of the copulatory performance in the female rat. *Neuroendocrinology*, **35**, 321–6.

Silverman, A. J. (1976). Distribution of luteinizing hormone-releasing hormone (LHRH) in the guinea pig brain. *Endocrinology*, **99**, 30–41.

Sirinathsinghji, D. J. S., Whittington, P. E., Audsley, A. & Fraser, H. M. (1983). β-endorphin regulates lordosis in female rats by modulating LHRH release. *Nature (London)*, **301**, 62–4.

Södersten, P. & Hansen, S. (1977). Effects of oestradiol and progesterone on the initiation and duration of sexual receptivity in cyclic female rats. *Journal of Endocrinology*, **74**, 477–85.

Södersten, P., Henning, M., Melin, P. & Lundin, S. (1983). Vasopressin alters behaviour by acting on the brain independently of alteration in blood pressure. *Nature (London)*, **301**, 608–10.

Sofroniew, M. V. (1979). Immunoreactive β-endorphin and ACTH in the same neurons of the hypothalamic arcuate nucleus in the rat. *American Journal of Anatomy*, **154**, 283–9.

Sofroniew, M. V. & Glasmann, W. (1981). Golgi-like immunoperoxidase staining of hypothalamic magnocellular neurons that contain vasopressin, oxytocin or neurophysin in the rat. *Neuroscience*, **6**, 619–43.

Steimer, Th. & Hutchison, J. B. (1981). Androgen increases formation of behaviourally effective oestrogen in dove brain. *Nature (London)*, **292**, 345–6.

Steinbusch, H. (1981). Distribution of serotonin-immunoreactivity in the central nervous system of the rat – cell bodies and terminals. *Neuroscience*, **6**, 557–618.

Stengaard-Pedersen, K. & Larsson, L.-I. (1981). Localization and opiate receptor binding of enkephalin, CCK and ACTH/β-endorphin in the rat central nervous system. *Peptides*, **2**, 3–19.

Stumpf, W. E. (1975). The brain: an endocrine gland and hormone target. In *Anatomical Neuroendocrinology*, ed. W. E. Stumpf & L. D. Grant, pp. 2–8. Basle: Karger.

Stumpf, W. E. & Sar. M. (1975). Hormone-architecture of the mouse brain with [³H]oestradiol. In *Anatomical Neuroendocrinology*, ed. W. E. Stumpf & L. D. Grant, pp. 82–103. Basle: Karger.

Stumpf, W. E. & Sar, M. (1981). Steroid hormone sites of action in the brain. In *Steroid Hormone Regulation of the Brain*, ed. K. Fuxe, J. A. Gustafsson & L. Wetterberg, pp. 41–50. Oxford: Pergamon.

Stumpf, W. E., Sar, M. & Keefer, D. A. (1975). Atlas of estrogen target cells in rat brain. In *Anatomical Neuroendocrinology*, ed. W. E. Stumpf & L. D. Grant, pp. 104–19. Basle: Karger.

Swanson, L. W. & Kuypers, H. G. J. M. (1980). The paraventricular nucleus of the hypothalamus: cytoarchitectonic subdivisions and organization of projections to the pituitary, dorsal vagal complex, and spinal cord as demonstrated by retrograde fluorescence double-labelling methods. *Journal of Comparative Neurology*, **194**, 555–70.

Swanson, L. W. & Mogenson, C. J. (1981). Neural mechanisms for the functional coupling of autonomic, endocrine and somatomotor responses in adaptive behaviour. *Brain Research Reviews*, **3**, 1–34.

Tennent, B. J., Smith, E. R. & Dorsa, D. M. (1982). Comparison of some CNS effects of luteinizing-hormone releasing hormone and progesterone. *Hormones and Behaviour*, **16**, 76–86.

Thomson, A. M. (1982). Responses of supraoptic neurons to electrical stimulation of the medial amygdaloid nucleus. *Neuroscience*, **7**, 2197–206.

Torres, I., Guaza, C., Fernandez-Durango, R., Borrell, J. & Charro, A. L. (1982). Evidence for a modulatory role of catecholamines on hypothalamic somatostatin in the rat. *Neuroendocrinology*, **35**, 159–62.

Toubeau, G., Desclin, J., Parmentier, M. & Pasteels, J. M. (1979). Compared localisation of prolactin-like and ACTH immunoreactivity within the brain of the rat. *Neuroendocrinology*, **29**, 384–94.

Ungerstedt, U. (1971). Stereotaxic mapping of the monoamine pathways in the rat brain. *Acta Physiologica Scandinavica* (Suppl. 367), 1–48.

Wang, B. C., Share, L., Crofton, J. T. & Kimura, T. (1982). Effects of intravenous and intra-cerebroventricular infusion of hypertonic solutions on plasma and cerebrospinal fluid vasopressin concentrations. *Neuroendocrinology*, **34**, 215–21.

Wardlaw, S. L., Wehrenberg, W. B., Ferin, M. & Frantz, A. G. (1980). Failure of β-endorphin to stimulate prolactin release in the pituitary stalk-sectioned monkey. *Endocrinology*, **107**, 1663–6.

Watkins, W. B. (1980). Presence of adrenocorticotropin and β-endorphin immunoreactivities in the magnocellular neurosecretory system of the rat hypothalamus. *Cell and Tissue Research*, **207**, 65–80.

Wehrenberg, W. B., McNicol, D., Wardlaw, S. L., Frantz, A. G. & Ferin, M. (1981). Dopaminergic and serotonergic involvement in opiate induced prolactin release in monkeys. *Endocrinology*, **109**, 544–7.

Weigand, S. J. & Terasawa, E. (1982). Discrete lesions reveal functional heterogeneity of suprachiasmatic structures in regulation of gonadotropin secretion in female rats. *Neuroendocrinology*, **34**, 395–404.

Wilkes, M. M., Watkins, W. B., Stewart, R. D. & Yen, S. S. C. (1980). Localization and quantitation of β-endorphin in human brain and pituitary. *Neuroendocrinology*, **30**, 113–21.

Wilkinson, M., Herdon, H., Pearce, M., & Wilson, C., (1979). Radioligand binding studies of hypothalamic noradrenergic receptors during the estrous cycle after steroid injection in ovariectomised rats. *Brain Research*, **168**, 652–5.

Wuttke, W., Mansky, T., Stock, K. W. & Sandman, R. (1981). Modulatory action of estradiol on catecholamine and GABA turnover and effects on serum prolactin and LH release. In *Steroid Hormone Regulation of the Brain*, ed. K. Fuxe, J. A. Gustafsson & L. Wetterberg, pp. 135–46. Oxford: Pergamon.

Yen, S. C. & Jaffe R. B. (1978). *Reproductive Endocrinology*. Baltimore: W. B. Saunders.

Zakarian, S. & Smyth, D. G. (1982). β-endorphin is processed differently in specific regions of rat pituitary and brain. *Nature (London)*, **296**, 250–2.

Zemlan, F. P., Leonard, L. M., Kow, L. M. & Pfaff, D. W. (1978). Ascending tracts of the lateral columns of the rat spinal cord: a study using silver impregnation and horseradish peroxidase techniques. *Experimental Neurology*, **62**, 298–334.

Zimmerman, F. A., Hsu, K. C., Fern, M. & Koslowski, G. P. (1974). Localisation of gonadotrophin-releasing hormone (GnRH) in the hypothalamus of the mouse by immunoperoxidase techniques. *Endocrinology*, **95**, 1–8.

Index